"This text highlights BAPT's gold level in competencies, providing a clear rationale about wh trained play therapist or BAPT recognized training (comprehensive guide providing insight into the clinical contexts in which play therapists work and invaluable information, support, and resources to all who are, or wish to become, involved in the field."

– **Eileen Prendiville**, Children's Therapy Centre, Ireland

"This book is a very comprehensive overview of the training, theory and practice of play therapy in the UK. All the contributors are highly experienced UK play therapists who give us an in depth presentation of current practice which is informed by cross-disciplinary theory and contemporary research. This book is quite remarkable in its depth and its breadth. A must-read for not only play therapists and students but also other related clinicians in the arts and psychotherapies, teachers in all forms of education and parents too. I am passionate about the importance of play, and reading this book was joyous and stimulating."

– **Professor Sue Jennings**, specialist in neuro-dramatic-play

Becoming and Being a Play Therapist

Becoming and Being a Play Therapist: Play Therapy in Practice presents a rich and illuminating account of current play therapy practice, with an emphasis on becoming and being a play therapist and on some of the varied clinical contexts in which play therapists work. Written by members of the British Association of Play Therapists, this book highlights the current complexity of play therapy practice in the UK and reflects the expertise of the collected authors in working with emotional, behavioural and mental health challenges in children and young people.

Divided into three parts, the book is designed to build on and consolidate the principles and professional/personal competences of play therapy practice. Key topics include:

- Training and establishing oneself as a play therapist in the UK, a comprehensive guide.
- The improvisational practitioner; therapist responses to resistance and aggressive play.
- Systemic considerations in play therapy with birth families and adopters; advantages and challenges.
- Case-study based explorations of play therapy across a range of service user groups, including childhood trauma, bereavement and sexual abuse, and agency contexts, including school and CAMHS settings.

Becoming and Being a Play Therapist will be relevant both for play therapy trainees and for qualified play therapists, as well as for related professionals.

Peter Ayling is a qualified play therapist and social worker who has specialised in working with children and young people within the care system for 25 years. He worked for 14 years within a Child and Adolescent Mental Health Service (CAMHS) for Looked After Children. Pete currently works as a Senior Lecturer in Social Work and maintains a small, private play therapy practice.

Harriet Armstrong obtained a Master's Degree in Play Therapy from the University of Roehampton in 2009. She has since worked as a play therapist privately and in schools with children who have suffered a wide range of trauma, disorders and difficulties. Harriet has been Chair of PR and Communications of BAPT and is currently Joint Vice-Chair.

Lisa Gordon Clark trained as a play therapist at Roehampton, following several years as a primary school teacher, and has since worked both in private practice and as resident play therapist at a Child and Family Centre in London. Lisa is currently Programme Convener of the Play Therapy MA at the University of Roehampton and Fellow of the HEA.

Becoming and Being a Play Therapist

Play Therapy in Practice

Edited by Peter Ayling, Harriet Armstrong and Lisa Gordon Clark

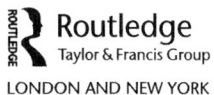
Routledge
Taylor & Francis Group

LONDON AND NEW YORK

First published 2019
by Routledge
2 Park Square, Milton Park, Abingdon, Oxon OX14 4RN

and by Routledge
52 Vanderbilt Avenue, New York, NY 10017

Routledge is an imprint of the Taylor & Francis Group, an informa business

British Library Cataloguing-in-Publication Data
A catalogue record for this book is available from the British Library

Library of Congress Cataloging-in-Publication Data
A catalog record has been requested for this book

ISBN: 978-1-138-56096-3 (hbk)
ISBN: 978-1-138-56097-0 (pbk)
ISBN: 978-0-203-71122-4 (ebk)

Typeset in Times New Roman
by Swales & Willis, Exeter, Devon, UK

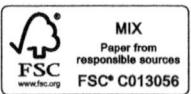

Printed and bound in Great Britain by
TJ International Ltd, Padstow, Cornwall

Peter: For my wonderful mum, Doreen, who taught me how to play, and for George, who keeps me playful still.

Harriet: I would like to dedicate this to my Dad, who always encouraged me and who I miss every day. And to my children, Austin, Alex and Connie who are amazing and bring so much joy to my life.

Lisa: For Rob – with thanks for his stalwart support, patience and tolerance, the nurturing meals and sustaining cups of Earl Grey as I grappled with this, and for his love. And for my Mummy, who would have been proud – and for Dad, Anya and Imogen who will be. Their love also keeps me going, always.

Contents

Figures

Contributors

Harriet Armstrong works as a self-employed play and filial therapist in schools and a specialist paediatric clinic. She has worked with children in different capacities throughout her adult life and qualified as a play therapist in 2009. As well as her direct work with children she also delivers training to other professionals and supervises other therapists. Harriet has sat on the Board of Directors for BAPT for a number of years, including in the position of Vice Chair for 3 years.

Peter Ayling is a social worker and play therapist who has worked with children in care throughout his professional life, initially within safeguarding contexts and then within specialist CAMHS services for looked after children. Peter served as Chair of the British Association of Play Therapists for 5 years from 2010–2015. Peter currently maintains a small independent practice in play therapy and clinical supervision, while working as a social work academic within higher education. Previous publications have focused on the role of creativity in supporting student learning and promoting play-based interventions for foster carers. Peter is currently undertaking PhD research around the use of empathy within social work practice with children.

Clare Carbis has a BSc Psychology (BPS accredited) and MSc Play Therapy (BAPT accredited). Clare works therapeutically with children who have experienced trauma, loss and bereavement, those with attachment difficulties, and those who have experienced neglect, physical, emotional and sexual abuse. Clare's training was in child-centred play therapy; however she incorporates integrative techniques into her therapeutic work with children and young people. Clare uses attachment based therapeutic techniques in her work with families, influenced by the work of Dan Hughes, Theraplay principles and Sensory Attachment Intervention (SAI). Clare completed SAI level 1 training in 2012 and Theraplay Level 1 training in 2014. Clare also provides therapeutic life story work interventions to children and young people and clinical supervision to play therapists. Clare has worked for Stepping Stones (Child Therapy Consultants) Ltd since August 2008 and continues to do this alongside being a senior lecturer and course leader for the MSc Play Therapy programme at the University of South Wales.

Trudi Cowper is a BAPT play therapist with an MA from Roehampton University, where she also co-delivers CPD courses on CPRT to play therapists. She has around 15 years' experience working with children, young people and families in a variety of settings such as schools, domestic abuse charities and services for looked after children. Trudi has delivered over 30 CPRT groups and one-to-one filial work to parents in the last five years. She also has training and experience in therapeutic horticulture and is a lecturer for the University of South Wales on the Master's in Play Therapy programme.

Stuart Daniel is a play therapist and researcher based in Devon, UK. Having a passionate interest in early communication, severe learning difficulties, and medical trauma, he has authored scientific and therapy articles in these areas along with co-editing the book: *Rhythms of Relating in Children's Therapies: Connecting Creatively with Vulnerable Children*, published by Jessica Kingsley.

Anne Fullalove is an advisory teacher, trainer, play therapist and Video Interaction Guidance (VIG) practitioner and supervisor, with 30 years of experience working with children and their families. Her most recent post was play therapist within the psychosocial team at The Children's Trust, a residential rehabilitation centre for children with acquired brain injury. Following a recent relocation, she now works in private practice. Her interests include working with children with developmental delay and social communication difficulties, and their parents. She has recently co-written a book, entitled *Innovations in Therapy for Paediatric Acquired Brain Injury* (ITP-ABI; London: Routledge), to be published in 2019.

Lisa Gordon Clark Having trained as a play therapist in the 1990s at what was then Roehampton Institute of Higher Education, Lisa is now programme convener for the Play Therapy MA at the University of Roehampton, where she also runs the annual 20-week Play Therapy Foundation Course. In addition, she is currently the external examiner for the Play Therapy Master's programme at Queen Margaret University, Edinburgh (in conjunction with WithKids, Glasgow). Alongside her academic roles she is also a clinical supervisor and freelance play therapist based in Wiltshire. She contributed a chapter on 'Play Therapy' to *The Handbook of Counselling Children and Young People*, edited by Pattison, Robson & Beynon (2014 – 2nd edition published 2018). Lisa has been editor of the *British Journal of Play Therapy* for the last 10 years.

Simon Kerr-Edwards is an independent play therapist, clinical supervisor and trainer and former dramatherapist who practices in Buckinghamshire, UK. He has a specialism in working with adopted children and their families as well as therapeutic ways of exploring children's early life-stories. His interest is in bringing creativity and improvisation into the clinical supervision relationship. He believes we are constantly evolving as practitioners through all our professional and personal activities and we bring that evolving self into the play room for therapeutic effect.

Ruth Lazarus is a BAPT play therapist and supervisor. She qualified as a play therapist in 2005 and a Filial therapist in 2007. Ruth has worked in CAMHS for the past 7 years and is currently in post as a creative therapist providing therapeutic interventions, duty and assessment work. Ruth also manages a therapeutic team in primary schools, which offers child and adult therapy, professional consultation and training. Ruth's passion for professional practice in play therapy inspired her to join the BAPT Board of Directors in 2011. Ruth is now the chair of Directors.

Debra May is an independent play therapist, accredited EMDR practitioner, registered social worker and drama teacher. Debra has over 20 years' experience working with children and families providing a range of assessment and therapeutic services, through the use of play, drama and EMDR. She specialises in working with a child individually, as well as with their parents/carers where there are attachment issues complicated by previous traumatic experiences for both the child and their parent.

Julie McCann completed her Master's in Play Therapy at Roehampton University and is a Full member of BAPT as well as a certified Theraplay practitioner. Her dissertation examined the views of experienced play therapists about their personal therapy and she went on to write a paper on the same subject for the *British Journal of Play Therapy*. Julie continues her interest in the divide and overlaps between supervision and personal therapy in her role as a supervisor. She currently works for TACT (an adoption and fostering agency), for a south London school and in a private practice.

Karen McInnes is Research Fellow at Norland College. Previously she was the joint award leader for the BAPT accredited MSc in Play Therapy and the MSc Play and Therapeutic Play at the University of South Wales. Whilst there she qualified as a BAPT accredited play therapist and has conducted the majority of her play therapy practice in schools with young children. She has a PhD in play and playfulness and has published widely in this field.

Sonia Murray holds a Diploma in Social Work and is a registered play therapist. She has over 25 years' experience as a practitioner in the fields of child abuse, social, emotional and behavioural difficulties, children's mental health, childhood trauma, parenting programmes and play therapy. Sonia trains nationally and internationally on topics related to play therapy, understanding behaviour, play, communicating with children, behaviour management and positive parenting. Sonia has also contributed to a number of publications, including *The Use of Therapeutic Stories*. Sonia served on the Board of Directors for the British Association of Play Therapists in a variety of capacities including treasurer and chair of Business and Research sub-committees for nearly 10 years.

Sharon Pearce is a registered play therapist with BAPT. Sharon works in CAMHS and she also has a private practice, where she has provided training for professionals interested in working therapeutically with children. She has many years' experience of working with vulnerable children and their carers and specialises in working with children placed in substitute care by their local authorities. She has a special interest in working with children with attachment and trauma issues along with their carers and wider networks. Sharon's previous publication 'Working with Narrative Play Therapy with Children experiencing Parental Divorce and Separation' was published in *Narrative Play Therapy* in 2011, Taylor de Faoite (ed.), published by Jessica Kingsley.

Carol Platteuw worked for many years as a social worker and Children's Guardian. Carol is now Director of Play Therapy Services Ltd, an adoption support agency which provides a range of therapeutic interventions for children and their families. Carol is a Certified Theraplay practitioner and runs a clinic for a local authority post adoption team where she offers bereavement work, therapeutic life story work, Theraplay and DDP. Carol delivers training for professionals focussing on effective communication with children and guest lectures on the MA in Play Therapy course at Roehampton. Previous publications include 'Play Therapy with Adopted Children' in *Narrative Play Therapy* (2011) Taylor De Faoite (ed.), published by Jessica Kingsley.

Linda St Louis has been working in the field of domestic violence and abuse for the past 25 years. Her early career with children and families involved the development and delivery of needs-led, community-based, family support services. She first graduated in Community Development and later trained as a play therapist at the University of Roehampton in 2010. She currently delivers play therapy interventions within her existing role with the London Borough of Ealing Council. Linda first became involved in BAPT as a member of the Training and Education Sub-Committee. Since 2014 Linda has been the Chair of Professional Conduct sub-committee where she has worked to review and revise the BAPT Complaints procedures. She is also a guest lecturer at University of Roehampton and has recently undertaken the BAPT accredited supervisors training course.

Jenny Reid completed her training in Non-Directive Play Therapy at the University of York, receiving an MA in 2006. She has greatly valued her involvement in BAPT throughout her career, particularly appreciating the opportunity to share experiences with other play therapists at the annual conference. She is now co-director of the Apple Tree Centre, a dedicated children and young people's therapy centre in Sheffield, where she provides play therapy sessions as well as Child Parent Relationship Therapy, clinical supervision and professional training.

Chris Stone has worked professionally with vulnerable children and families for over 40 years, in both the statutory and voluntary sectors. With a background in residential child care, couple and family therapy, child advocacy, counselling and play therapy, she has particular expertise where issues of bereavement and loss are a primary concern, including consultancy to schools in 'Critical Incidents'. Self-employed for eight years, Chris is also a BAPT approved clinical supervisor. Her practice is integrative, underpinned by person-centred principles, attachment theory and systems theory. Chris offers non-directive play therapy, utilising a more directive approach when appropriate.

Berni Stringer After qualifying to teach, Berni continued her career working for some years in secure provision with young people, finally re-training as social worker. In this role she worked in the community with children and their families, until she moved into the field of Child and Adolescent Mental Health as a social worker and trained as a play therapist. In the latter part of her career, Berni worked for the British Association for Adoption and Fostering, delivering training and consultation to Local Authorities and Agencies and set up a network of therapists who could offer interventions to children in care and or in adoptive placement. For the last 3 years, Berni has been an independent play therapist, working almost exclusively with children who have experienced abuse and are fostered or adopted.

Carrie Waldron is a registered BAPT play therapist. She qualified as a play therapist in 2004 and later as a Filial Therapist. Carrie has worked for CAMHS since 2008 in a generic post as a Specialist CAMHS Practitioner with a specialism in play therapy. Before this Carrie worked as a senior social worker with Children and Families. Carrie's other current work roles are as a trainer for the Early Years Service in East Sussex and an independent social work assessor. Before social work, Carrie trained and was employed as a Registered Mental Health Nurse.

Lisa Waycott In addition to play therapy training, Lisa has a Master's degree in Social Work and was a senior lecturer at the University of South Wales between 2007 and 2015. Lisa has also undertaken level 2 training in Theraplay. Lisa has also worked therapeutically with children and young people in a variety of settings and with regard to a wide range of needs. Her work has included working with severely traumatised and vulnerable children and young people with complex histories. Lisa is also the Clinical Director of Stepping Stones (Child Therapy Consultants) LTD which is an independent agency which supplies therapeutic services for children and young people, training and consultancy. Lisa has established strong links with a range of international experts and academics in the field of child therapy. Lisa has been instrumental in the delivery of the first accredited play therapy training course in Wales, as recognised by the BAPT.

Tim Woodhouse is an advanced and certified Sensorimotor Psychotherapist, Enactive trauma therapist, registered non-directive play therapist, Filial therapist, EMDR practitioner, Jungian and Integrative sandplay therapist and an ABE approved social worker. He worked on the NSPCC child sexual abuse consultancy for 16 years, was a founding member of St. Mary's children's sexual assault referral centre in Manchester, was an investigator on the Waterhouse inquiry and vice chair of BAPT. He was principal tutor on the Liverpool Hope MA course in play therapy and is a visiting lecturer to Manchester Universities 2nd Year MA social work programme. He is the Director of Tiptoes Child Therapy Service, a provision for children and families affected by sexual harm and developmental trauma launched in 2010. He is a published author, keynote speaker, consultant, trainer, clinical supervisor and has been a governmental advisor on a number of research programmes.

Abbreviations

BAPT   British Association of Play Therapists
CPRT   Child Parent Relationship Therapy
DDP   Dyadic Developmental Psychotherapy
DoE   Department of Education
DoH   Department of Health
EMDR   Eye Movement Desensitisation Reprocessing
NDPT   Non Directive Play Therapy
PSA   Professional Standards Authority
PTSD   Post Traumatic Stress Disorder
WTSC   Working Together to Safeguard Children

Foreword

This book, which was conceived by members of the British Association of Play Therapists as they celebrated the association's 25th anniversary, is remarkable in several ways. The most notable way is that this enthusiasm actually turned into a lengthy and valuable book for the play therapy profession! The book is also remarkable because it demonstrates how BAPT itself has functioned over all these years, with members generously giving both their time and expertise to a demanding project. This book also parallels my own personal experiences of BAPT: that elected professional and lay members give their time and considerable energy voluntarily because they are dedicated to providing children and their families with the best play therapists possible. All of BAPT's core competences and values embodied in ethical practice are very creatively and effectively illustrated in this book.

I am honoured that the editors have asked me to write the foreword for this ambitious book. It is written with gratitude to everyone who has helped BAPT to develop and maintain its reputation at home and internationally. It is with pride that we members can belong to an organisation that is recognised for its standards in accrediting training programmes and in play therapy practice. Not only play therapists, but most of all, the children, teens and families worked with by BAPT therapists, have gained much from having such an effective professional organisation.

The wellbeing of children is solidly at the heart of this book, and it serves well the two audiences it is intended for – first, those who are at the beginning of their careers, and second, those who are qualified, experienced practitioners. This book is particularly helpful for practitioners and trainees who enter new settings, or encounter unexpected challenges in their work. For example, a play therapist in a school setting, faced for the first time with a child who has had a medical trauma, can read about familiar issues encountered in school settings in a couple of chapters, and read new material on working with children who experienced medical traumas, in order to absorb essential new information and ideas to overlay onto the familiar. Or an experienced play therapist who feels somewhat overwhelmed by a particularly aggressive child, can read about aggression and traumatic reactions, illustrated with several case examples in various chapters. This can help engender confidence and improvisation in practice with this child's difficult behaviour. Other play therapists, who decide to leave current employers and launch their independent practice, will find several chapters relevant, in addition to the chapter on independent practice, including the chapters on ethics and time-limited interventions. The book also serves to inform readers about training requirements on courses accredited by BAPT, and to stimulate experienced play therapists to search out new training and reading, and to communicate with members who have similar values, yet different experiences from their own.

It is difficult to choose certain chapters to comment on in this foreword. It is partly because I like the book's diversity so much. It has been inspiring to read about members' practice from so many perspectives, and emotionally satisfying to read about their thoughts and practice from a child-centred stance. I was also curious about what contributors I know personally would write, as I started to read, and intrigued by what members wrote whom I do not know. I found myself having internal dialogues with contributors, jotting down references that I would like to read, and in general having a wonderful time learning much more about everything to do with UK current thinking and practice in play therapy.

In addition to enriching play therapists' practice by contributors linking their play therapy practice to their research, or to others' research and theory, the book also is a rich source of hypotheses for future research. For example, as I read, I began thinking about promoting play therapists' wellbeing, which is alluded to in several chapters, and becomes more concrete in the chapter on independent practice. That chapter can be an excellent starting point for a qualitative research project with play therapists on their case loads, types of referrals, professional supports, and their personal strengths and challenges. Another research project comes to mind on improvisation in child-centred play therapy, which could examine the key moments play therapists recognise as improvising, and devise ways to investigate whether this affected the child's progress in play therapy. These kinds of research questions, and others from a quantitative research perspective, can help play therapists and trainees to practise in new ways, and to confirm what works best for them as therapists in their current situations. Readers will have many more research ideas as they read this book.

Now that BAPT is very well-established, it is important for our profession to accumulate a body of UK play therapy research to support the good practice promoted by BAPT. It is exciting that this type of research is now beginning to emerge as qualified play therapists embark on research projects at doctoral level. Hopefully the editors will consider a second book, once they recover their energy. There is so much more to say and do!

Dr. Virginia Ryan

Introduction

Peter Ayling, Harriet Armstrong and Lisa Gordon Clark

The idea for this book was conceived as the British Association of Play Therapists (BAPT) celebrated its 25-year anniversary at the BAPT annual conference. As we relaxed together in the bar after dinner, we recognised the wealth of experience and innovation in terms of play therapy practice amongst the members in the room around us. Those initial discussions were the inspiration for this project and helped to shape the final structure of this book, spurred on by the enthusiasm of our fellow contributors. As we hope the book demonstrates, play therapy practice in the UK is flourishing, informed by a wide range of theoretical approaches and research evidence that support the use of play and creativity within therapy.

Indeed, play therapy practice in the UK has developed significantly over the last three decades, building on the work of influential pioneers in the field, such as Dr Ann Cattanach (1994), Dr Sue Jennings (1999), and Dr Virginia Ryan (Wilson & Ryan, 1992; Ryan & Wilson, 2000). The first British-based play therapy training courses at Holborn, London in the early 90s, led by respected dramatherapists Jennings and Cattanach, created an interest in play therapy as a separate and unique approach in its own right. This, in turn, led to the establishment of the British Association of Play Therapists (BAPT) in 1992, a professional body aiming to support the growing interest in the practice of play therapy in the UK, by promoting clear standards for ethical practice and developing training pathways for those interested in becoming play therapists. As the first professional body for play therapy in the UK, BAPT has since achieved national and international recognition for the standards of our accredited training and professional practice.

BAPT is an association of practitioners, led by elected members and appointed lay-members, who serve as Directors of the Board for an elected period. Like many such associations, we are an eclectic and increasingly diverse group, united by our passionate belief in the value of play as a therapeutic modality which supports children's – and adults' – emotional wellbeing and health, facilitating development and recovery. As interest and awareness of play therapy has grown in the UK, BAPT has supported the accreditation of a number of play therapy training programmes, delivered in partnerships by experienced play therapy practitioners and well-respected regional universities. As a members' association, the BAPT register of qualified play therapists is accredited by the Professional Standards Authority (PSA) who review and quality assure our practice standards annually, for the protection and safety of the public. (You can find out more about the PSA on their website www.professionalstandards.org.uk/)

In line with other creative arts therapy trainings within the UK, BAPT play therapy training is currently delivered at Master's level, to ensure our members are trained in both theoretical understanding and clinical application for practice, to a high standard. For more information about current programmes you can visit the BAPT website at www.bapt.info. (See also Chapter 1 by Gordon Clark in this volume for detailed guidance on play therapy training.)

Play therapy has its origins in the work of Carl Rogers (1951) and, in particular, Virginia Axline (1964, 1989), who applied Rogers' humanistic and person-centred approach to therapeutic practice with children. Fundamental to play therapy practice is a belief in the child's capacity for healing and development, for moving towards health and integration. Play therapists view the therapeutic relationship with the child as the primary vehicle to support the child's growth and healing (Landreth, 2012) and utilise play and creativity as the primary form of self-expression within the therapeutic process.

BAPT defines play therapy as

> the dynamic process between child and Play Therapist in which the child explores at his or her own pace and with his or her own agenda those issues, past and current, conscious and unconscious, that are affecting the child's life in the present. The child's inner resources are enabled by the therapeutic alliance to bring about growth and change. Play Therapy is child-centred, in which play is the primary medium and speech is the secondary medium.
>
> (BAPT, 2018a)

Significantly for BAPT members, while contemporary practice may be informed by a number of theoretical orientations and models, it remains fundamentally child-centred, ensuring that the child's voice and wishes are honoured within the therapeutic process and represented effectively within decision making forums. Equally apparent within this volume is the importance of a systemic perspective (Dallos & Draper, 2015) within play therapy practice. As well as the individual work with the child in the therapy room, play therapists regularly collaborate with birth and adoptive parents and other substitute carers, as well as with wider professional networks who are supporting the child. Increasingly, play therapy interventions will form part of a coordinated, multi-agency and interdisciplinary plan, developed as a response to identified safeguarding, family support or mental health needs and responding to changes in the wider systems around a child. Play therapists need to be able to take a flexible approach here, to sustain effective working relationships with a wide range of professionals, whilst ensuring the wellbeing and privacy of the child.

Building on these foundations, BAPT has developed a set of Core Competences (see Appendix 1), which inform and underpin the training and practice of play therapy by our members. Play therapists need to be sufficiently skilled to adapt their practice to the needs of individual children, integrating knowledge of child development and understanding of the impact of past life experiences, whilst also responding sensitively to the identity needs and cultural practices of a diverse population of children and young people. We have highlighted these competences throughout the book, to illustrate their integration within our practice. Similarly, BAPT members abide by the ethical principles for practice found within our *Ethical Basis for Good Practice in Play Therapy* (BAPT, 2018b) and this framework is also explored in some detail within this volume.

The book will service as a handbook for those who are interested in, or currently undertaking, their play therapy training, as well as a resource for more experienced play therapists. There are three distinct sections. In Part I, 'Becoming a play therapist' we explore a number of key issues for play therapy trainees and seek to provide a valuable resource for therapists at the beginning of their play therapy careers. Gordon Clark outlines some important considerations for anyone considering applying to undertake a BAPT-accredited training programme, while chapters by both McCann and Platteuw explore the dual expectations of personal therapy and clinical supervision, with which all our play therapists will engage during their training. In her chapter on the physical space, Fullalove explores the significance and symbolic potential of the physical environment to support the therapeutic process and relationship, while Armstrong outlines a range of practical and ethical issues to consider when establishing an independent play therapy practice.

Part II is designed to consider a range of issues relating to the experience of 'Being a play therapist' and asks the questions – what does it mean to be ethical, to be creative, to be playful, to respond to emotions, to set limits and to design plans for short-term interventions? St Louis outlines the ethical framework which supports safe and effective play therapy practice and highlights some of the most common dilemmas for practitioners in relation to recording, consent and maintaining confidentiality. McInnes provides an important overview of the developmental functions of play and play theory before considering the relevance of 'playfulness' as a key characteristic for play therapists, while Kerr-Edwards considers the importance of improvisation as a skill for practice and discusses the importance of therapist self-awareness. These two chapters share an emphasis on the play therapist's capacity for creativity, spontaneity and flexibility within their practice. Ayling's chapter considers the role of the therapist in containing and regulating the child's emotions within the play relationship and explores how therapeutic limits can support this process. Finally in this section, Reid's chapter considers the benefits and challenges of working within short, time-limited play therapy interventions and highlights principles for good practice in this context.

Part III 'Play therapy in practice' moves on to provide examples of contemporary play therapy practice across the UK, within a wide range of practice contexts. Play therapists currently work with an increasingly diverse client group, including children, adolescents, parents and carers and, in some cases, adult clients. As this volume illustrates, they practice in a broad variety of health, education and social care settings, demonstrating the growing recognition of play therapy as a therapeutic approach. Each chapter in this section includes a case example to illustrate play therapy practice within the specific context. The reader will also note the explicit consideration in many of the chapters around engaging with parents and carers to support the child's individual therapeutic journey.

The first chapter, by Lazarus and Waldron, gives an account of practice within a Child and Adolescent Mental Health Service (CAMHS) and details some of the challenges for practitioners within this context. Murray's chapter explores the challenges and advantages of developing a play therapy service in schools, whilst Pearce's chapter discusses the benefits of using a group narrative play therapy model within a school context to support pupils' emotional and academic development. The chapter by Woodhouse explores play therapy practice with children and adults who have experienced sexual harm and considers the use of video-recording within this specific context. Stone discusses the value of play therapy when working with children who have experienced bereavement and loss, and stresses the importance of working with parents within this process.

The next three chapters focus on aspects of working with traumatic experience and offer a range of contrasting models for work in this field. Waycott and Carbis present their integrative model of working with children who have experienced abuse and neglect, informed by theories of attachment and developmental trauma. Daniel, working within the field of medical trauma, explores the relevance of polyvagal theory for understanding and responding to children's play and behaviour within the therapy process. May's chapter demonstrates the integration of child centred play therapy with Eye Movement Desensitisation Reprocessing (EMDR) to support a child experiencing post-traumatic stress following a serious car accident.

The final two chapters in this section focus on work with parents and carers and explore different approaches to bringing the parent into the therapeutic process with the child. Stringer, working with foster and adoptive parents and carers, proposes a model to support parental understanding of the child's therapy through observation, education and relational engagement with both adults and child together in the therapy room. In contrast, Cowper presents her experience of delivering Child Parent Relationship Therapy (CPRT) groups with parents, identifying the potential to promote learning and emotional support through peer interaction within the filial therapy-informed group programme.

It should be apparent from this brief outline that play therapy practice is thriving within the UK, as practitioners apply their professional training across a broad spectrum of challenging practice contexts. BAPT seeks to support members to maintain and refresh their knowledge base through the annual conference, approving post-qualifying training and by setting continuing professional development (CPD) requirements for members. As can be seen from the scope of this volume, many BAPT therapists continue to undertake professional training in a wide variety of other therapeutic approaches and models including filial therapy (VanFleet, 2013), Theraplay[1] (Booth & Jernberg, 2010), and attachment informed models (Hughes, 2007). Play therapy practice continues to evolve as practitioners integrate new theoretical learning from neuroscience and the fields of attachment, trauma and loss within their practice, or develop their own new, integrative models adapted for their particular context.

The regulatory framework in the UK surrounding therapeutic and safeguarding practice also continues to develop and to place increasing demands on play therapy practitioners. Indeed, even as we were preparing the final chapters for publication, crucial new legislation in the form of the GDPR regulations on data protection came to the fore (ICO, 2018), reinforcing the fact that the context of our work is continually evolving and we cannot ever become complacent about our professional practice. Given this rapidly changing landscape, membership of an established and respected professional association plays an important role in helping practitioners keep up to date, while also providing opportunities for a collective professional voice to respond to wider policy and political issues affecting therapy practitioners.

Like many therapeutic models, play therapy has experienced a period of rapid change and development from its original conception, informed by the emerging body of evidence from neuroscience and from the study of trauma around the world. These findings include significant challenges for therapy practitioners, but also offer support for the deliberate use of creative and playful approaches within therapeutic practice. BAPT is committed to continuing to support play therapists in promoting the highest standards of play therapy practice within the UK. One area of ongoing focus is to build the research and evidence base for play therapy practice, in order to demonstrate the relevance and effectiveness of play therapy, alongside other modalities. Looking to the future, BAPT will continue to promote the safe and ethical practice of play therapy, within this increasingly complex professional environment. We hope that this book helps to illustrate the variety and flexibility of contemporary play therapy practice within the UK.

Note on confidentiality

Please note, to preserve the anonymity and confidentiality of service users, all case material in the book has been altered and pseudonyms are used throughout. Where actual case material is used, explicit permission for this has been given by service users and is stated within the text. In other cases, composite case material has been developed, reflecting the therapist's experience of working with a large number of children, rather than with any specific child.

Note

1 Theraplay is a registered service mark of The Theraplay Institute, Evanston, IL, USA.

References

Axline, V. (1964) *Dibs: In Search of Self.* London: Penguin.
Axline, V. (1989) *Play Therapy.* London: Churchill Livingstone.
Booth, P.B. & Jernberg, A.M. (2010) *Theraplay: Helping Parents and Children Build Better Relationships through Attachment Based Play.* (3rd ed.) San Francisco: Jossey Bass.
British Association of Play Therapists. (2018a) *General Information – Definition of Play Therapy* [online]. Available at www.bapt.info/ [Accessed: 19/06/2018]
British Association of Play Therapists. (2018b) *Ethical Basis for Good Practice in Play Therapy* [online]. Available at www.bapt.info/play-therapy/ethical-basis-good-practice-play-therapy/ [Accessed: 19/06/2018]
Cattanach, A. (1994) *Play Therapy: Where the Sky Meets the Underworld.* London: Jessica Kingsley Publishers.
Dallos, R. & Draper, R. (2015) *An Introduction to Family Therapy: Systemic Theory and Practice.* Maidenhead: Open University Press/McGraw Hill.
Hughes, D. (2007) *Attachment Focused Family Therapy.* New York: W.W. Norton & Co.
Information Commissioner's Office. (2018) *General Data Protection Regulation 2018* [online]. Available at https://ico.org.uk/for-organisations/guide-to-the-general-data-protection-regulation-gdpr/
Jennings, S. (1999) *Introduction to Developmental Play Therapy: Playing and Health.* London: Jessica Kingsley Publishers.
Landreth, G.L. (2012) *Play Therapy: The Art of the Relationship.* (3rd ed.) New York: Routledge.
Rogers, C. (1951) *Client Centred Therapy.* London: Constable & Robinson.

Ryan, V. & Wilson, K. (2000) *Case Studies in Non-directive Play Therapy.* London: Jessica Kingsley Publishers.

VanFleet, R. (2013) *Filial Therapy: Strengthening Parent-Child Relationships through Play.* Sarasota: Professional Resource Press.

Wilson, K. & Ryan, V. (1992) *Play Therapy: A Non-Directive Approach for Children and Adolescents.* Oxford: Balliere Tindall.

Part I

Becoming a play therapist

Chapter 1

Training issues

Before, during and after

Lisa Gordon Clark

Chapter overview

This chapter will explore issues around play therapy training at pre-qualifying, qualifying and post-qualifying stages. I will offer guidance to those interested in pursuing a play therapy training programme with advice on what prior qualifications and experience are sought by admissions teams as well as the personal attributes that contribute to a suitability to train. I will describe core curriculum content of the BAPT-accredited Master's courses, University-validated programmes, which all integrate crucial strands of theoretical/academic learning, clinical/professional skills and personal development. I will also discuss Continuing Professional Development pathways, and outline various further training avenues which aim to consolidate, deepen and broaden learning for qualified play therapists.

What makes a suitable candidate for training as a play therapist?

I believe that the training providers are the gatekeepers to the play therapy profession and thus careful and conscientious selection of potential trainees is critical to its future integrity. In my own role on the admissions panel at the University of Roehampton I take this responsibility very seriously, as do staff on each of the BAPT-accredited programmes. I am often asked by interested candidates if I think their qualifications and experience make them suitable to apply. I tend to reply that each training applicant's merits are considered quite holistically and decisions are usually based on all components of the admissions process, including the personal statement and references as well as presentation at interview. Nevertheless, there are stipulations about suitable candidates made in the latest course accreditation criteria produced by the British Association of Play Therapists (2016). First, it is stated therein that the Master's level programmes are aimed at either:

a   professionals with a relevant qualification and/or degree in a related discipline, together with a minimum of two years' post qualifying experience in, for example, social work, teaching, educational psychology, clinical psychology, nursing

or

b   those with a minimum of five years' relevant prior experience and learning. Relevant experience means working face-to-face with children, young people and their families/carers.

According to these professional body criteria, applicants will normally be required to hold a good undergraduate degree at Honours level (2:1 or above), or its equivalent for overseas applicants. In most cases this degree will be in a relevant discipline such as psychology, education, early childhood studies or social sciences, or perhaps in a creative modality such as art, drama or performing arts. Appropriate clinically related disciplines for graduate-level professional qualifications include teaching, paediatric nursing, mental health nursing, social work and occupational therapy. Further to this baseline academic qualification specification, applicants are expected to have adequate appropriate experience which might include working with children with behavioural or developmental challenges, learning difficulties, child mental health, etc. This can either be on a voluntary or an employed basis, although, because of the inherently competitive nature of the admissions process, regularity and longevity of this work, experience can play a factor; those who can only claim to have done regular babysitting or volunteered at a weekly youth club, for example, are unlikely to be selected at the first stage in the process. Sometimes those who have considerable experience as foster carers or as nannies are also considered if this is combined with an adequate academic qualification. Applicants may need to evidence that they can meet the academic demands of a Master's degree, and, in certain circumstances, programmes might require candidates to submit a brief written report to support their application.

But suitability to train as a play therapist is more than possessing a strong academic CV and having an extensive work experience record. In addition to meeting these quantifiable criteria, applicants to the BAPT-accredited programmes need to demonstrate a maturity of personality and self-awareness compatible with training as a therapist. Admissions teams therefore seek to ascertain an appropriate measure of emotional literacy, robustness and an ability to be self-reflective. I often advise that the personal statement on the application form is not just about what the candidate has done prior to applying to train, but what they have learned and gleaned from what they have done, i.e. how their qualification(s) and experiences have helped them better understand children, and themselves. A cursorily written personal statement which does not contain adequate evidence of a capacity to be thoughtful and reflective may take the candidate no further in the applications process.

There are other factors that may determine whether a candidate is successful in being invited to the interview stage, and beyond. One is the standard requirement for two references, normally: one that comments on the applicant's academic suitability, and another on their clinical/personal suitability for the programme. Mature candidates who have been out of education for many years before deciding to retrain may find it impossible to track down university lecturers, etc., who can vouch for their academic prowess. In such circumstances, recent or current employers typically supply an appropriate reference instead. Very out-of-date references, written generically, may lead to a request for a more recent or programme-specific document. It can be rather off-putting to admissions teams when the reference alludes to applying for a different course of study altogether!

Finally, again in line with BAPT criteria, the minimum level of competence in the English language at the point of application is an IELTS (International English Language Testing System) score of 6.5, with no component score below 5.5. This baseline competence and confidence in English means that not only are students able to follow complex theoretical content in lectures and their academic reading and to write coherently in course assignments, but that on clinical placements – which start early in the programme – they can communicate with assurance with referrers, placement managers, parents and carers, as well as, of course, the children themselves. Being able to engage constructively with those around the child at the assessment stage and beyond, understanding their concerns and articulating clearly what play therapy is would be hampered if speaking and listening skills were inadequate from the outset of the training.

If these various entry conditions have been evidenced with the written application, we will invite applicants to a face-to-face interview. In the case of overseas candidates this may be via a video link, but, whenever possible, physical attendance is preferred. On the interview day, which typically contains both group and individual components, admissions teams will look more at the personal qualities, values and attitudes of the applicants, such as empathy and acceptance; at their existing knowledge base of play therapy and of the therapeutic relationship (although this is not expected to be comprehensive); and at evidence of the nascent skills required to be a student play therapist. Some programmes may ask the interviewees to talk in detail about a child that they have worked with, including background information, details of the work carried out with the child, the outcome of the support and reflections on the work undertaken. The way in which the candidate thinks about children, their ability to form relationships with children, and their understanding of the significance of this, are crucial. Other programmes may send out a play therapy-themed article in advance of the interview or provide a moral tale to read on the day, and may ask candidates to discuss in a small group their response to the paper or examine the attitudes and issues in the tale. The purpose is to discern their capacity to think critically, but also to observe their contribution to the group discussion: we on the interview panel will be trying to perceive whether candidates can listen to others and express and tolerate different opinions, and hope to get a sense of whether potential trainees are able to make their own voice heard without dominating the discussion.

Interview panels will also examine applicants' preparedness for embarking on this demanding course, not only with regard to their academic readiness but also emotionally, financially and in terms of their time. Deeper questioning may explore the emotional robustness and resilience of candidates, with sensitive exploration of how they have handled and resolved past traumas or dealt with mental health challenges, and consideration of the support networks around them. It is essential for a professional training of this nature, which prepares students to become grounded and secure therapists working with vulnerable client groups, that applicants are not still struggling themselves with unresolved issues likely to be triggered by aspects of the course. Sometimes a suggestion may be made following interview that an applicant takes time to make use of personal therapy before reapplying for the programme another year, once feelings are less raw and overwhelming. In any case, all students must be prepared to enter mandatory ongoing personal therapy for the duration of the programme: another crucial aspect of the BAPT-accredited training courses.

For other creative arts therapies, such as music therapy or art psychotherapy, proficiency in the focus discipline is an essential criterion in assessing suitability for postgraduate training. A portfolio of artwork or a musical audition may form part of the application process for those programmes. Play skills are evidently harder to evaluate for potential play therapy trainees. Nevertheless, some programmes do seek to ascertain playfulness and creativity at interview, with an activity which aims to evaluate applicants' capacity to use metaphor: a key tool of the play therapy approach.

Feedback from the interview panel may suggest that an applicant who shows potential but is perceived to be not quite 'ready' for the Master's training first completes an Introductory Day, Summer School or Foundation Course in Play Therapy, where this is available. Such preliminary-level, non-qualifying courses offer students a valuable insight into many of the core skills and basic theory of the play therapy approach. Such insight will not only serve to enhance their subsequent application but will ensure that they have a really clear concept of the nature of the training and are genuinely committed to pursuing it before investing the considerable time, energy and finances the full training entails. Those students who have first undertaken one of these preliminary courses have anecdotally expressed to me that it really helped them to 'hit the ground running' when it came to commencing study at Master's level.

What the training entails and what to expect

Once students have been successful in gaining entry to a BAPT-accredited training, demands are intense and rigorous. The present course accreditation documentation from the British Association of Play Therapists is at Master's level, comprising of a two-year, full-time academic programme or a block or part-time delivery programme carried out over three years. BAPT also specifies a minimum 100 hours of clinical play therapy practice overall during the course, plus a minimum of 50 hours of clinical supervision and 60 hours of personal therapy.

BAPT-accredited courses are expected to provide a balanced learning experience for trainees, of which approximately 60 per cent should be theoretical and 40 per cent experiential. The latter will include hands-on familiarity with a range of toys and play resources, for example, the use of clay, sensory materials, sand worlds, miniatures, art and role-play. In addition to the specified contact hours, trainees are expected to undertake a minimum of 1,200 hours of independent study over the duration of the programme. Independent study includes assessed work, child observations, written records associated with clinical practice and preparation for supervision. This all adds up to a demanding training experience, and the impact on the student is not to be underestimated – but, those who are fully committed to the course and prepared to invest substantial time, energy and effort will reap the rewards. For some, it is a 'rollercoaster', but one they consider very well worth the ride once they reach the end of track. For those who do wobble on the rails or encounter some unexpectedly steep inclines, there is a benefit to being on an accredited programme where the staff are practising therapists: we do aspire to role-model excellent pastoral care for our students and ensure that we provide nurturing support and sensitive, empathic containment throughout their journey. Certainly, a well-supported trainee makes for a more resilient practitioner.

Whilst BAPT states it does not wish to be prescriptive about the exact format of the courses that it accredits, it is a requirement of accreditation that each Master's programme can evidence that the Core Competences are all met within the curriculum (see Appendix 1 for the full list of these). It proposes that the following subject areas be used as a baseline in the syllabus, learning outcomes that cover BAPT's essential *Knowledge and Understanding* competences.

Child development

By the end of their training, Play Therapy Master's students should understand some of the key theories of typical child developmental processes within the context of familial and social diversity. They should also demonstrate an understanding of how life events and circumstances, including family and ethnicity, the experience of trauma, physical and mental health/ill-health may impact on development.

The core syllabus stipulated by BAPT covers the following aspects of child development:

- an introduction to theory of child development and normal developmental processes;
- attachment theory;
- knowledge of the child's physical, social, emotional, cognitive, linguistic and spiritual development;
- the effects of disability, poverty, illness, race and gender on child development;
- abuse and neglect, and their effects on a child's development;
- separation and loss, for example, divorce, death and separation from family of birth;
- the impact of trauma on child development, for example, accident, civil conflict;
- an understanding of child mental health diagnoses.

Focus on these learning outcomes, which draw on the knowledge base of normal and abnormal developmental psychology, helps the play therapy trainee to put their clients' needs into context and perspective, and develops a capacity to adapt their therapeutic method appropriately to work effectively with a range of client groups. Keeping up with fast-evolving research in development psychology, such as recent illuminating advances in neuroscience (Music, 2016), can make this an exciting topic for students.

Child observation

All students on BAPT-accredited Master's courses are required to undertake a minimum of 30 hours of child observation. There is scope for some variety in how the accredited training courses manage this, with at least one – the University of Roehampton – stipulating that all 30 hours be with the same child, preferably a baby under 6 months of age. BAPT suggest, more flexibly, that a minimum of 20 observations are of the same child under three years of age, and that the remaining hours be made from other categories such as a school-age child or a sibling pair.

All the accredited courses provide academic support for these child observations, for example, group discussions or regular seminars, with clear links to the theory of child development. The impact of the first days, weeks and months of life on every child's subsequent development and well-being is increasingly recognised (Gerhardt, 2004), so it is essential for play therapists to have an in-depth understanding of this and of the growth of the infant's relationship with their caregiver. But another vital dimension to this aspect of the training is that students learn to hold the role of observer. This combines objective information-gathering with an awareness of how the subjective impact of children's behaviour on the feelings of the receptive observer can be used as a source of clinically relevant information. Part of this includes tolerating factors which students encounter within their observations and thinking how this might inform their understanding of the infant's emotional and cognitive development. Reflective self-awareness is key – as is a keen retentive memory, which this observation experience serves to hone.

Play and play therapy

The syllabus proposed by BAPT includes a comprehensive knowledge of the literature relating to the practice of play therapy, its historical development and the stages and development of play. Central components include:

- theories of play;
- stages and development of play;
- play as a therapeutic metaphor;
- an examination of the difference between play therapy, therapeutic play and direct work with children;
- the theory of the specific model of play therapy promoted by the course and an overview of other play therapy approaches;
- the ability to evaluate critically a range of theoretical frameworks and therapeutic approaches other than play therapy in relation to practice. This necessitates understanding of the history and development of therapeutic work with children, for example, Psychoanalytic (Klein, Freud, Jung, Winnicott); Social Construction Theory; Person-Centred (Rogers, Axline) and Gestalt (Oaklander);
- the context of play therapy within other therapeutic and assessment provisions for children, for example, hospitals, schools and clinics;
- the process of therapy: assessment, therapeutic stages, evaluation, liaison with family and others, endings;
- the impact of play therapy on the child, family and other support systems.

In addition to these central aspects of the play therapy training curriculum, BAPT also advocates learning outcomes appertaining to:

- *Families, care systems and wider networks,* including the child's social context, i.e. family, school, environment and race; general attitudes and beliefs towards children and family life, plus different types of families and care systems.

- *Legal and Statutory Framework* entailing knowledge of the Children Act 1989 or the Children (Scotland) Act 1995, and other relevant legislation, an understanding of the roles and relationships between the statutory, voluntary and private/independent sectors, including the role of social services and child-oriented voluntary agencies, as well as the role of the play therapist vis-à-vis the courts. It is essential that play therapists are aware of their statutory responsibilities in line with the most recent inter-agency safeguarding procedures – currently Working Together to Safeguard Children document in the UK (HM Gov, 2015).
- *Other therapeutic approaches.* It is helpful for the trainee to be aware of other methods of working with children within the family, for example, cognitive behaviour therapy, family therapy, counselling, group therapy, art psychotherapy and dramatherapy, etc. This enables them as therapists to identify problems that can be helped by other methods as well as those outside their own limits of expertise.
- *Professional issues* such as record-keeping, confidentiality, ethics, the impact of therapeutic work on the play therapist, setting up in independent practice, equal opportunities issues and a commitment to anti-discriminatory and culturally sensitive practice.
- *Research.* Since training to be a BAPT-registered play therapist is now at Master's level, there is a significant credit weighting given to research, partly to ensure that students' eventual therapeutic practice is evidence-based. This includes an awareness of current research into play therapy and allied disciplines, an ability to evaluate critically relevant research findings, the ability to use academic libraries and databases and to carry out a literature search, and sufficient knowledge of research methodologies to be able to plan and carry out a piece of research relevant to the field.

The breadth and depth of these substantial syllabus topics inevitably necessitates a huge amount of reading and independent study in addition to the required contact hours. We do impress upon our students the benefit of keeping abreast with their background reading and those who fall behind can struggle to catch up. A well-organised conscientious work ethic is a major advantage.

While obviously hugely important, these various strands of theoretical/academic learning outcomes which address the first nine Core Competences (those subtitled 'Knowledge and Understanding', see Appendix 1), form just one dimension of the comprehensive syllabus of the BAPT-accredited training programmes. Equally crucial components, running in close parallel, are those of which cover the other two categories of Competences: *Personal Development* and *Practice Skills*. These vital aspects differentiate these professional training programmes from many other standard academic postgraduate courses, since they are about developing clinical skills and also focus on the very personhood of the fledgling play therapist. The training bodies all recognise that learning to be a competent play therapist is not just the acquisition of theoretical knowledge and techniques but that 'who the therapist is and the way the therapist relates may be as important as what the therapist says' (Rowan & Jacobs, 2002: 88).

Clinical practice and supervision

It is within the clinical placements that each student must synthesise, integrate and apply all aspects of their learning. BAPT specify that a minimum of 100 hours of play therapy practice is required during the training period, closely supervised by a qualified, accredited play therapist at a ratio of 1:2 supervision hours to clinical hours. Some courses provide internal group supervision for the first placement as part of the tuition fees, but externally accessed individual supervision, with close liaison with the programme staff, is more the norm. Practice-based learning entails assessing for, setting up, maintaining and processing about five play therapy cases, usually carried out in two separate placement contexts. The first two placement cases (total duration 30 clinical hours) need to be at a low level of need appropriate to the level of skill development of the trainee. For the second placement, one case should be a long-term intervention of 30 hours duration, at least 25 hours of which need to be face-to-face work with the child, allowing five hours for assessment, parent meetings, reviews, etc. With increasing recognition of the importance of careful assessment and of working systemically, each student is required to participate in the assessment process of potentially appropriate referrals before commencing any therapeutic work. Identification of which referrals to proceed with may involve collaborative discussions with both their placement manager and their clinical supervisor – liaison which is very helpful for trainees in preparing them for subsequent systemic and interdisciplinary practice.

For the BAPT-accredited Master's programmes it is now recommended that all sessions be video-recorded (with full informed consent from both parent and child, and stored/destroyed in careful compliance with Data Protection procedures in the 2018 GDPR) and that seven hours of video clips be presented to the clinical supervisor. I regard this as an essential training aid and imperative for promoting and ensuring ethical play therapy practice and the protection of the public. The recordings also provide a valuable resource for the trainee by helping them to develop clinical practice skills, self-reflexivity and the ability to become an observer to their practice. Watching back the footage in the supportive presence of their clinical supervisor enables trainees to review and consider their own strengths and limitations and thus to operate and practise efficiently within their own levels of competence. I know that many students report finding it uncomfortable viewing at first as their vulnerabilities and learning edges are exposed on screen, but all soon come to appreciate its incomparable value as a way of honing their skills and ultimately of developing their own 'internal supervisor.'

Most students express the view, perhaps unsurprisingly, that this opportunity to implement and integrate their theoretical learning into real hands-on experience on placement is the most valuable aspect of the training. Literally putting into practice what they have been learning – and continue to learn – in the classroom and from books is by turns daunting, exciting, scary, affirming and challenging, but always skill-enhancing. As I found in my own training, it was only by experiencing the power of play therapy 'for real' and for myself that I could begin to do what I now always urge trainees to do: trust the process.

Personal development

As alluded to above, the ability to recognise the limits of one's personal expertise, skills and approach is essential to safe and effective practice, as is the awareness of personal development processes and a capacity to use such insights in therapeutic, reflexive ways. Accordingly, a minimum of 60 hours of personal therapy is mandatory during the BAPT-accredited Master's programmes. This ongoing personal therapy also provides emotional support, a context in which students can explore the roots of personal issues arising during training/client work, and has the further benefit of enabling students to gain experience of being in the client role, to experience the therapeutic relationship 'from the other side', as it were.

Personal therapy, along with other experiential learning opportunities in training such as 'the process group' or 'practice exchange group' provided by some courses, is instrumental in the developing awareness for students of their introjected beliefs about the self and how these influence their self-concept and behaviour, and can impact on their work with clients. As one of my Roehampton colleagues puts it:

> To use ourselves in our work, to use the *self* as an agent of change, requires by definition a confidence and knowledge in who we are … how we use ourselves and bring our own self-awareness into the therapeutic relationship is ultimately the most important and uniquely significant element of the process.
>
> (Le Vay, 2016: 2)

Furthermore, therapy also facilitates the development both of a sufficiently strong sense of personal identity to resist being drawn into the client's pathology, and of 'self-acceptance' – or at least a significant movement in that direction. Similarly, the personal development aspect of the accredited trainings enhances the student play therapist's awareness of self in relation to others, such as enduring patterns in their own interpersonal behaviour and the needs and fears upon which these patterns are based. Hopefully this leads to a reduction of personal prejudices, which can inhibit the achievement of mutuality in therapeutic relationships. Indeed, when working therapeutically with vulnerable young clients and their families it is essential that students are alert to any potential blocks with respect to the expression of the therapeutic conditions of empathy, unconditional positive regard and congruence (Rogers, 2003), which, if unrecognised, could lead to them being susceptible to clinical over-involvement or under-involvement. This aspect of training encourages a disposition of openness to experience, an acceptance of responsibility for one's own behaviour and learning and the capacity to self-appraise openly and accurately, all of which I believe significantly strengthen the calibre of new recruits to the play therapy profession. (For further reading about the value of personal therapy both during and post-training, see Chapter 2 by McCann.)

What happens once qualified?

I am a fervent exponent of the view that learning to be a play therapist – or learning to become a better one – does not stop at graduation. In order to retain BAPT full membership status, qualified play therapists need to meet minimum requirements for continuing professional development (CPD) in line with the government impetus to monitor standards of professional training, performance and conduct.

There are three sections to BAPT's CPD requirements:

1) training or activities directly related to play therapy, which could include attendance at relevant conferences, supervision training, post-qualified play therapy research including writing articles/papers/books, attendance at local play therapy support group meetings, etc.;
2) indirect CPD activities, such as providing clinical supervision, personal therapy, peer group discussion, reading articles, other training, e.g. child protection, supporting parents, and other teaching/workshops related to play therapy for other professionals;
3) ongoing clinical supervision, the frequency of which will vary according to the extent of post-qualifying experience, levels of monthly caseload and the intensity of the work. The clinical supervisor remains crucial for the play therapist well beyond training and throughout their professional career (see also Chapter 3 by Platteuw for more on the role the clinical supervisor).

Much of this CPD activity not only ensures retention of full professional body membership, and thus inclusion on the Professional Standards

Authority (PSA) approved register, but will also enhance the quality of the service that the qualified play therapist can offer. Remaining up-to-date with professional learning, beyond the need to meet approved learning outcomes on training, is crucial for upholding the standard and integrity of our profession. Furthermore, attendance at the annual conferences, CPD workshops and at informal local support groups is a great way to 'network' and feel part of the wider play therapy community. Personally, I always find these opportunities to touch base with like-minded colleagues so affirming, inspiring and re-motivating: every bit as important in a way as the formal content of the lectures and workshops themselves.

There are also some specialist follow-up training courses available for qualified play therapists wishing to further or broaden their career. Many choose to pursue training in filial therapy (Van Fleet, 2005) or in child parent relationship therapy (CPRT) (Landreth & Bratton, 2015), helping parents and carers to acquire and utilise some of the core child-centred play skills to build and strengthen relationships with their own children. There is increasing recognition of and demand for such systemic approaches that empower parents to be the 'agents of change' and that can leave a tangible enduring legacy of our professional input. Similarly, there are qualified play therapists who find the Theraplay approach fits well with their way of working, again using play techniques to enhance attachment relationships. These further professional pathways are perhaps particularly valid and appreciated for Looked After Children and, accordingly, some play therapists who opt for adding these additional strings to their skill bow find a good source of work through the Adoption Support Fund.

Alternatively, or additionally, many play therapists with adequate post-qualifying experience opt to progress to the role of clinical supervisor and recent years have seen the emergence of a few approved training courses to prepare therapists for transition to this responsible professional role. The more the play therapy profession grows the more need there will be for clinical supervisors to support the next generation and ensure their practice is safe and effective. It is an essential rung on the play therapy career ladder … as indeed is supervision of supervisors!

Finally, for some qualified play therapists the appetite for further academic study does not abate and they are drawn to pursue a research trajectory. The number of those undertaking PsychD or PhD research in the UK is growing rapidly and their contribution to an enhanced and rigorous evidence base for our practice can only bode well for the reputation, status and secure future of our profession: an evidence base that provides material for subsequent generations of trainees and for the benefit of all.

Summary

- Criteria for what makes a suitable candidate for training as a play therapist were discussed including appropriate prior qualifications, relevant experience and personal aptitude. An insight into the admission process was provided.
- Core curriculum content of the BAPT-accredited Master's level training programmes was outlined with links drawn to the BAPT Core Competences and a rationale was provided for video-recorded and supervised practice-based learning as well as for personal therapy on training.
- Possibilities and opportunities for post-qualifying career progression were raised, including further training routes, supervision and research.

To find out more about the Master's programmes currently accredited by BAPT

England: University of Roehampton
  www.roehampton.ac.uk/postgraduate-courses/play-therapy/
Scotland: Queen Margaret University, Edinburgh
  www.qmu.ac.uk/study-here/postgraduate-study/2018-postgraduate-courses/msc-play-therapy/
Wales: University of South Wales http://courses.southwales.ac.uk/courses/639-msc-play-therapy

References

Gerhardt, S. (2004) *Why Love Matters: How Affection Shapes a Baby's Brain*. (2nd ed.) London: Routledge.
HM Gov. (2015) www.gov.uk/government/uploads/system/uploads/attachment_data/file/592101/Working_Together_to_Safeguard_Children_20170213.pdf. Accessed 9/2/018
Landreth, G. & Bratton S. (2015) *Child Parent Relationship Therapy (CPRT): A 10-Session Filial Therapy Model*. New York: Routledge.
Le Vay, D. (2016) To be or not to be? The therapeutic use of self in child-centred play therapy. In Le Vay, D. & Cuschieri, E. (eds) *Challenges in the Theory and Practice of Play Therapy*. London: Routledge. pp. 1–17.
Music, G. (2016) *Nurturing Natures*. (2nd ed.) London: Routledge.
Rogers, C. (2003) *Client Centred Therapy: Its Current Practice, Implications and Theory*. (3rd ed.) London: Constable & Robinson.
Rowan, J. & Jacobs, M. (2002) *The Therapist's Use of Self*. Maidenhead: Open University Press.
Van Fleet, R. (2005) *Filial Therapy: Strengthening Parent-Child Relationships through Play*. (2nd ed.) Saratosa, FL: Professional Resource Press.

Chapter 2

The play therapist's personal therapy

Julie McCann

Overview

In this chapter, I will put forward the rationale for BAPT's requirement for all students to undergo personal therapy and for its approval of personal therapy as part of continuing professional support and development. I will examine the views of therapists in general and play therapists in particular about their experience of personal therapy, both during training and throughout professional practice. Within this, I will point towards research into the impact of personal therapy on the practitioner as well as the clients and the difficulties in carrying out such research. I will also raise some of the current issues in the field of therapy training about whether or not mandatory personal therapy should be continued.

Untangling the knots

> Below the surface of our conscious awareness a vast unknown rootage determines our actions .... We become aware of the patterns of blindness and obsession which unknowingly drive us.
>
> (O'Donohue, 1997:118–119)

In training and in developing as a play therapist, the exploration of my own psyche is an ever deepening, spiralling path towards glimpsing and challenging these unknowns. When alongside a young client and in relating to the family members, school staff, social workers and others who form the system around that client, I am frequently attracted to, repelled by and tossed about by a jumble of feelings, judgements, urges and responses. How do I untangle this often complex knot of reactions and relationships? How do I provide the core conditions of empathy, congruence and unconditional positive regard (Rogers, 1957)? As a student and now as a practising play therapist, I am immensely grateful for the practice of personal therapy which continues to enable me to unpick and bring into knowing some of the depths of myself that resonate when with my clients.

What is BAPT's rationale for personal therapy?

The dynamic nature of non-directive/child-centred play therapy means that who I am as a person matters greatly to the child and it is vital that I know, understand, accept, and care for myself in ways that allow me to relate to my young clients whilst neither being overwhelmed by or unknowingly dominating their play with my own issues. In play therapy, the 'success or failure of therapy ... rests on the development and maintenance of the therapeutic relationship. It is the relationship with the child that becomes the vehicle for sustainable change and growth by the child' (Landreth, 2012:11). This means that my conscious understanding of myself, my childhood, relationships and patterns of behaviour can have an immense impact on how I work.

Whilst BAPT requires all play therapy students to undergo personal therapy during training, there is currently no rationale given for it in BAPT documentation. Instead, each training institution gives students its own rationale for personal therapy in course materials and in lectures which focus on personal development, self-awareness and the use of self within the therapeutic relationship. There are three overarching rationales common across all training institutions:

1. Personal support – Trainers recognise that their courses are demanding and rigorous, both emotionally and academically; 'This journey that you have embarked on is not an easy one. You will find many challenges along the way' (Roehampton University, 2017:3). Some students are returning to academic study after many years, there are financial, time and travel commitments to negotiate as well as new relationships with fellow students, the stresses of learning about trauma, being faced with parts of ourselves we have hidden or forgotten. Having external, unconditional support from a personal therapist throughout training is regarded by all of the institutions as vital.

2. Personal issues – Trainers advise that students need to be aware of their personal areas of conflict, blocks, or habitual responses that may constrict their contribution to the peer process groups and supervision, and which may interfere with a child's therapy process. When on placement seeing children, students may encounter issues that resonate with their own, and personal therapy is seen as a context within which students can recognise, explore the roots of, and resolve their personal issues which are still eliciting distress. This high level of self-awareness allows play therapists to be 'better able to work with clients and to cope with the stresses of learning on the course without undue interference from internal conflict' (Queen Margaret University, 2016/17:21) and to recognise and contain their own unresolved problems or blind spots, so that they are aware of 'what's mine and what's the child's' and do not inadvertently impact on the child's therapeutic journey.

3. Therapist as a model/experience of being the client – Trainers want students to have a direct experience of a therapeutic relationship and of the processes involved in personal therapy. Although the mode of therapy is different to that which the student offers children, students experience a dynamic, person-centred therapy for themselves and can use their personal therapist as a model for how they can practise. Of course, students need also to be self-aware enough not to presume that their clients experience therapy in the same way as they do and to be alert to when a child's communications through play are resonating with their own issues.

What are the requirements?

The training of BAPT play therapists in the UK developed from a Certificate to a Master's qualification, and the requirement for personal therapy hours has gradually increased over time. Currently BAPT's Training and Education Sub-Committee mandates for a minimum of 60 hours of personal therapy, spread equally through the two or three years of training. The financial commitment is a substantial one and students are urged to budget for this alongside fees and other study costs when considering accepting a place.

Choosing a therapist

Training institutions advise students on selecting a therapist who must be accredited to a professional body such as BACP or the United Kingdom Council for Psychotherapy (UKCP) and have a minimum number of years' experience. Some institutions offer a list of recommended therapists, although there are no specified 'training therapists', and the personal therapist is not part of the teaching team, as is the case in some psychological trainings.

For students who have previous experience of personal therapy, some continue to see their current therapist, others return to a previous therapist and some choose to find a new therapist from a different modality to 'try something new'. Students are expected to remain with the same therapist throughout their training to experience a long-term intervention and develop a supportive therapeutic relationship. Any change in therapist during the course is discussed with course directors to explore why the student feels this change is necessary. Such discussions may alert staff to the student's avoidance of difficult issues or there may be a genuine mismatch or inadequacy of the personal therapist in question.

Modality of the personal therapist

Although one of the main reasons for undertaking therapy is for the personal therapist to act as a model, it is not particularly recommended that students undergo play therapy. This is because play is considered to be the primary form of communication for children, allowing them to describe and resolve their thoughts, feelings and perceptions. 'When children speak about trauma metaphorically in their play, although they may be depicting horrors, they are simultaneously *playing* with what is depicted' (McCarthy, 2012:29). As adults, we generally use spoken language and creative tools in therapy to 'play' with the material that interests or disturbs us. It is the therapeutic relationship, the dynamic between therapist and client, that is the most vital component for change and so students should seek a therapist who practises within a humanistic, psychodynamic or person-centred orientation.

A recent online survey, entitled 'Personal therapy – have your say!' (McCann, 2017), showed that most BAPT play therapists, whether during training or after qualification, seek out a therapist who works through 'talking' (79%). A significant number choose a creative therapy such as art psychotherapy (18%) and small numbers have undertaken play therapy (9%) or sand tray therapy (4%). Play therapists clearly value having personal experience of a non-directive mode of therapy, one in which the therapeutic relationship is central and the focus is on 'tolerating uncertainty' (Cayne & Loewenthal, 2007:375), sitting with the unknown, examining themes, tussling with dynamics and allowing subconscious feelings to emerge, rather than solution-based therapy or counselling, in which the focus may be on strategies or theories being studied.

Recording personal therapy during training

Students are required to submit a personal therapy registration form, signed by their therapist, to confirm that the therapist's qualifications, professional orientation and experience meet the requirements of the training institution. At the mid-point and end of their training, they gain their therapist's signature as proof of the hours undertaken and an affirmation that he/she considers the student an appropriate person to work with children.

Each training institution requires some form of reflective feedback from students and embeds the personal therapy competence within its own learning framework. Students may be required to keep a private reflective log which includes comments on their personal therapy and how it relates to their learning and practice. While the details of personal therapy remain confidential, students are expected to integrate their experience of personal therapy into all aspects of their learning so that the impact on their personal development and self-awareness can be alluded to and referenced in any written assignment. Some institutions specifically teach their rationale for personal therapy and require students to submit written work on the topic.

The training institutions acknowledge that the benefits of personal therapy during training may not be obvious, for example: 'The personal development needs of students go beyond personal preferences and initial opinions.

The development needs of the student are often broader than those s/he might immediately identify' (University of Roehampton, 2017:24). I would have valued opportunities within my course to comment on, discuss and draw understanding from my personal therapy, especially in relation to my clinical placements, and am encouraged that current training includes open reflection and written assignments on personal therapy.

Links with core competences and self-care

Students and qualified play therapists are made aware that personal therapy is considered to be a valuable ongoing intervention for self-care, personal development and professional practice. BAPT's Core Competences for play therapists are divided into three areas, the second of which is 'Personal Development' (see Appendix 1). Section 14 of this promotes the 'Utilisation of personal therapy and support for development' through integrating 'personal therapy and development support in an appropriate and effective manner' and demonstrating the 'ability to be self-reflective and to integrate learning into therapeutic practice to ensure effective and ethical standards of practice and promote public safety'. Students are required to demonstrate their skills in these areas through the 'Competence Log', making reference to personal therapy in relation to their clinical practice.

The Core Competences also include a list of Personal Qualities which, whilst they do not directly refer to personal therapy, can be seen to support this form of development both in training and during professional practice:

Self-Awareness: To assess, review and consider own competences, strengths and weaknesses as a Play Therapist.

Self-Responsibility: To operate and practise efficiently within own level of competences.

Critical Reflection: To critically reflect upon the emotional, social and psychological world of clients, significant others and the Self and to integrate reflection into practice.

Commitment to personal development: To be reflexive, to integrate personal insights into future practice, to continue personal development in a responsible and effective manner.

Qualified play therapists are required to meet high standards of Continuing Professional Development (CPD). Up to six hours of personal therapy can be counted as CPD indirectly related to play therapy (BAPT CPD Section 2) and therapists are required to give a brief account of how the activity has enhanced professional practice. Play therapists, like others who have careers that can impact profoundly on psychological and physical well-being, seek out a range of strategies to support and sustain professional practice. In my interview study of four play therapists (McCann, 2012) the interviewees, whose names were changed to protect identity, were invited to speak about the self-care strategies that support their work:

> Masses! Gosh, the things I need are: I need my hands in the earth or on clay. I do pottery and I've got an allotment ... and I do stained glass as well ...
>
> (Pauline)

> Music still, of course, is a huge part of my life. And weekends, going for walks in the countryside. That's a big thing that has to happen, so I'm always making space for that! It instantly, instantly lifts me. It is incredibly restorative.
>
> (Anna)

The 2017 online survey was my attempt to gather a broad picture of the experiences and views of BAPT play therapists regarding personal therapy before, during and after training. I found that 32% of respondents reported they continue personal therapy immediately after training and 55% seek it out at some point during their professional life. The time given to personal therapy post-qualification ranges from short-term interventions of fewer than twenty sessions to long-term analysis over more than fifteen years. A large number of play therapists report three separate periods of personal therapy overall and the highest overall average is for around five years. This indicates that accessing personal therapy throughout the career of a BAPT play therapist is common.

How open are play therapists about their personal therapy?

While it is clear that personal therapy remains a significant source of self-care and support throughout professional life, from personal conversation and the interview study, I find that there can be a reluctance to openly acknowledge this. Play therapists who trained some time ago were not required to make explicit connections between their personal therapy and professional development in the more direct ways that current students can be asked to do. Consequently, in the survey I asked to what extent play therapists talk about their own therapy.

Many (94%) share with colleagues and close friends the fact that they are or have been undergoing personal therapy. A variety of reasons are given, including: helping to demystify therapy, normalising the process, and lending empathy for the client's process.

Likewise, in the interview study (McCann, 2012) all participants were open, to some extent, about the actuality of their own therapy:

> My whole family would know … And all my friends actually … It's not at all a taboo topic … It's just one of those things you do if you think it's good for you.
>
> (Anna)

However, some were reticent to share the fact of undergoing personal therapy, especially in work environments where colleagues might see it as a weakness rather than a strength:

> I remember a colleague of mine going through a very, very difficult time … I was quite open I was in therapy and found it helpful and I said had she thought about it and she just looked really aghast.
>
> (Greta)

One participant brought up the element of shame and how rarely friends and colleagues, in her experience, talk about personal therapy:

> It's almost a feeling of 'Should I be doing this?' There's still that feeling that there's some guilt and perhaps shame … people don't talk about it, do they?
>
> (Clare)

It seems, from the survey, that while the vast majority of play therapists let a few people know that we are undergoing personal therapy post-qualification, very few share the *content* or details. Reasons given not to do so include: identifying too much with the client, wanting to keep professional boundaries and potential shame in sharing too much personal information. One interviewee, however, was unusual in her openness in sharing the themes and details of her personal therapy:

> Oh, very open about it because I just think it's all life experiences and if my experiences can help someone else – I talk about anything really. Even the abuse … So I'm probably more open than other people would be.
>
> (Pauline)

I wonder if more recently trained play therapists will speak about it with more openness and approach a return to therapy with a less hidden attitude than their colleagues who trained when there was no explicit teaching around the impacts of personal therapy.

How do we know the impact of play therapists' personal therapy?

It is difficult to examine the impact of personal therapy on play therapists since, to my knowledge, there is only one piece of published research (McCann, 2012) which specifically relates to the experiences of play therapists. My searches indicate that there is no research that examines the impact of personal therapy on therapists working primarily with children, such as child psychotherapists. I find this frustrating and surprising, especially as over 70 years ago writers such as Bornstein (1948) were proposing that responses from the therapist towards the client are stronger and more immediate in therapeutic work with children compared to similar work with adults, leading to the opinion that it is more imperative for child therapists to be self-aware to protect the child as well as the self. The issue was raised again by Littner and Schour in 1971 at a time when specialised study for psychotherapy work with children was rare (usually it was an adjunct to generic adult training). Here the authors point out

> a serious obstacle to the mastery of this [profession] … is the student's own unconscious resistance. Since he is required to study about some of the identical conflicts that he himself is trying to keep repressed, unconsciously he may try to avoid knowing what consciously he is struggling to learn.
>
> (Littner & Schour, 1971:265)

I would argue that personal therapy is one avenue for developing such a high level of self-awareness as would be needed for this young client group, a view echoed in several UK play therapy books and manuals (Cattanach, 2003; Jennings, 1993; Le Vay & Cuschieri, 2016; West, 1992) where there is also a promotion of the benefits of ongoing periods of personal therapy (Landreth, 2012; Le Vay & Cuschieri, 2016; West, 1992).

In the absence of studies of play therapists, I have looked to the research on therapists from a wide range of modalities, most of whom are working with adults but some, it can be presumed, also have children and young people as their clients. Therapists (including psychologists, counsellors, and psychotherapists) have been surveyed since the 1960s through large-scale quantitative surveys, most of which have come from the USA (e.g. Henry et al., 1973; Norcross & Prochaska, 1986; Orlinsky et al., 2005). Since such research relies on self-reported views, it is subjective and does not gather the views of the client, the client's family members, or the therapist's professional colleagues. How, then, do we know that personal therapy for the play therapist has a positive impact on clients? Indeed, is the impact on clients important? This is an ongoing debate and the question explored by many researchers, including Sandell et al. (2006), Chaturvedi (2013), Curtis and Qaiser (2005) and Rizq (2011).

In the 2017 survey, I found 100% of respondents reported that personal therapy (including the mandatory period and post-qualification) had/has a positive impact on the therapists' *professional* role. Within that, 68% rated the impact as 'greatly positive'. These figures are very similar to the reported impact on *personal* lives, with 100% positive impact and, within that, 66% 'greatly positive', indicating that play therapists give slightly higher overall positive regard for personal therapy than that reported by therapists in general studies, such as those by Williams et al. (1999) (87%) and Grimmer and Tribe (2001) (94%).

Why do play therapists rate personal therapy experience so highly? Why are there no reports of a negative impact of personal therapy? Perhaps the high financial cost and considerable time commitment, as well as the historical presumption that 'it's a good thing', mean that play therapists feel compelled to view personal therapy as beneficial. It is also possible that those therapists who would rate personal therapy negatively did not respond to the survey. Others' research shows that a small but significant percentage of therapists report a negative impact, with reasons including: starting therapy coinciding with the start of training (Williams et al., 1999), dislike of the therapist, insensitivity from the therapist, time constraints, power struggles, increased distress and confusion over shifts from client to practitioner (summarised in Rizq, 2011:177).

When asked, 'In your experience, what do you consider the main benefits for personal therapy whilst training?', play therapists selected any number of motivation suggestions based on the training institutions' rationales:

> Helps to identify one's own issues including those that appear in clients' play: 96%
> Experience the process that clients experience: 88%
> Use of the therapist as a model for one's own role as therapist: 67%
> Gain support while in training: 54%

Anonymous, self-reported surveys such as this seek to examine *whether or not* personal therapy has a beneficial impact rather than on *how*, especially on *how* it affects client outcomes. In more recent years, there has been a move towards small-scale, qualitative interview studies where the narrative content of the responses is examined and gathered into main themes (Ciclitira et al., 2012; McCann, 2012; Oteiza, 2010; Rizq & Target, 2008a, 2008b). These small-scale studies 'give voice' to the findings of the surveys, and the themes which emerged include increased personal awareness, influence on professional self-identity, positive effects on personal and professional relationships and awareness of the connection between personal therapy and supervision.

One of the sub-themes that emerged in my study of BAPT play therapists (McCann, 2011, 2012) was the support students gained during training from their personal therapy. The detailed responses from the small group of participants were similar to the above survey results. Whilst finding it very challenging, all four interviewees said how much their personal therapy was a solid bed of support.

> I didn't predict how unravelling the therapeutic training would be just by doing the experiential things ... I was very glad to have [personal therapy] parallel to my training as ... a lot got unearthed that I felt I couldn't quite handle without having this external person waiting for me, week after week with an attentive presence.
>
> (Anna)

All of the participants commented on how their personal therapy during training, and since, helps them to separate their 'own stuff' from that of the child in the playroom.

> It's so imperative that we keep our own stuff separate and that we're aware of what is boiling in our own heads so that we can leave it at the door.
>
> (Pauline)

Interviewees emphasised the benefits to personal development and relationships which, in turn, they perceived to have an impact on their levels of self-awareness and empathy when with a client.

> I think by going deeper into therapy and feeling more robust and developing more of a sense of security ... I'm much more confident ... I can tune in more ... and maybe help children.
>
> (Greta)

Personal and professional life impacts

As with the general population, the motivation for seeking personal therapy among therapists is for personal issues rather than professional issues (e.g. Bike et al., 2009). BAPT play therapists report that 70% had sought personal therapy prior to training and, when returning for further periods of personal therapy, cite general self-care (60%), specific life events including bereavement (47%) and relationship difficulties (27%) as the prime motives. Issues directly relating to client work, including child issues, secondary trauma and viewing the therapist as a model for professional practice, are rarely the motive (5–12%). An aspect of professional life not explored in the survey, but one which is particularly complex in work with children, is the system around the child, i.e. school staff, family members, social care professionals. Not only must play therapists be aware of a child's conflicts, resistances and myriad emotions, they must work with other people in the child's life who 'may revive his own anger, guilt, and competition' and so 'must be able to prevent his own unconscious problems from being triggered' (Littner & Schour, 1971:263).

Should personal therapy be mandatory for all play therapy students?

There is an ongoing dialogue regarding mandatory personal therapy for trainees both within the professional bodies of UK play therapists and in therapy training generally. The decision in 2005 of the British Association for Counselling and Psychotherapy (BACP) to remove the requirement for compulsory therapy for its accredited courses generated considerable debate. Arguments against a mandatory training therapy include: starting personal therapy at the same time as starting training could be an additional strain on the student (in Thorne & Dryden, 1991); students who have undergone therapy prior to training may not wish to re-engage in it, especially when emotional disturbances brought up may interfere with the learning process (Kumari, 2011:213); it is a 'financial scam' which keeps a significant number of therapists in work, blocks places from patients without access to a mental health service and potentially excludes applicants who would find the cost prohibitive (Mearns et al., 1998).

Since 70% of BAPT students undergo personal therapy by choice *prior* to training, they negate the 'jolt' of beginning to explore their own emotional processes alongside the start of training. Part of the rigorous selection process for BAPT training involves seeking to ascertain that applicants are no longer seriously troubled or damaged by past traumas and losses. Indeed, BAPT course directors view previous personal therapy in a positive rather than negative light and explore to what extent the applicant can express insights about past experiences to ensure that the impacts have not remained raw and unresolved. Von Haenish reported that therapists in training 'enjoyed exploring issues around their self-awareness but most of them were by no means seriously troubled or damaged by their childhood experiences' (2011:153). Of course, personal therapy is not the only route for resolving the past and building emotional strength, but for those training to be therapists I believe it is fundamental to our development to have someone stay with us through the 'not knowing' and to have our unease contained without rescue or solutions. 'The greater our level of self-awareness and personal insight the greater our confidence in our practice as therapists' (Le Vay & Cuschieri, 2016:13).

The phenomenon of the 'wounded healer' is a well-known one (see Carl Jung in Dunn, 2000). As the therapist, I should be consciously aware of my own wounds and open to when these are activated in being with a child in play therapy, especially when the child is bringing up issues similar to my own. With conscious awareness, I acknowledge these similarities to myself, challenge the disturbance, and continue to play with the child, exploring what meaning the activity has for this child, on this day without presumptions from my past. 'It is contended that we stand a better chance of making an authentic relationship with those we seek to help if we are prepared to celebrate our scarred, glorious, mis-shapenly successful, and often faulty selves for what we are' (Martin, 2011:10).

Despite the BACP's decision to drop the requirement for personal therapy, most therapy training bodies in the UK do still require an element of personal therapy (up to 4–5 times weekly for child analysts) and some also require students to have up to two years of personal therapy before entering a course (Tavistock Child and Adolescent Psychotherapy Doctorate). Alternative models include personal therapy being optional or for it to be required for only some students when 'issues arise during the course that impede the student's ability to work with children' (Play Therapy UK website). Rizq suggests future research to 'compare the experiences and clinical outcomes of those undertaking mandatory therapy and those whose training specifies it as a voluntary activity' (2011:183) which would provide rich material for the debate, especially among UK play therapists.

I welcome the slant in current courses towards requiring students to make specific connections between personal therapy and therapeutic practice. Several of my student peers struggled with the compulsory nature of personal therapy. It was, in their eyes, a burdensome necessity to meet the course requirements and not the supportive and developmental experience it is intended to be. Conversely, some students accepted unquestionably this element of training, believing it must be a 'good thing' simply because they are being told to do it and senior play therapists had done it too.

Cross over and boundaries between personal therapy and clinical supervision

Clinical supervision, explored elsewhere in this volume (see Platteuw, Chapter 3), is distinct from personal therapy and differs from it in being an ongoing, compulsory requirement for all play therapists. In drawing up the supervision agreements, supervisors are careful to describe the contrasts between supervision and personal therapy indicating that the supervisor may need to direct the supervisee towards personal therapy when particular issues arise. Likewise, personal therapists may advise a play therapist to discuss issues regarding child clients with the supervisor. I have certainly experienced both the boundaries and the crossovers between these relationships in my professional practice. Often, I have shared details of a child's play session with my personal therapist in order to gain insight into the feelings that emerged for me and what blocks I may be putting in the child's way because of my own past. My relationships with adults in the system around the child also bring up many issues that can be challenging and need reflection. I am explicit about not allowing an exchange in therapy to become advice on how to be with a child although inevitably, once I am conscious of what comes from me and what is being projected by others, I am released to be more empathic and congruent towards the child's own meanings. All my interview study participants reflect on how personal therapy and clinical supervision are often intertwined:

> It is difficult to distinguish between therapy and supervision. Not because they're the same in any way but it's difficult to know which one gives you the ability to work well with the children.
>
> (Clare)

> It's so much more ... interwoven. It's actually not that clear cut at all. Quite a sliding trajectory ... Everything is so much more complicated!
>
> (Anna)

Conclusion

I have no doubt that discussions about the benefits of personal therapy for the therapist and for clients will continue, and that play therapists will have varying views about the extent to which they find the experience helpful in their personal and professional lives. Overall, BAPT play therapists identify this part of their training and professional support as worthwhile and greatly valuable, if challenging. It seems that current research in the wide arena of psychotherapy training is moving towards a focus on examining the outcomes of clients in relation to their therapist's personal therapy experience and on whether or not only some students should be advised to enter therapy for themselves. For now, I am content to be as fully present in the playroom with a child as I can be, with all that I know (so far) of myself and bear witness to the play that the child entrusts me with. 'Our knowing that [the play] has meaning is even more important than knowing what that meaning is' (McCarthy, 2012:29).

Summary

- BAPT play therapy training requires all students to undergo personal therapy.
- The rationale for therapy during training is for personal support, to explore personal issues and to have a professional role model.

- BAPT play therapists are very positive about their experience of therapy and see it as a vital part of their training.
- There is an ongoing debate within the psychotherapy profession about the benefits or hindrances of mandatory training therapy.

Further reading

Daw, B. & Joseph, S. (2007) Qualified therapists' experiences of personal therapy. *Counselling and Psychotherapy Research.* 7(4) pp. 227–232.

Galbraith, V.E. (2010) Developing self-care and resilience. In Woolfe, R., Strawbridge, S., Douglas, B. & Dryden, W. (eds.) *Handbook of Counselling Psychotherapy.* (4th ed.) London: Sage. pp. 213–227.

Macaskill, N.D. (1998) Personal therapy in the training of the psychotherapist: Is it effective? *British Journal of Psychotherapy.* 43 pp. 219–226.

Norcross, J.C. & Connor, K.A. (2005) Psychotherapists entering personal therapy – Their primary reasons and presenting problems. In Geller, J.D., Norcross, J.C. & Orlinsky, D.E. (eds.) *The Psychotherapist's Own Psychotherapy: Patient and Clinician Perspectives.* New York: Oxford University Press. pp. 192–200.

Norcross, J.C., Bike, D., Evans, K. & Schatz, D. (2008) Psychotherapists who abstain from personal therapy: Do they practice what they preach? *Journal of Clinical Psychology.* 64(12) pp. 1368–1376.

Poal, P. & Weisz, J.R. (1989) Therapists' own childhood problems as predictors of their effectiveness in child psychotherapy. *Journal of Clinical Child Psychology.* 18 (3) pp. 202–205.

References

Bike, D., Norcross, J. & Schatz, D. (2009) Processes and outcomes of psychotherapists' personal therapy: Replication and extension 20 years later. *Psychotherapy: Theory, Research, Practice, Training.* 46(1) pp. 19–31.

Bornstein, B. (1948) Emotional barriers in the understanding and treatment of young children. *American Journal of Orthopsychiatry.* 18 pp. 691–697.

Cattanach, A. (2003) *Introduction to Play Therapy.* Hove: Brunner Routledge.

Cayne, J. & Loewenthal, D. (2007) The unknown in learning to be a psychotherapist. *European Journal of Psychotherapy and Counselling.* 9(4) pp. 373–387.

Chaturvedi, S. (2013) Mandatory personal therapy: Does the evidence justify the practice? In debate. *British Journal of Guidance and Counselling.* 41(4) pp. 454–460.

Ciclitira, K., Starr, F., Marzano, L., Brunswick, N. & Costa, A. (2012) Women counsellors' experiences of personal therapy: A thematic analysis. *Counselling and Psychotherapy Research.* 12(2) pp. 136–145.

Curtis, R.C. & Qaiser, M. (2005). Training analysis: Historical considerations and empirical research. In Geller, J.D., Norcross, J.C. & Orlinsky, D.E. (eds.) *The Psychotherapist's Own Psychotherapy: Patient and Clinician Perspectives.* New York: Oxford University Press. pp. 365–378.

Dunn, C. (2000) *Carl Jung: Wounded Healer of the Soul: An Illustrated Biography.* New York: Parabola Books.

Grimmer, A. & Tribe, R. (2001) Counselling psychologists' perceptions of the impact of mandatory personal therapy on professional development – An exploratory study. *Counselling Psychology Quarterly.* 14(4) pp. 287–301.

Henry, W.E., Sims, J.H. & Spray, S.L. (1973) *The Public and Private Lives of Psychotherapists.* San Francisco: Jossey-Bass.

Jennings, S. (1993) *Playtherapy with Children: A Practitioner's Guide.* Oxford: Blackwell Scientific.

Kumari, N. (2011) Personal therapy as a mandatory requirement for counselling psychologists in training: A qualitative study of the impact of therapy on trainees' personal and professional development. *Counselling Psychology Quarterly.* 24(3) pp. 211–232.

Landreth, G. (2012) *The Art of the Relationship.* (3rd ed.) New York: Taylor & Francis.

Le Vay, D. & Cuschieri, E. (eds.) (2016) *Challenges in the Theory and Practice of Play Therapy.* London: Taylor & Francis.

Littner, N. & Schour, E. (1971) Special problems of training psychotherapists to work with children. In Holt, R.R. (ed.) *New Horizons for Psychotherapy: Autonomy as a Profession.* New York: International Universities Press. pp. 260–293.

Martin, P. (2011). Celebrating the wounded healer. *Counselling Psychology Review.* 26(1) pp. 10–19.

McCann, J. (2011) *I'm Not Such a Strange Creature after All.* Unpublished dissertation, Roehampton University.

McCann, J. (2012) I'm not such a strange creature after all. *British Journal of Play Therapy.* 8 pp. 50–65.

McCann, J. (2017) *Personal Therapy – Have Your Say!* Unpublished online survey, Survey Monkey.

McCarthy, D. (2012) *A Manual of Dynamic Play Therapy: Helping Things Fall Apart, the Paradox of Play.* Philadelphia: Jessica Kingsley Publishers.

Mearns, D., Dryden, W., McLeod, J. & Thorne, B. (1998). £1,200 personal therapy: Financial scam. Letter to the editor. *Counselling: The Journal of the British Association for Counselling* 9 (2) p. 83.

Norcross, J.C. & Prochaska, J. (1986) Psychotherapist heal thyself: I. The psychological distress and self-change of psychologists, counselors, and laypersons. *Psychotherapy: Theory, Research, Practice, Training.* 23(1) pp. 102–114.

O'Donohue, J. (1997) *Anam Cara: Spiritual Wisdom from the Celtic World.* London: Bantam Press.

Orlinsky, D.E., Rønnestad, M.H., Willutki, U., Wiseman, H. & Botermans, J. (2005) The prevalence and parameters of personal therapy in Europe and elsewhere. In Geller, J.D., Norcross, J.C. & Orlinsky, D.E. (eds.) *The Psychotherapist's Own Psychotherapy: Patient and Clinician Perspectives.* New York: Oxford University Press. pp. 165–176.

Oteiza, V. (2010) Therapists' experiences of personal therapy: A descriptive phenomenological study. *Counselling and Psychotherapy Research.* 10(3) pp. 222–228.

Queen Margaret University. (2016/17) *Clinical Process and Practice Modules: Practice Education Handbook for MSc Play Therapy.* Edinburgh: Queen Margaret University Division of Occupational Therapy and Arts Therapies.

Rizq, R. (2011) Personal therapy in psychotherapeutic training: Current research and future directions. *Journal of Contemporary Psychotherapy.* 41 pp. 175–185.

Rizq R. & Target, M. (2008a) 'The power of being seen': An interpretative phenomenological analysis of how experienced counselling psychologists describe the meaning and significance of personal therapy in clinical practice. *British Journal of Guidance and Counselling.* 36(2) pp. 131–153.

Rizq, R. & Target, M. (2008b) 'Not a Mickey mouse thing': How experienced counseling psychologists describe the significance of personal therapy in clinical practice and training. Some results from an interpretative phenomenological analysis. *Counselling Psychology Quarterly.* 21(1) pp. 29–48.

Rogers, C.R. (1957) The necessary and sufficient conditions of therapeutic personality change. *Journal of Consulting Psychology.* 21(2) pp. 95–103.

Sandell, R., Lazar, A., Grant, J., Carlsson, J., Schubert, J. & Broberg, J. (2006) Therapist attitudes and patient outcomes III: A latent class analysis of therapists. *Psychology and Psychotherapy: Therapy, Research and Practice.* 79 pp. 629–647.

Thorne, B. & Dryden, W. (1991) *Training and Supervision for Counselling in Action.* London: Sage.

University of Roehampton (2017) *MA Play Therapy Programme Handbook.* London: University of Roehampton.

Von Haenish, C. (2011) How did compulsory personal therapy during counseling training influence personal and professional development? *Counselling and Psychotherapy Research.* 11(2) pp. 148–155.

West, J. (1992) *Child-Centred Play Therapy.* (2nd ed.) London: Hodder Arnold.

Williams, F., Coyle, A. & Lyons, E. (1999) How counselling psychologists view their personal therapy. *British Journal of Medical Psychology.* 72 pp. 545–555.

Websites

www.bapt.info/play-therapy/play-therapy-core-competences
www.playtherapy.org.uk/PTUK

Chapter 3

The role of clinical supervision in play therapy practice

Carol Platteuw

Chapter overview

This chapter will explore the practice of clinical supervision for play therapists. I will consider different theoretical frameworks for supervision, various creative approaches that supervisors could use within supervision sessions and finally key responsibilities that supervisors hold. Exploration of some of the practical issues relating to supervision will also be included.

What is clinical supervision?

'Supervision' is defined by Cambridge Dictionary as 'the act of watching a person or activity and making certain that everything is done correctly, safely, etc.' 'Supervise' is defined by Oxford Living Dictionaries as 'Observe and direct the execution of (a task or activity). Observe and direct the work of (someone). Keep watch over (someone) in the interest of their or others security'.

The above definitions suggest a one-dimensional, hierarchical, rather authoritarian role for supervisors. Within this chapter I will suggest that while the play therapy supervisor does have responsibilities for ensuring good practice and safeguarding the child's welfare, she can draw on various theoretical stances alongside bringing a playful and creative element to supervision which enriches both the supervisee's and supervisor's practice.

Play therapy training universally requires students to undertake supervision as part of the practicum leading to a qualification. Once certified, the requirements vary from country to country and one professional body to another, in relation to how much supervision, if any at all, is required in order to practise.

Clinical supervision requirements

The British Association of Play Therapists (BAPT) stipulates that both students and qualified play therapists *must* undertake supervision as a condition of registration. The supervisor would usually be a qualified play therapist, or in cases of unavailability, play therapists may also be supervised by appropriately qualified and experienced therapists with specialist experience of working with children and young people. *The Ethical Basis for Good Practice in Play Therapy*, available on the BAPT website (www.bapt.info), sets out expectations of BAPT members in relation to supervision.

Under the section 'Starting to practice – Subsection 1.4 Supervision' it states:

- All play therapists, including supervisors, are required to receive ongoing, appropriate, formal and regular supervision independently of their managerial relationships.
- Supervisors have a responsibility to maintain the good practice of supervisees and to protect clients from harm and bad practice.
- Supervision must be provided by an appropriately qualified and experienced play therapist, except where no such play therapist exists in the geographical region. In such circumstances the play therapist must receive supervision from an appropriately qualified and experienced child therapist.
- Supervision must involve face to face contact, except in circumstances where physical distance between the play therapist and an available supervisor precludes such contact.
- Play therapists must receive supervision adequate to maintaining their level of competency, functioning and good practice.

These requirements are reconfirmed under 'BAPT Play Therapy Core Competence 13: Maintenance and effective use of clinical supervision' (see Appendix 3).

Definition

BAPT defines clinical supervision in play therapy on the BAPT website www.bapt.info under the 'Clinical Supervision' section, as:

> A formal and mutually agreed relationship between two play therapists where the supervisor is a significantly more experienced and competent play therapist than the supervisee. The aim of this supervision is to monitor, develop and support the supervisee's play therapy practice. This supervision will be independent of all managerial relationships.

BAPT specifies different formats of acceptable supervision. Clinical supervision will usually involve face-to-face supervision, except where geographic location significantly precludes this. In such circumstances, telephone or webcam supervision will be accepted. Group supervision and peer supervision are acceptable under certain stipulations.

The importance is emphasised of supervisors having supervision on their own supervision. This may also be through individual, group or peer supervision, depending on geographical constraints.

BAPT stipulates the number of supervision hours a therapist must undertake in order to remain a member of the professional body. This varies according to experience. Student supervision requirements are one clinical supervision hour for every two hours of clinical practice. Newly qualified play therapists undergo a probationary period for twelve months from the point of beginning practice. During this twelve-month period of play therapy practice, BAPT requires a minimum of 24 hours clinical supervision for newly qualified members. Qualified and experienced play therapists should receive different amounts of supervision according to the level of their workload and the intensity of the work. Guidelines are provided regarding minimum number of hours of supervision for safe play therapy practice.

Theoretical models

Three different theoretical models will be described and considered from the author's personal experience.

The Integrative Developmental Model of Supervision is a model proposed by Stoltenberg and McNeill (2010) whereby the therapist commences as inexperienced and uncertain and progresses to a more confident, assured, competent and knowledgeable therapist. There are four different levels of progression. In Level 1 the therapist is unsure of their practice and wishes to be guided and taught to hone their therapeutic skills by the supervisor. In Level 2 the therapist begins to feel more confidence as a practitioner and their focus moves from anxiety about the self to a focus on the client and their needs. The therapist begins to feel less dependent on the supervisor and more comfortable with their therapeutic skills. In Level 3 the therapist attains more autonomy. This is evidenced by independent thinking, as the therapist gains more experience and becomes aware of different behavioural challenges and also her response to different client groups. In Level 3i the therapist is the 'master therapist', her therapeutic skills are well developed, she is able to assess the client's needs and take into account relevant research. This integration of ideas and skills comes with continuing experience and self-reflection. In Level 3 and 3i the supervisee uses supervision more as a consultancy role.

As a supervisor who has guided many students and continued to supervise them as they become established in their play therapy career, this model resonates for many of my supervisees. An example was one student who stayed at Level 1 for much longer than expected. I will call her Anna. Anna is a competent, warm and engaging woman but lacked confidence in her own abilities, having come to play therapy later in life and not having the same level of academic qualifications as other students on her course. Anna needed a high level of teaching, guidance and encouragement. An unexpected event helped move her from Level 1 to Level 2. Anna worked in a school and returned from an Easter break to discover the play room had been flooded and was unusable. She had four child clients that day. She managed to find another room, she went around the school borrowing play materials from various sources and set them out for her clients. She said all the children were unsettled by the change of venue and the lack of familiar play materials – however, she was appropriately able to reflect their feelings and some children went on to play out or describe other difficult changes in their lives. At our next supervision session Anna was a different therapist. She had managed to contain her own anxieties and had been able to focus on the children and their needs. This increase in confidence continued, Anna became more autonomous in her thinking and it was a pleasure to see her flourish and develop her play therapy skills.

A second model that I find helpful in my own supervision practice is *The Seven-eyed Supervision Model* by Hawkins and Shohet (2012), which provides guidance to the supervisor from different perspectives.

Eye One is the *seeing eye*: looking in detail about what happens in a session, how the client presents and how the therapist responds.

Eye Two is the *how to manage different situations eye*: looking at practice – assessment, planning the therapeutic intervention, closure and any other procedural issues that arise during the work. In my experience, Eye One, Eye Two and Eye Seven are frequently used with students and inexperienced therapists.

Eye Three focusses on *the therapeutic relationship*: what is happening between the therapist and the client consciously and unconsciously and how this is affecting the client and the therapist. The supervisor may explore the issue of transference using this eye. Freud (1923) described how unconscious processes can affect emotions, behaviours and impact on relationships. He used the term 'transference' to describe unconscious feelings that someone may have about one person which becomes transferred towards another. For example, a child may have unconscious feelings about a grandmother and if working with an older female therapist may attribute actions, thoughts or expectations onto her.

Eye Four follows on from Eye Three by focussing on *counter transference* which may impede the therapeutic process. Here the supervisor concentrates on exploring the emotional impact of the client on the supervisee. Counter transference is the redirection of a therapist's feelings toward a client. Freud (1923) cautioned that this could impede a successful intervention and suggested the therapist should seek their own therapy. In my opinion, this is a useful issue to discuss in supervision. For example, if a play therapist dreads seeing a particular child client as the child is extremely controlling, these feelings may originate from the play therapist's past experiences of an abusive parent and in this case it would be appropriate for the play therapist to seek their own therapy. However, after talking with the child's network, the play therapist may learn that this child's strategy to feel safe is to take control of adults and/or situations and thinking about enhancing a sense of safety might be a more helpful way forward.

Eye Five is where the supervisor looks at the *relationship between the supervisor and supervisee.* The supervisor ponders whether anything within the supervisory relationship is mirroring anything within the supervisee/client relationship that could provide insight.

Eye Six is where the supervisor looks *at any possible counter transference for herself* within the supervision session. In my experience, Eyes Five and Six are often needed when the play therapist and/or the supervisor are under pressure, from home or work, and their emotional focus is compromised. Eyes Five and Six also indicate the importance of a supervisor having their own clinical guidance.

Eye Seven is where the supervisor looks at the *overall context* in which the therapy is occurring and any stresses that may impact on the process: the client's wider family, community, overall support situation, any issues within the venue where the therapy occurs or administrative issues regarding referrals and funding difficulties.

Hawkins and Shohet suggest that supervisors can use different eyes at different times according to the supervisee's level of experience and/or the complications or challenges the supervisee is facing.

A further theoretical model for supervision is *The Play Therapy Dimensions Model* developed by Yasenik and Gardner (2004). Chapter 9 in their book is titled 'Utilising the Play Therapy Dimensions Model in Supervision'. The model conceptualises the play therapy process according to two primary dimensions: *Directiveness* and *Consciousness*. The *Consciousness dimension* reflects the child's representation of consciousness in play and is represented by the child's play activities and verbalisations. The *Directiveness dimension* refers to the degree of immersion and level of interpretation by the play therapist. The model is depicted visually by the two dimensions intersecting to make four quadrants: 1. Active Utilisation, 2. Open Discussion and Exploration, 3. Co-facilitation, and 4. Non-Intrusive Responding.

Non-Intrusive Responding (where the child leads the play and the play therapist is a non-intrusive responder) and *Active Utilisation* (where the child leads the play, but the play therapist occasionally makes interpretive comments) are quadrants on the *Non-Directiveness* side of the continuum. *Open Discussion and Exploration* (where the play therapist plays a more directive role, selecting activities and openly discussing issues with the child) and *Co-facilitation* (where the play therapist is directly involved in the play at the child's invitation but the interpretations 'stay within the play') are quadrants on the *Directiveness* side of the continuum.

The model is integrative: play therapists are encouraged to view their interventions as a continuum of directiveness and consciousness, whatever their theoretical stance. The use of self is explored which enables the play therapist to reflect on the ways they intervene within particular approaches and with different client groups. Yasenik and Gardner suggest that supervisors can invite supervisees to look at the four quadrant diagram in supervision and consider questions such as:

• What quadrant are you working in?
• What play therapy approach are you using?
• What quadrant did you begin to work in?
• Did you consciously choose to remain working in this quadrant or move to a different one?
• What factors influenced your decision to shift?

In my experience, Yasenik and Gardner's model is a useful tool to use when working with supervisees who use a different theoretical model or work with different client groups to those with whom the supervisor is familiar. A case example of this is provided later in the chapter.

The supervisor's own theoretical model

The supervisor's personal theoretical model will influence their supervisory style and practice. My own theoretical stance is integrative, tailored to the child client I am working with. Schaefer and Drewes (2014) suggest the term 'trans-theoretical play therapy', which entails selecting and adding to your repertoire the best change agents from amongst all the major theories of play therapy. As my main client group has become fostered and adopted children, *Theraplay*[1] (Jernberg & Booth, 2010) is my preferred intervention. Theraplay is an attachment-based intervention, working with parent and child together, enhancing four key dimensions within the relationship. The parent is helped to provide – and the child helped to receive – adequate *Structure, Nurture, Engagement* and *Challenge*. In Theraplay the therapist enhances the parent's capacity in the domain of *Structure* to set limits and to provide an appropriately ordered and safe environment; in the domain of *Engagement*, to engage the child in playful interactions while being attuned to the child's state and reactions; in the domain of *Nurture*, to meet the child's need for comfort, calming and care, and finally in the domain of *Challenge*, to support and encourage the child's efforts to achieve at a developmentally appropriate level.

These dimensions provide a useful framework for supervision and fit neatly around the 12 duties of a clinical supervisor as defined by BAPT.

The supervisor should provide *the Structure* around supervision, the provision of a reliable space and the external focus on ensuring that the supervisee's practice is ethical by:

- providing a clear contract regarding fees and services provided in clinical supervision;
- advising, guiding and monitoring the supervisee's practice and conduct in all areas of play therapy practice;
- ensuring the supervisee's practice and conduct conforms to BAPT's Ethical Basis for Good Practice in Play Therapy;
- ensuring the supervisee's practice is competent, ethical and appropriate.

In relation to *Engagement*, the quality of the supervisor/supervisee relationship is crucial to the supervisory process in

- facilitating the on-going supervisory relationship;
- offering clear and honest information regarding the supervisee's play therapy and supervisory experience and training;
- supporting the supervisee.

Supervisors should provide a *Nurturing* environment for supervisees and be mindful of issues such as secondary trauma. Information regarding this issue can be accessed through the website www.childtrauma.org. Also

- enabling the supervisee to delineate between supervisory issues and personal therapy issues.

Finally, supervisors should provide the appropriate level of *Challenge* for supervisees based on Stoltenberg and McNeill's (2010) model described earlier, in

- undertaking clinical supervision appropriate to the supervisee's experience, competences and ability;
- undertaking supervision training and any other related professional development activities that enhance the quality of supervisory practice;
- facilitating the supervisee's learning and awareness of strengths and weaknesses;
- facilitating the supervisee's personal and professional development.

Theraplay is a relational approach using the four dimensions described above to enhance attachments. The use of a Theraplay informed approach in providing clinical supervision fits well with Stoltenberg and McNeill's model, the supervisor continuing to be the safe base for the supervisee, whatever their level of competency.

Creative approaches

Various authors have suggested that supervision can be enhanced by the use of creative interventions alongside traditional talking supervision. Mooli Lahad's (2000) book *Creative Supervision* contains a range of creative interventions including drawing, use of stories, letter writing, use of therapeutic cards and use of small objects. Lahad suggests encouraging supervisees to use the creative, intuitive, more holistic right hemisphere of the brain, as opposed to staying with the verbal, logical, analytical left hemisphere of the brain, thus enabling a greater understanding of the processes of therapy, intervention and support. Lahad suggests that use of expressive materials can enable both the supervisor and supervisee to better understand the child's world and can help in situations where the supervisee feels stuck.

Examples of Lahad's interventions include the *Colour, Shape and Line technique*. The supervisee is asked to take three pieces of paper and some crayons. On the first paper he is asked to draw the problem or issues he feels are at the core of the case in colours, shapes or lines. Next, he is asked to draw the problem solved and on the third paper draw what will happen in the middle. Lahad suggests that when discussing and observing the three drawings, innovative solutions may emerge. Another example is Lahad's suggestion of using a *Small World* technique where the supervisee is invited to use miniatures in a sand tray to show what is happening in the therapist/client relationship. The supervisor and supervisee then have a visual image to reflect on together.

The Six-Shape Supervision Structure devised by Anna Chesner (2014) is a projective supervisory tool which is based on the six-part story making method (Lahad, 1992). The supervisee is asked to make six irregular shapes on a large piece of paper. The supervisee is asked to formulate a supervisory question and then in shape one make an image of the person, persons, group, team or organisation that is the focus of the question. The supervisee is then asked to focus on the supervisory question in relation to the client. Is there a goal, a difficulty or a preoccupation? In shape two the supervisee is invited to make an image to represent this. For the third shape, the supervisee is asked to create an image which shows what gets in the way of achieving the goal or overcoming the difficulty.

The supervisee is then instructed to put their thinking head aside and just focus on their feelings about the situation. They are invited to make an image to represent this feeling in shape four. For shape five the supervisee is asked to put back on their thinking head and consider what they know (the context and causes) about the situation they are exploring. The supervisee is again invited to make an image to represent this. Finally, for shape six the supervisee is invited to review the process thus far:

> Have a look at the five shapes and what you have marked in them. You
> have been on a journey of exploration and reflection, identifying the client,

the goals of the work, what is in the way and how you feel about that and what you know. When you are ready make an image of a next step.

This final part enables the supervisee to find a possible solution, or explore their thinking to consider future options with their supervisor.

Using creative approaches within supervision can help when supervisees and/or supervisors become stuck, want to change the energy in the room, need additional challenge or just need to be playful! BAPT competence 27, 'Inter-personal communication through use of creative media' (see Appendix 3) requires play therapists to *demonstrate and facilitate a range of verbal, non-verbal and symbolic communication using a variety of play and creative media with children, young people and families.* Using creative approaches in supervision could also provide an opportunity for the supervisee to demonstrate their skills to their supervisor.

Roles and responsibilities

When agreeing to supervise a play therapist, a play therapy supervisor should have several years' experience in practice and ideally have undertaken a short course on supervision to ensure they are knowledgeable regarding various theoretical models of supervision and different creative approaches that can be used during supervision sessions. But most importantly they need an awareness of the main responsibilities of play therapy supervisors, which in my opinion are:

(a) The child's welfare – the supervisor's prime responsibility

The child's welfare should always be paramount within play therapy and within the supervision process. The supervisor herself should ensure she is fully updated regarding current safeguarding practices and legal frameworks. This is specified in BAPT competences 8 and 23 (see Appendix 3).

Within supervision the supervisor should be vigilant regarding any possible safeguarding issues. Verbal disclosures of abuse from the child should be reported immediately to the relevant authorities. Play therapists should be cautious about reporting disclosures to the parent, as this may impede the safeguarding process.

Case study

As a student play therapist, I was working with a 6-year-old girl in foster care. During a session when we were using clay, the child made a sausage shape (in a similar shape to a penis). She then stated, 'my brother asks me to suck his willy at night'. My immediate reaction was to tell her that her brother should not be asking her to do this and I would talk to her foster carer after the session to ensure her carer kept her safe. In my naivety, I did so, and the carer's response to the child's statement was 'She's a liar – he would never do such a thing like that'. She then told the child never to repeat such lies again. I immediately reported the content of the session to the child's social worker and subsequently the child was removed from the placement. I was then a Level 1 supervisee as in Stoltenberg and McNeill's (2010) model. When subsequently – and belatedly – discussing the incident in supervision, my supervisor challenged my actions and educated me regarding how my instinctive and well-intentioned reaction to keep the child safe and inform the carer had actually placed the child in an invidious position and potentially jeopardised the safeguarding process. In such circumstances, immediate consultation with your supervisor is good practice.

Themes of play which are indicative of abuse should be carefully recorded and discussed within supervision. If such themes are repeated three or more times the supervisor could suggest a meeting of professionals involved with the child to ensure the network is working protectively.

Case study

I supervised a student play therapist working in a school – Level 1 in Stoltenberg and McNeill's (2010) model. She was working with an 8-year-old child about whom she had several concerns: the child always presented as unkempt, tired and pale. The mother stated the child was missing her father who had been imprisoned some weeks earlier. The child made no verbal statements within therapy sessions; however, within her play the child repeatedly, in every session, played out scenarios involving a small figure on her own in a dangerous world. I was concerned about the material the child was presenting but the play therapist was inexperienced and anxious. She did not want to infer anything without a verbal disclosure. I suggested the play therapist request that the school convene a professionals meeting to share information. At this meeting the child's teacher stated the child almost fell asleep on occasions in lessons and it appeared the child came to school on her own. The playground supervisors stated the child was isolated and appeared sad. A safeguarding referral was made to Children's Services who subsequently discovered the child's mother had started working nights, was leaving the child alone at home each evening and expecting the child to make her own way to school.

This second case example serves to emphasise how inexperienced/ hesitant supervisees often benefit from the more objective overview of an experienced supervisor who can instil in them the courage to act appropriately on their concerns to safeguard a child. It also demonstrates the importance of working closely with the child's network in accordance with BAPT competence 28 (see Appendix 3) whereby a play therapist is expected to collaborate and communicate with other professionals for the benefit of children, young people and families.

(b) The supervisee's theoretical and practical development

Stoltenberg and McNeill's model reminds us that the supervisor will be proactive in guiding and/or educating students or newly qualified therapists. However even very experienced therapists, on occasions, can be challenged in relation to theory or practice.

Case study

I supervised a play therapist who was working with a 4-year-old boy who had just been removed from his birth family having suffered profound neglect. The child had spent lengthy periods of time in a room on his own with no toys. He did not know how to play. In play therapy he was frozen, sitting in a centre of the therapy room, seemingly overwhelmed by the materials surrounding him. The supervisee was an experienced child-centred play therapist and had always waited to follow the child's lead in the therapeutic process. She was most comfortable with a non-directive approach working with children who play within metaphor. In Yasenik and Gardner's (2004) model she felt most comfortable in the 'Non-intrusive Responding' quadrant. In supervision we reflected whether the child had the capacity to make choices, based on his early experiences. Using Yasenik and Gardner's model, we thought about how the play therapist could become more active and directive to meet this child's needs. We considered developmental levels of play (Jennings, 2005) where a child moves from embodiment play, to projective play to role play. I invited the play therapist to consider providing and demonstrating the use of sensory materials so the child could begin to get in touch with his physical senses. Once the play therapist began starting the sessions in this way the child began to engage and the therapeutic process commenced.

This case example demonstrates how helpful Yasenik and Gardner's model is for considering the child's needs and the play therapist's use of self.

(c) The supervisee's personal well-being

Although it is not the supervisor's role to be a therapist to the supervisee, inevitably personal issues impact on a supervisee's practice. Supervisors should be alive to such issues, be a nurturing presence and supportively reflect upon these, if appropriate, within supervision. When required a supervisee should be encouraged to resume personal therapy.

Case study

I supervised a male play therapist who was assisting in caring for his elderly father. His father yo-yoed in and out of hospital and each time the package of care promised on his return home never worked out. In one supervision session we were discussing an adopted child who had complex needs. The play therapist angrily stated his frustration at the professional network who appeared not to be taking his advice and he wondered what the point was in continuing the work. I was mindful that this reflected the therapist's own situation with his father. Using Eye Four in Hawkins and Shohet's (2012) model I reflected how difficult it is not to be listened to and how powerless one feels. The therapist immediately made the link with his personal situation and resolved to continue to be an advocate for both his father and his child client. He also prioritised resuming personal therapy.

Supervisors should also be alive to the issue of Secondary Trauma in professionals. Play therapists work with children who have experienced extremely traumatic early lives and, consequently, some of the material within the sessions can be disturbing.

Case study

I supervised a therapist who was working with an 8-year-old boy who had been sexually abused by his siblings. In sessions the child would sometimes unexpectedly rub himself against the therapist's back in a highly sexualised manner. In supervision the therapist stated she dreaded sessions with this child and had begun to dream about him tormenting her. Being mindful of Eye Three in Hawkins and Shohet's model, we explored how the therapist could feel safer both within sessions, by implementing firmer boundaries by stating explicitly: 'My job is to keep you safe, I will not hurt you and I will make sure there are no hurts when we are playing together', and outside sessions by increasing her level of self-care.

(d) Monitoring the supervisee's practice to ensure it meets good practice guidelines and to protect the public from harm

Notes of supervision should be carefully made to reflect issues discussed. Some supervisees take a copy of their supervisor's notes away after the session. Supervision notes can be used to support the supervisee, if required. On occasions I have written a supportive statement to a social worker – confirming the therapeutic plan made within supervision. Supervisors should also be mindful that supervision notes will be important if the therapist is made subject of a complaint or if the child becomes subject of court proceedings.

The supervisor should always ensure that a contract is drawn up between supervisor and supervisee. The contract should make reference to the therapist's code of ethics as a basis for good practice, the requirement to have adequate indemnity insurance and the need to remain registered with a professional body. See sample contract – Appendix 3.

Ensuring a therapist gains adequate consent prior to commencing therapy is a recurring issue in supervision when parents have separated. If both parents have Parental Responsibility I advise supervisees to obtain both parents' consent. This safeguards the therapist from a deceitful parent who states they do not know where the other parent is, when the parent is in fact contactable and has a right to know the child is undertaking therapy. (See also Chapter 6, 'Being an Ethical Play Therapist').

Prior to the work starting, it is essential, particularly in training, to use supervision to think carefully about whether a play therapy intervention is appropriate. Two factors are crucial: the child needs to be in a safe place and the child's carer needs to be supportive of the intervention.

The Therapeutic Touchstone model (Prendiville, 2014) recommends explicitly telling the child that the therapist is aware of their history – by outlining the events leading up to why they have been referred for therapy. This removes the pressure on the child of wondering whether the therapist knows their story. How to sensitively set out this narrative is another factor that can be considered in supervision prior to work starting.

The rewards of being a supervisor

In my opinion, supervision is a privilege for supervisors. To be involved and responsible for another play therapist's work enables supervisors to have ethical guidelines in mind at all times, to learn new techniques and interventions, to hear about different client groups in different contexts, all of which result in the supervisor's own practice being enriched. I therefore encourage experienced play therapists to consider taking the step to become supervisors and assure you that your own practice will be enhanced as a result.

Summary

* This chapter has considered how, in order to provide effective and safe supervision, supervisors should ensure they are aware of different theoretical models of supervision. As an attachment-based therapist I find Yasenik and Gardner's (2004) model invaluable as, regardless of the supervisee's approach, it focusses on the child's presentation, play and needs and the play therapist's use of self to best meet those needs.
* As is the case for play therapists, supervisors should be able to describe their theoretical practice and how this impacts on their supervision. As a Certified Theraplay practitioner I can clearly see how this model influences my practice and how my belief that strengthening *Structure, Engagement, Nurture* and *Challenge* in all relationships (including the supervisory relationship) is beneficial.
* This chapter has also considered different creative interventions. As play therapists we have a toolbox of techniques at the ready at all time – so why not use them within supervision to aid reflection and insight?
* Finally, this chapter considered roles and responsibilities of a supervisor. Ultimately supervisors have a duty to protect the public from harm by ensuring the supervisee's practice is safe and the child's well-being is paramount.

Note

1 Theraplay is a registered service mark of The Theraplay Institute, Evanston, IL, USA.

References/further reading

BAPT Code of Ethics. Available at www.bapt.info/play-therapy/ethical-basis-good-practice-play-therapy/

Cambridge Dictionary. Available at https://dictionary.cambridge.org [Accessed: 26/01/18]

Chesner, A. (2014) The Six-Shape Supervision Structure. In Chesner, A. & Zografou, L. (eds.) *Creative Supervision across Modalities*. London: Jessica Kingsley Publishers. pp. 71–85.

Cost of Caring: Secondary Traumatic Stress and the Impact of Working with High Risk Children and Families. Available at www.childtrauma.org

Freud, S. (1923) *The Ego and the Id*. London: Hogarth Press.

Hawkins, P. & Shohet, R. (2012) *Supervision in the Helping Professions*. (4th ed.) Maidenhead: Open University Press.

Jennings, S. (2005) *Creative Play with Children at Risk*. London: Routledge.

Jernberg, A. & Booth, P. (2010) *Theraplay: Helping Parents and Children Build Better Relationships through Attachment Based Play*. San Francisco: Wiley.

Lahad, M. (2000) *Creative Supervision*. London: Jessica Kingsley Publishers.

Oxford Living Dictionaries. Available at https://en.oxforddictionaries.com [Accessed: 26/01/18]

Prendiville, E. (2014) The Therapeutic Touchstone. In: Prendiville, E. & Howard, J. (eds.) *Play Therapy Today*. Oxon: Routledge. pp. 7–28.

Schaefer, C. & Drewes, A. (2014) *The Therapeutic Powers of Play*. Hoboken, NJ: Wiley.

Stoltenberg, C.D. & McNeill, B.W. (2010) *IDM Supervision*. (3rd ed.) New York and London: Routledge.

Yasenik, L. & Gardner, K. (2004) *Play Therapy Dimensions Model. A Decision Making Guide for the Integrative Play Therapist*. London: Jessica Kingsley Publishers.

Chapter 4

The play therapy room

Why it matters

Anne Fullalove

Chapter overview

Within play therapy literature many references are made to the importance of the physical space in supporting effective therapeutic provision, but there is an absence of research on the degree of its significance. In the light of research from other fields, I will consider how the setting can positively impact the specific functions of play therapy and support the holding environment of the therapeutic relationship. I will propose the need for a researched knowledge base to inform the design of dedicated spaces which optimally support therapeutic work and offer a better level of service to clients.

The impact of the physical setting: what do we know?

I have yet to meet a play therapist who has not recounted an anecdote about how the physical therapeutic space has influenced the quality of their service delivery. Developing and managing the play therapy room is one of the BAPT core competences (Competence 29, Appendix 1). As well as establishing health and safety standards, this competence also includes ensuring privacy and preserving confidentiality for the client. Without rigorous groundwork in the selection of materials and the set-up of the room, optimal support for the child can be significantly compromised.

There is considerable agreement amongst play therapy theorists that the physical setting has wide implications for the efficacy of the work. It impacts the quality of expression of the child, as well as their relationship with the therapist. However, Wilson and Ryan (2005:163) reflect a general consensus that 'although the physical setting should be carefully considered, it is not an overriding factor, and lack of optimum surroundings should not of itself be reason for foregoing therapy'.

Landreth (2012:138) presents the therapeutic relationship, 'the emotional climate that develops as a result of the therapist's attitude, the use of her own personality and the spontaneous interaction between therapist and child', as the most significant aspect in facilitating a successful play therapy intervention. The purpose of this chapter is not an attempt to refute this perspective, but rather to invite play therapists to undertake a closer examination of the impact of the physical setting on both the child and the therapist. Play therapy interventions may be missing aspects of qualitative service delivery by not evaluating environmental factors more thoroughly.

Spaces communicate

Architects suggest that our instincts and our unconscious mind are very responsive to the spaces we inhabit. Lawson (2001) asserts that architecture, as the discipline that designs spaces for us, has the important function of using the language of design that humans implicitly understand. Organised physical space can guide our behaviour, change our moods, and help us to delineate between activities.

Pallasmaa (2012:76) agrees that architecture 'initiates, directs and organises behaviour and movement'. He asserts that we are in a constant dialogue with our environment, and goes so far as to say that it is impossible to separate our sense of self from our environmental experience or physical situation. He quotes the poet Noel Arnaud: 'I am the space, where I am' referring to his belief that physical and mental space form an 'indivisible continuum' (Arnaud, 1950, cited in Pallasmaa, 2012:69).

The human geographer Tuan (2001) explains that space communicates directly to the senses and the unconscious mind, and that it has a powerful, symbolic communication that does not need the medium of language to convey its messages. Given that symbolic communication is a core component of play therapy, it can be assumed that children will also be sensitive to the symbolic projections of the physical space itself. Play therapist and theorist Garry Landreth (2012:125) acknowledges the 'critical importance' of the physical setting as it is the first thing the child encounters. He speaks of it as communicating important messages to the child, and it should say: 'This is a place for children. You are free to use what is here. Be yourself. Explore'.

Within my own practice I frequently witness striking verbal and non-verbal responses from children to the physical space upon entering my therapy room. It seems to offer an unspoken invitation for children to explore and connect with themselves, before connecting with me. The architect Eberhard (2007) believes that recent findings from neuroscience can help us investigate the impact on emotion or state of mind when a person enters a space. Functional brain imaging technology can be applied to understanding the effect that a building's visual properties have on people's unconscious reactions. There is real potential here for fascinating research into identifying positive design details from how children respond when they enter play therapy rooms. I would welcome research that analyses initial responses from children, and how these may impact future sessions and outcomes.

Spaces have purpose

Environmental psychologists believe that because of this intrinsic human response to the physical environment, the design of spaces should consider client need and be used to influence the dynamics of interaction. When this is done well it creates a 'congruence' between people's actions and the physical and social setting. Wright (1954) states that the fundamental task for human beings, and also for architecture, is to aim for integrity. This echoes the emphasis the play therapist places on authentic or congruent responses to the expressions of the child: a key personal quality within the core competences that BAPT requires of its practitioners. Thus, the design of the space could reinforce aspects of the psychological principles of the therapeutic provision.

There is evidence of congruence between buildings and interaction everywhere in society, as personalised design principles are used to influence participation. These principles are used to full effect in the design of theatres and the composition of stage and props for performances. McAuley (1999) acknowledges that the physical presence of the actors and their behaviour is of central importance, but also gives significant weight to the centrality of the design and layout of the staging that help to articulate the meaning of the play and influence how meanings are received by the audience.

Trustman (2013), a dramatherapist, asserts that on approaching and entering a theatre, audiences immediately begin a kind of transformation process, out of the ordinary world into the non-ordinary world. This is supported by their knowledge and felt experience of the structure and rituals of the theatre. He believes this principle can be positively exploited in the field of creative arts therapy. Manipulation of the space and materials can create a facilitating environment that is a space apart from everyday life. This space can support the therapist in taking the client safely through a process of engaging with the reflective self to access challenging emotional material. In my experience, as well as benefiting the client, the structure, layout and materials of the room orientate me towards my role as play therapist and support me in my improvisation.

The communicative and purposeful functions of play therapy

Pallasmaa (2012) concurs that space should have integrity in the service of the needs of those who inhabit it. In pursuit of the idea that having a dedicated, designed space can enhance levels of engagement, a consideration of the needs of both client and therapist in the context of the principles and goals of play therapy is essential.

Child-centred play therapy is based upon the development of a therapeutic relationship built on trust. This is facilitated by the personal qualities of the therapist: unconditional positive regard, congruence and empathy (Rogers, 1951). This trusting relationship will foster the child's expression of feelings at their own pace and direction. The respectful acceptance of these feelings and the non-directive nature of the intervention activate the child's inner resources. This leads to expressions of competence from the child. Thus, for the purposes of this chapter, I have selected three overarching functions of play therapy for consideration:

1   Establishing a therapeutic relationship built upon trust
2   Facilitating, accepting and containing the expression of feelings
3   The promotion of self-efficacy.

How the physical environment can support the therapeutic relationship

Winnicott (1989) spoke of the mother's emotional and physical holding of the infant that gives the child a reliable and predictable experience of being cared for. This holding is crucial to their mental development and psychological well-being. Lanyado (1991) believes that the therapeutic relationship has much in common with this and is supported through the external therapeutic environment we provide. Klein (1949), in her early psychoanalytic work with children, discovered that this consistent and predictable holding should be reflected in the setting for the work, as she noted over time how sensitive children were to even the slightest changes. Play therapy theorists such as Wilson and Ryan (2005) echo the therapeutic importance of creating an environment that is familiar, consistent and well designed. This is harder to achieve if one is working in a disorganised setting and can create anxiety in the child.

In my own practice I have worked in a variety of settings, including in rooms with shared use. I have noticed how difficult it is for the child to attend to their process if the allocated room is not suitable for purpose, resources are not easily accessible, or have been moved or altered in some way in between sessions. Children in therapy have less time and energy available to attend to their process whilst they are accommodating to any distracting demands or discomforts of the space.

A number of studies reflect that therapists are also susceptible to the influences of their physical surroundings. A mixed methods study by Backhaus (2008) into the design of psychologists' offices revealed that certain design features were prerequisites for a healthy, therapeutic environment and for positive outcomes. The layout of the furniture in the room, the quality of the sound acoustics, the lighting and colours used, as well as furnishings were all considered to be important to both clients and therapists.

They impacted feelings of safety, as well as comfort, and therefore the ability to relax and engage within the therapeutic work. Studies by environmental psychologists such as Anthony and Watkins (2002) have shown that because therapists spend a lot of time in their therapy rooms, an unappealing environment can also have a significant negative influence on their mood and their responses to the client.

Being a therapist requires a very focused level of attention and attunement, and I notice that in certain settings it takes a greater effort to achieve this, which can impact my ability to attend to the client and create a consistent emotional holding environment.

Privacy and the therapeutic relationship

The maintenance of confidentiality and privacy for clients and their families is a BAPT core competence, and this aspect is often referred to by theorists in relation to the physical environment. Landreth (2012) states that if parents or other children hear what is going on in the playroom, the child may feel that their privacy has been violated and the relationship will suffer. Therapeutic provision often occurs within environments where room availability is an issue, let alone the provision of carefully planned and designed spaces. Even when the room itself is a suitable design, its position within the building can be problematic. Topf (1994:289) examined the impact of what he termed 'ambient stressors'. These can be any uncontrollable and therefore inescapable aspects of the surrounding environment, such as unwanted sounds, that can result in stress.

Therapy rooms often have adjacency to other rooms or public spaces, including corridors or waiting areas. Soundproofing or complete isolation is desirable but often not attainable. Sound interruption may appear trivial, tolerable and even acceptable to a degree, as a reflection of daily life. However, these distractions can all have a negative impact on a child's ability to be psychologically available for therapeutic work. They can also be difficult to tolerate for a child with symptoms of trauma, such as hypervigilance. Ideally, therapy rooms should be places apart from everyday interruptions, in which emotional concerns can be given highest priority.

Some of these issues can be difficult to resolve, but often good communication can reduce their impact. In one setting I requested that no chairs were placed outside my room, so that it could not be used as a waiting area. When my sessions were in progress (indicated by a clear sign on the room door), any persons passing by or using the space were requested to do so quietly. An important message to widely deliver is that the child exiting a session must not be informed, even playfully, if they have been overheard.

Visual privacy can also be compromised. In schools it is often a policy to have window panels in internal doors so that the safety of participants can be monitored from the hallway. This has implications for children in therapy inside the room, who may create visual depictions of their process with small world toys, or through art or role play. These can be representations of intense inner struggles they are attempting to resolve, and they may be in touch with vulnerable emotional states. If the child is conscious that people can see into the room, then it is reasonable to assume that they would feel a reduced freedom to express themselves. This can also apply to the therapist who could be distracted from their attunement to the child's process, or their engagement in role play with the child.

Some of my colleagues have addressed this issue by providing screens on these windows with narrow visual access at the top, for use by informed and trusted staff members, thus ensuring that the focus on the child's process remains undisturbed.

Sometimes other adults may need to be available to assist the child and can therefore become a part of the physical environment. In my work within a residential rehabilitation facility for children with acquired brain injury, some of my clients have required close attendance by nurses. For each one we have had to undertake detailed risk assessments to determine whether confidential therapy could be offered. I was able to successfully work with some very physically vulnerable children through carefully adapted room design, the use of alarm systems, and training from the medical team to identify warning signs of health issues, along with close proximity of nurses outside a closed door.

On other occasions I have been required to work with interpreters in the room. This has also required very careful preparation, including training about the approach, the strict observance of confidentiality, and the necessity of faithful representation of both client and therapist language. It also includes issues for the interpreters such as where to position themselves in the room, and how to maintain their impersonal stance within and outside of the therapeutic space. Interpreters have also needed ongoing access to support as they can be exposed to very challenging emotional material.

Working effectively in different settings is another core competence for the play therapist (Competence 30, Appendix 1). This includes a consideration of the dilemmas of integrating play therapy practice within a variety of organisational contexts. Practitioners need to have clear knowledge of their approach and the needs of their clients. Effective communication within the system is essential in order to provide an acceptable working environment and practices that do not contravene the health and safety requirements or general policies of the organisation.

How the physical environment can support the expression and containment of feelings

Whilst healing lies in the therapeutic relationship, the physical space that promotes the child's physical as well as verbal expression needs to be considered. Once the therapeutic relationship is established, and the child feels accepted through congruent, respectful and empathic responses, the child in play therapy can then use the safety of this relationship to express him or herself more fully. Stacey (2008) states that through being held in the safe therapeutic space by the therapeutic relationship and engaging creatively through play, internal material can be embodied and projected into the outside world. Cattanach (1994) sees play as the symbolic transformation of experience and, whilst playing, the child can process difficult feelings and material through indirect expression.

Joseph (1998) underlines how therapeutic work with children is more dependent on action than on words, and consequently demands that the therapist needs to consider seriously the nature of the physical space in which the therapeutic interactions occur. The therapist needs to feel relaxed to promote a sense of trust and safety in which children feel free to express emotions. In order to maintain a containing stance for these expressions, the therapist needs to be free from anxiety and concern about how the room can support this.

If the therapist feels anxious in any way, it can potentially interrupt the therapeutic relationship as the therapist will no longer feel able to focus on accepting the child's need to freely project. This links again to the therapist's ability to maintain their child-centred stance; any lack of comfort on the part of the therapist could be sensed by the child, which they could interpret as a lack of unconditional positive regard from the therapist.

Landreth (2012:530) suggests that 'every playroom should have some inexpensive items that are for smashing, breaking, or throwing, or to be stacked and kicked over, jumped on, smashed, broken apart, thrown and painted'. Ray (2011) supports this premise that for children who have a need to project aggression, the physical environment needs to convey a sense of control and containment, thus avoiding contributing to their feelings of inner chaos and lack of safety.

It is a BAPT core competence to include a variety of play and creative media to facilitate a range of verbal, non-verbal and symbolic communication (Competence 27, Appendix 1). Unstructured materials such as sand, clay, slime and water have a high therapeutic value, as is increasingly evidenced by recent advances in neuroscience. Schore (2003) and Perry (2009) state that children need to work at the sensorimotor level to activate neural network growth essential for symbolic play and verbalisation. Landreth (2012:142) shares the view that sensory materials such as sand and water are potentially the most therapeutically useful play media for children, but goes on to say that 'they can be the least likely to be found in play therapy settings, perhaps because these materials are more challenging for the therapist to contain within a physical space'.

This statement is a clear indicator of the need to consider the importance of a carefully designed space. Some materials can be managed through appropriate limit setting, whereas others may be more challenging, and alternatives may have to be found. I choose to provide sequins and glitter glue, but not glitter, as my concerns about the management of it would take my attention away from attending to the child. Many therapists find glitter to be a therapeutically useful resource, but I find it invasive, remaining distractingly in evidence on every surface it encounters for prolonged periods of time. A wide range of expressive media is important, but therapists need to be aware of their own sensory preferences and what they can tolerate.

How the physical environment can support the promotion of self-efficacy and competence for the client

Rogers (1951) states that the impetus for any change must originate from within the client for the change to be authentic. Therefore, in play therapy, it is particularly important for the therapist to be committed to promoting self-directed change. Cochran et al. (2010) use a stage theory to track the processes of change in a child in play therapy. They name the final stage the 'Mastery' stage, in which elements of their growth achieved throughout the process become an integral part of the child's self-expression. These elements are evidenced through positive demonstrations of self-efficacy and competence, along with a mastery over their interaction with the environment and the tools within it.

Central to this idea is the importance for the child of having control over what they do or say within the setting, which has immediate implications for the set-up of the room. Environmental psychologist Maxwell (1996), in her study of pre-school children, found that there is a relationship between the physical environment and a child's self-identity, self-esteem and academic performance. She acknowledged the primacy of the care-giving relationships for children, but claimed that children are also very responsive to environmental cues. They can be socialised by their physical environments as well as by the people in their lives. She concluded that when children understand the specific physical characteristics of a space, they can respond more effectively, which positively impacts their self-esteem.

Studies by Blau (2000) attribute such importance to this spatial understanding that they recommend that any evaluation of the quality of child care must include an assessment of the physical environment. Given what we have established about the emotional and therapeutic dividend for a child in achieving competence as a key goal of play therapy, studies in this area are valuable. As Landreth (2012:137) states, children in need of play therapy have poor self-images, so accessible materials need to be provided which can be mastered and manipulated easily, necessary for building up a feeling of, 'In here, I can do things for myself. I can be successful'.

There are many features that contribute to preparing an environment for children that promotes competence. Trancik and Evans (1995) recommend providing opportunities for the child to perform independently at a level appropriate for their developmental stage, and having a wide range of materials and equipment so that children can interact with the environment at a self-determined level of challenge. Good visual access and appropriate adjacency of materials and equipment were also identified as necessary. Evans et al. (1991) call this a 'legible' environment and agree that these features contribute to children's development of competence as they make it easier to predict and make decisions about how to use a space.

Evans et al. (1991) identify the importance of reducing constraints on behaviour caused by having furniture and equipment that is either not easy to access or is of an inappropriate scale for the ease of use of the child. Supplying furniture and play items that can be easily rearranged by children to meet their needs during the course of play activities gives children a sense of environmental control, resulting in increased feelings of competence.

Another aspect to promote competence is to offer the child some control over their level of interaction. Altman (1975) states that children need a dedicated private area, or at least the provision of materials so that a child can construct their own. If a therapist can provide an environment that respects this need for privacy, this will also enhance trust in the relationship. With opportunities for the child to engage and disengage, the room can support the therapist in maintaining their containing child-centred stance.

For this purpose, I have used fabric canopies hanging from the ceiling, or provided material that children can use to make their own simple dens, hide underneath, or cover their heads with. Net fabrics can be very effective also, offering a sense of being apart without full isolation. Other therapists have used small pop-up tents.

Kaplan (1995) concurs that privacy through environmental control is important, and opportunities for 'restoration' from feelings of fatigue through engagement in activities that do not require focused interactive attention should be provided. I have found the inclusion of toys with high visual or tactile interest such as kaleidoscopes, containers with slow-moving coloured oils or sand, and hand-held stretchy toys useful. They can have a calming effect upon children who need a break from processing difficult emotional material, or even from the challenge of initiating interaction with words. These can also be very useful at the beginning of a session to help a child transition into the space, or at the end, to prepare for re-integrating back into a public space.

All these studies suggest a positive relationship between the physical environment and competence in children. To ensure equality of opportunity, these environmental issues need to be considered even more carefully when working with specific populations of children. Self-expression can be greatly hindered for those with learning disabilities, illness, restricted mobility, motor difficulties, or sensory processing difficulties. These children inevitably have 'fewer opportunities for the self-directing play which is central to the development of a sense of autonomy' (McMahon, 2009:142). This brings into play a further BAPT core competence relating to anti-discriminatory practice: ensuring that children and young people in a diverse society have equal opportunity (Competence 9, Appendix 1).

In my experience the best environment will provide opportunities to flexibly re-arrange the play therapy space between sessions. Height-adjustable tables and chairs are extremely useful, as are tables with a cut-away semi-circular space at the front that can comfortably accommodate wheelchairs. Opportunities to work at floor level should also be offered, supported by comfortable carpeting and cushions. For children who can be adversely affected by too much visual stimulation, neutral fabrics can be quickly arranged to cover surfaces or screen off areas of a large or cluttered room.

Further considerations and challenges

Whilst some organisations do offer dedicated spaces for service delivery in which we can experiment with some of the design principles discussed, therapists encounter many challenges in the world of peripatetic creative arts provision.

Art psychotherapist Wood (2000) suggests that external socio-economic and political issues have influenced the availability of dedicated creative art therapy spaces within organisations. Economic cuts and policy changes (such as the model of psychiatric care in the community) have fostered a re-consideration of the principles of art psychotherapy towards a focus on the psychotherapeutic relationship rather than the freedom of expression through art materials.

Wood does acknowledge that successful therapeutic interventions can be achieved without a designated, well designed studio. She cites the work of two other art psychotherapists, Kalmanowitz and Lloyd (1997), who used basic portable studios in difficult environmental circumstances in former Yugoslavia and in South Africa. Nevertheless, she argues that due to the demanding nature of psychotherapeutic work, a consistent and contained space in which to work is important for the psychological well-being of the therapist. She concludes that whilst attention in art psychotherapy has moved from the studio room to the therapeutic relationship, the studio is still the best setting in which to work with clients.

Dramatherapist Boutell (1979) asserts that because of the pressures for room space in organisations such as schools, therapists respond by changing their levels of expectation, and adapt to increasingly restrictive compromises for fear of losing their position. Boutell argues that in order to preserve the excellence of our practice we must not become the victims of these reduced standards.

Within the field of play therapy, Cattanach (1994) asserts that the challenges of the physical space can be overcome by changes of technique. She believes that her portable approach, using a mat to delineate the space, transforms a room into a safe, boundaried, therapeutic area. However, Cattanach does acknowledge that one of the tasks of the therapist is to ensure a feeling of security for the child and to maintain the safety of the play space. This desirable component is much more difficult to achieve in this portable model wherein there is a greatly reduced degree of environmental control, and which is often based on luck. It is certainly an undesirable factor to have to rely on chance to provide the best environment for the well-being of a child who has already suffered from the lack of an emotionally supportive holding environment.

Conclusion

In comparison with a wealth of studies from other fields demonstrating significant impacts upon the health and well-being of child clients in health and child care settings, research from the field of play therapy is hard to find. The absence of such evidence is perhaps of concern, considering that the therapy room is a place in which clients need to feel sufficiently safe and relaxed in order to be able to explore and process their challenging emotional concerns.

As play therapists we all need to take some responsibility for undertaking, contributing to, or at the least, requesting research into areas of our practice. It is a core competence to enhance the evidence base for play therapy and apply research evidence to our practice to increase effectiveness and assure quality of service delivery (Competence 10, Appendix 1). This chapter is my contribution to encouraging further work in this area. I am constantly aware of the ebb and flow of the interaction between the child, myself and the room. There are times in which the human relationship takes precedence, and others when this becomes more of a minor role to the greater dramatic encounter of the child and the room that the child inhabits and fills with so much meaning. There is much to explore within what is for me a fascinating area and unmined seam of potential gains. Even if the physical attributes of a space were only to play a small part in influencing behaviour, it is still advisable to examine any influences in order to capitalise on positive effects.

Research could provide theoretical clarity and evidence which could persuade organisations to offer more adequate, and more visible spaces for our service delivery. This in turn could have an important impact on raising the profile of play therapy in our communities. It is perhaps time that we no longer rely on our expertise in dealing with often mediocre spatial compromises, and strive for optimal reparative experiences in supportive and inspiring spaces that our heavily disadvantaged clients and our society deserve.

Summary

- Research from related fields and other disciplines evidences that physical space has a communicative function outside of language that can influence the dynamics of interaction.
- A carefully designed setting could potentially support the relationship principles and goals of play therapy:

  - A consistent physical environment reflects and supports the reliable emotional holding of the therapeutic relationship
  - A safe and containing space creates increased therapeutic opportunities for physical exploration and expression from the child
  - Developmentally sensitive design features promote independent exploration for the child, resulting in self-efficacy and competence.

- The presence of carefully designed, dedicated play therapy rooms could raise the profile of the work and create more opportunities to offer therapeutic support where it is needed.

Further reading

It has been beyond the remit of this chapter to comprehensively consider the vital importance of valuing and reflecting cultural diversity. It is crucial that play therapists take responsibility for being fully informed about factors such as ethnicity, gender, disability and religious belief, and how the play therapy setting can represent and promote equality of opportunity for all members of society. This is another area in which more research is needed. Please refer to the following paper for a useful consideration of diversity issues:

O'Connor, K. (2005) Addressing diversity issues in play therapy. *Professional Psychology.* 36(5) pp. 566–573.

For more information on the selection of play therapy materials and toys:

Cochran, N. H., Nordling, W. J. & Cochran, J. L. (2010) *Child-Centred Play Therapy: A Practical Guide to Developing Therapeutic Relationships with Children.* New York: John Wiley & Sons. Chapter 5.

Landreth, G. L. (2012) *Play Therapy: The Art of the Relationship*. (3rd ed.) New York: Brunner-Routledge. Chapter 7.
West, J. (1996) *Child Centred Play Therapy*. (2nd ed.) London: Arnold. Chapters 7–8.

For further evidence on the importance of sensorimotor play:

Ogden, P., Minton, K. & Pain, C. (2006) *Trauma and the Body*. London: W.W. Norton.
Rothschild, B. (2000) *The Body Remembers*. New York: W.W. Norton.

References

Altman, I. (1975) *The Environment and Social Behaviour*. Pacific Grove, CA: Brooks/Cole.
Anthony, K. H. & Watkins, N. J. (2002) Exploring pathology: Relationships between clinical and environmental psychology. In Bechtel, R. & Churchman, A. (eds.) *Handbook of Environmental Psychology*. New York: John Wiley & Sons. pp. 138–140.
Backhaus, K. L. (2008) *Client and Therapist Perspectives on the Importance of the Physical Environment of the Therapy Room: A Mixed Methods Study*. Denton, TX: Texas Woman's University.
Blau, D. M. (2000) The production of quality in child-care centers: Another look. *Applied Developmental Science*. 4(3) pp. 136–148.
Boutell, C. A. (1979) The shrinking space. *Dramatherapy*. 2(2) pp. 1–3.
Cattanach, A. (1994) *Play Therapy: Where the Sky Meets the Underworld*. London: Jessica Kingsley Publishers.
Cochran, N. H., Nordling, W. J. & Cochran, J. L. (2010) *Child-Centred Play Therapy: A Practical Guide to Developing Therapeutic Relationships with Children*. New York: John Wiley & Sons.
Eberhard, J. P. (2007) *Architecture and the Brain: A New Knowledge Base from Neuroscience*. Atlanta, GA: Greenway Communications.
Evans, G. W., Kliewer, W. & Martin, J. (1991) The role of the physical environment in the health and well-being of children. In Schroeder, H. (ed.) *New Directions in Health Psychology Assessment*. New York: Hemisphere Publishing. pp. 127–157.
Joseph, B. (1998) Thinking about a playroom. *Journal of Child Psychotherapy*. 24(3) pp. 359–366.
Kalmanowitz, D. & Lloyd, B. (1997) *The Portable Studio: Art Therapy and Political Conflict: Initiatives in Former Yugoslavia and South Africa*. London: Health Education Authority.
Kaplan, S. (1995) The restorative benefits of nature: Toward an integrative framework. *Journal of Environmental Psychology*. 15(3) pp. 169–182.
Klein, M. (1949) *The Psychoanalysis of Children*. London: Hogarth.
Landreth, G. L. (2012) *Play Therapy: The Art of the Relationship*. (3rd ed.) New York: Brunner-Routledge.
Lanyado, M. (1991) On creating a psychotherapeutic space. *Journal of Social Work Practice*. 5(1) pp. 31–40.
Lawson, B. (2001) *Language of Space*. Oxford: Architectural Press.

Maxwell, L. E. (1996) Multiple effects of home and day care crowding. *Environment and Behaviour.* 28(4) pp. 494–511.

McAuley, G. (1999) *Space in Performance: Making Meaning in the Theatre.* Ann Arbor, MI: Michigan University Press.

McMahon, L. (2009) *The Handbook of Play Therapy and Therapeutic Play.* (2nd ed.) Hove: Routledge.

Pallasmaa, J. (2012) *The Eyes of the Skin: Architecture and the Senses.* New York: John Wiley & Sons.

Perry, B. (2009) Examining child maltreatment through a neurodevelopmental lens: Clinical applications of the neurosequential model of therapeutics. *Journal of Loss and Trauma.* 14 pp. 240–255.

Ray, D. (2011) *Advanced Play Therapy. Essential Conditions, Knowledge, and Skills for Child Practice.* New York: Routledge.

Rogers, C. R. (1951) *Client-Centered Therapy: Its Current Practice, Implications and Theory.* Boston, MA: Houghton Mifflin.

Schore, A. (2003) *Affect Regulation and Repair of the Self.* New York: W. W. Norton & Company.

Stacey, J. (2008) The therapeutic relationship in creative arts psychotherapy. In Haugh, S. & Paul, S. (eds.) *The Therapeutic Relationship: Perspectives and Themes.* Monmouth, Wales: PCSS Books. Vol. 18. pp. 217–229.

Topf, M. (1994) Theoretical considerations for research on environmental stress and health. *The Journal of Nursing Scholarship.* 26 pp. 289–293.

Trancik, A. M. & Evans, G. W. (1995) Spaces fit for children: Competency in the design of daycare center environments. *Children's Environments.* 12(3) pp. 311–319.

Trustman, M. (2013) *Dramatherapy.* Play Therapy in Context PLT020L614. 18 March 2013. Lecture at University of Roehampton, London.

Tuan, Y. F. (2001) *Space and Place: The Perspective of Experience.* Minneapolis, MN: University of Minnesota Press.

Wilson, K. & Ryan, V. (2005) *Play Therapy: A Non-directive Approach for Children and Adolescents.* (2nd ed.) London: Elsevier Ltd.

Winnicott, D. W. (1989) *Playing and Reality.* London: Routledge.

Wood, C. (2000) The significance of studios. *Inscape: The Journal of the British Association of Art Therapists.* 5(2) pp. 41–53.

Wright, F. L. (1954) *The Natural House.* New York: Horizon Press.

Chapter 5

Setting up in independent practice as a play therapist

Harriet Armstrong

Chapter overview

This chapter will seek to provide a comprehensive guide for those considering working as a self-employed play therapist, addressing the key aspects of BAPT Core Competence 16 (see Appendix 1). I will explore a range of professional considerations for those wishing to set up as a freelance therapist or running their own private practice. I will discuss possible settings for practice, establishing yourself as a therapist, legal considerations, financial matters, your play therapy kit and sources of support. I will also refer to ethical guidelines, although this is covered elsewhere within this volume in more detail (see Chapter 6 by St Louis).

Location of work

Setting up in private practice can feel exciting and daunting wherever you are in your career. There are a number of different working environments which you may want to consider. In discussions with my BAPT colleagues I have found that many play therapists work within a variety of places.

Working in the child's home

When play therapy was a new profession in this country many therapists went into people's homes to provide therapy, and this is still the preferred location for some therapists. There can be benefits to seeing a child within their own home: they can feel safer and more relaxed and therefore find the beginning process of therapy easier. When entering a child's home you immediately have insight into the environment in which they live. You are able to get a better perception of the relationships between the family members, parenting styles and parents' ability to maintain boundaries. The child and parent do not have to travel, meaning it is easier for them, especially as there may be reasons that make travel difficult (e.g. parental illness or disability, other siblings, lack of a car or public transport links). Another advantage is that a parent is readily available after a difficult session for the child, in contrast to the school setting in which this can prove difficult. However, there are a number of potential issues to consider: protected space and confidentiality within the home, intrusion of therapy into the home for some children, travel time and cost for yourself, transportation of a play therapy kit and your personal safety. It is important to help the parents/carers understand that when the therapy is taking place within the home the boundaries of confidentiality still need to be the same as in a clinical context. Equally some children may find having therapy at home intrusive and may feel they want it separate from their everyday life and own family space. Other children may find it difficult to stay in the room especially if they hear familiar sounds outside of the room. Once a child wanted to finish early because they heard their grandparents arrive for a visit. This is fine of course but not as a frequent occurrence. Furthermore, as the therapist we have little control over the wider contents of the room changing, such as furniture being moved, and having a space for play therapy may be impossible in some houses: there just may not be a suitable room where a parent could not overhear or a sibling would not be able to crash in. In circumstances such as these, many therapists approach the child's school or a local children's centre (with the parent's consent) as an alternative location. For the therapist travelling to different homes a working day is more tiring, time consuming and costly. However, if you put a realistic limit on the number of clients per day then the time between homes may allow you to process and prepare mentally for the next one.

Working in schools

Play therapists are increasingly to be found working in schools, many now even having a play therapist in residence, especially in major cities where more therapists are available. The way the play therapist functions within different schools can be dependent on the school's knowledge of play therapy, the understanding of the senior leadership and the size and demographic of the school. I have found it helpful to provide whole school training on play therapy, where I talk about the interaction between emotions and behaviour, what children may be experiencing, our expectations of them, how we can support them and how play therapy can help. Whenever I begin working with a child I ensure I meet with the teacher, partly to gain knowledge of the child and how they present in school, but also to give an overview of play therapy and how it works in schools. The more we all do this the more play therapy is understood. I have worked in my current school for nearly 10 years and I recently heard the magic words 'it doesn't matter what time he has his session, play therapy is more important'.

Disruptions to sessions are a difficulty which many therapists encounter in the school context. In some schools this is never overcome despite signs on doors and endless reminders – I remember a headteacher coming into a group session to tell a child that he needed to see him afterwards (to discipline him for behaviour at lunch time). The so-called safe space for all the children in the group was immediately compromised. I had previously discussed with the head about not having interruptions and thought I had explained the importance of why. After this incident I went to him asking if I could help in any way with the child and gain some further details of the behaviour. Within this conversation I conveyed how the children had begun to feel safe in the group, that they had begun to open up to each other and gain support from one another, that this had been a place of sanctuary for them in a tough world, in a tough school. It was as if a light had been turned on and he suddenly understood the therapeutic space and we thought together about how and when children could be spoken to regarding issues with their behaviour. These important interactions with school staff are a core skill for a play therapist to develop, as identified in the competence *Maintenance of effective inter-professional relationships* (BAPT Core Competence 28, see Appendix 1). (See also Chapter 12 by Murray for further considerations on working in schools.)

Multidisciplinary team setting

Working as part of a specialist team within a clinic or Child and Adolescent Mental Health Services (CAMHS) team can have many benefits. Layered working is often more commonplace in these types of setting whereby therapists can pass on cases to other members of the team where appropriate (Padmore, 2016). This could range from just having another colleague's viewpoint on an assessment, to being fully supported by another team member. Another professional may focus on a different aspect of a child's difficulties such as speech and language, sensory processing or parent counselling, leaving the play therapist to focus solely on the emotional impact of their difficulties. One example was a play therapy client whose school was not able to understand her difficulties despite dialogue between myself, school and parent. Staff were unable to perceive that she had greater levels of need than those she was displaying on the surface. The educational psychologist, who was also a neuropsychology specialist, could map out a plan with the school for transition with which they felt comfortable and seemed to understand more. Thus a multi-disciplinary plan was put in place for the child, whereby she continued with play therapy as her safe space to explore non-directively, with a specialist teaching assistant employed to support her at school, and a limited number of sessions with the educational neuropsychologist, specifically focussing on psycho-education regarding her anxiety and social difficulties. Another benefit when being part of this type of team is that there is increased opportunity to ask colleagues questions and hold case discussions. At the clinic we have monthly CPD evenings including such case study discussions. Working with the other members of the team gives me further insight into the world of the child and family, what they may be experiencing, coping with or can do. I have found being part of this type of team a favourable way of working and it means I feel less isolated in my role as play therapist.

Renting a play therapy space

As with any setting there are positives and negatives about renting your own space. Compared with working within a school, child's home or established clinic, renting your own space will have more outlay such as rent, electricity, gas, water and insurance. Some places will offer you an hourly, day or half-day rate, or you may want to have a long-term let with the scope to make changes for your benefit (such as painting walls or putting up shelves). Some tenancies may include repairs and maintenance but others may not, so do look in detail at what you are being offered. The control you have over when you open and close/take holiday breaks are much better if you are the sole tenant. You are completely in charge of how you want to run your service without having to fit into another person's ideas. I experienced several difficulties in one place where I wanted to work on a Saturday. This was fine at first in the September I started, however in school holidays and on several other occasions I found that the main building had limited opening hours and the caretaker was employed in split shifts at times to cover evening events. This had not been communicated clearly to me and therefore there were several occasions when I had to cancel or alter sessions.

Wherever you choose or get an opportunity to work, BAPT Core Competence 29 of *Developing and managing a play room/play therapy environment* is vital (see Appendix 1 and Chapter 4 by Fullalove). You need to take responsibility for the development and safe management of the play therapy room, in line with health and safety standards. Helpful places for guidance on health and safety legislation are HSE (www.hse.gov.uk/) and NICE guidelines (www.nice.org.uk/guidance). You will need to carry out a risk assessment of the environment and take appropriate steps to ensure continuing safety such as awareness of trip hazards or electrical sockets.

Many therapists work in several different settings over the week and I have found this variety suits me well. The nature of play therapy means I never have two sessions the same but the mix of client difficulties plus different settings across a week means I experience an even wider range of issues which the children and families bring. For example, in one setting I have been referred many children who have witnessed domestic violence and in another setting many of my clients have physical disabilities or learning difficulties. Being in different work environments can mean avoiding the office politics (benefit) but you may also feel less of a sense of belonging (downside). The latter issue can feel difficult for some therapists but I find having lunch in the staff room and getting to know my colleagues, involving myself in staff meetings and attending staff social events really helps to feel part of the team.

Often when we start out as a therapist we do not have the luxury of choosing our ideal place of work – we may have to take whatever is offered. It is important to consider what the best fit is and if you are compromising too much on what you want then perhaps try to find an alternative. The next section may help with ideas of how to find employment.

Getting established as a play therapist

Getting work can feel very difficult when you first set out and deciding when and how to spend budget in this area is important.

First, make the most of your professional body membership. BAPT members can ensure they are listed on the 'Find a therapist' database which is held on the BAPT website (www.bapt.info/find-therapist/). Ensure you have as much information as possible on here to give potential clients enough knowledge to make a decision. Give a guide to the fees you charge as parents often report that transparency in this area is a key factor in their choice.

Second, design yourself a website. This does not have to be expensive and initially you may just need a few pages to ensure you are visible on the internet. Especially important to include would be an explanation of what play therapy is, what you can offer in terms of individual child sessions, filial therapy/family or group sessions. List areas of expertise you have or types of difficulties you are willing to work with and your location. Once you have seen some children perhaps you could include testimonials to help give parents reassurance.

Local support groups can also be a good source of work: where one therapist may not have capacity for a referral or indeed where it may not be their area of expertise or be too far to travel, it might be just right for you. Therapists happily pass on cases to others in my local London group, with prior parental consent to do so. It is important to network to get established in your local community as well as the 'play therapy world' so you could attend conferences and relevant events, contact local GPs, schools, children's centres and children's services. I have found that once I have supported one child, I am frequently offered further work from that team.

You can advertise in local listings such as community newspapers and on websites such as the counselling directory (www.counselling-directory.org.uk/). Put up postcards in children's centres, libraries and community noticeboards. I have found it particularly successful to offer free training to local schools. Within the clinic, most of our work comes via word of mouth but whenever we provide training (both free of charge and at cost) we have an influx of referrals afterwards.

Legal and ethical matters

There are a range of legal and ethical issues to consider as a therapist in independent practice. Thorough understanding of these legal matters will ensure you can carry out your practice as ethically as possible (BAPT Core Competence 12, see Appendix 1). The more informed you are the better protected you will be if something goes wrong. You will need to write and have available your own policies and procedures such as child protection procedures, health and safety policies and complaints procedures. (Please refer to Chapter 6 by St Louis for more on ethical compliance.)

Formal contracts are important to show what you will be providing as a service as well as setting boundaries for your clients (French & Klein, 2012) (BAPT Core Competence 19, see Appendix 1). Contracts with parents/referrers should include a brief description of play therapy, the agreed day and time therapy will take place and a statement about confidentiality. Ensure that you are clear in your contracts that information will be kept confidential between you and the child except when you are concerned about their safety or that of others.

Child protection

Child protection should be in the forefront of every therapist's mind and when you write your child protection policy include details of who to contact if you feel a child may be in danger of harm. Refer to the latest *Working Together to Safeguard Children* document (DES, 2017) for guidance. Your policy should state very clearly what you will report. Your local authority will have a referral and assessment department where there will always be a duty manager from whom you can gain advice. There should always be a secure record of all child protection concerns.

Record-keeping and data protection

As a play therapist I need to keep a record of the clients I have seen, however it seems less clear as to what should be included in those notes. Helpful guidance can be found in Bond and Mitchels' (2014) book on the topic. We have to record attendance of a child at therapy sessions. If your notes are identifiable as a particular child or person they are subject to data protection law. When training we are taught to record a factual description of the play and toys used, what the child says, and information such as positioning in the room, proximity to therapist, usually with a separate section containing the therapist's reflections on the meaning, themes and process. Records held about a child need to be available for that child (or their parent) to see, should they request. These notes can be requested by the police, social care, or certain other officials. The request for information should be made in writing and the records should be given within a month of this free of charge. In line with the latest General Data Protection Regulations (GDPR) you need to ensure that you are clear in your contracts for what purpose you collect data, how you store it securely and how long you will keep the records. There is no law on retention, however professionally and ethically the consensus is until the child is 25 years old, giving them an opportunity to request information for up to 7 years after they become an adult.

As well as case notes we hold information about clients such as name, address, DoB, medical conditions, details of GP and possibly financial details, and GDPR states we need explicit consent to hold this sensitive personal information. Any written records should be in a locked cabinet within a lockable room (when vacant). This means if you keep any written records in your play therapy room, this room should be locked when not in use. Do not make unnecessary copies of written records and avoid removing these records from your office. Ensure the keys to your office and filing cabinet are kept secure. If you have employees, only allow them access to client records if necessary, ensure they understand confidentiality and ensure they sign an agreement regarding this. If you use electronic records make sure your computer is password-protected. Back up your all information on your computer and keep your back-up secure and in a different place. When sending letters or reports via email these should be encrypted and saved as PDF files in order that they cannot be edited by other people/agencies. Do not forget to add disclaimers to your emails stating the confidentiality of information within.

In order to comply with the GDPR if you hold any client information on your computer then you need to register with the Information Commissioner's Office (ICO). Any breaches of data (e.g. a break-in at your place of work where you store files or a stolen laptop from your home) must be reported to the ICO within 72 hours. You will need a professional executor who would be able to take care of your data should you be taken ill or are unable to return to work. Your professional body, GDPR and the ICO website (https://ico.org.uk/) can offer help and guidance on data protection.

When working for yourself it is important to have a professional living will drawn up. This is a document stating your wishes in the event of death, disappearance or disability rendering you incapable of seeing clients or dealing with your practice. It will include the name/s of persons who will inform your clients and families of your unavailability. Those persons will need to ascertain the client's need for referral on to an alternative therapist and provide support for this. It will also detail where you keep both hard copy notes and electronic information and will state how to gain access to these. Insurance and accountant information should be included on this document. I found reading through an actual example of the document very helpful (Ragusea, 2008) to ensure I had covered everything.

Financial matters

Charges

When considering what to charge, start by calculating your own costs: how much are you paying in rent on your play therapy room, what are your travel costs, how much do you spend on consumables (paper, playdough) etc.? You need to factor in expenses for electricity, phone bills/broadband, special email address, printing, insurance, clinical supervision, professional body membership etc. Then you need to think about the amount of time you spend. A session may last 45/50 minutes but you need additional time to set up beforehand and tidy afterwards, to write up your notes, answer emails and have phone calls with parents. Therapists typically charge for sessions with the child, meetings with parents or teachers and then some administration time (or this may be included in the session/hourly rate). Reports for school, social care and other agencies are usually charged at an hourly rate. Have a look at guidance produced by BAPT on the members' area of the website: www.bapt. info/members/resources/.

Insurance

Deciding what kind of insurance you need can feel like a bit of a minefield when you are setting up in independent practice and it is also dependent on where you work. *Public liability insurance* refers to insurance which covers you if a member of the public (a child you are seeing or parent) suffers an injury or damage to their property when in your place of practice. For example, if a parent tripped on a loose carpet in your waiting area and the injury temporarily stopped them from working, with loss of income, they could take you to court for damages and your public liability insurance would cover this. If you work out of a rented space you would definitely need this, whereas if you are working in a school or clinic they should already hold this type of insurance. If you work out of your own home, you would also need home business insurance. *Professional indemnity insurance* refers to the service you provide as a therapist. Should someone feel you have not delivered what you agreed or that you have done something wrong, then this insurance should cover legal advice and representation if needed. If you wish to set up practice in a room within your own home you will need to gain permission from your mortgage provider. You also need to consider whether you need extra car insurance if you travel for work. Car insurance companies are able to advise you on this.

Tax

When you are self-employed you need to file a tax return yearly. As the January deadline approaches each year I start to feel pretty sick about completing my tax return. As I fill it in I worry if I have answered questions correctly (I am almost 100% certain I have!) but I also realise how little time it takes in the end. I usually spend more time worrying about it than actually doing it. You could employ an accountant to do the legwork for you, but it is fairly straightforward if you have one or two sources of income (i.e. billing private clients and one weekly employment day). There are plenty of notes on the government website to help (www.gov.uk/self-assessment-tax-returns/get-help) and there are also YouTube videos on how to complete your tax return. One thing I would recommend though is filling it in as soon as you receive it, usually April each year. You then have until 31 January the following year to pay any tax you owe. I also suggest you budget carefully for paying your tax, putting money aside each month so you do not end up with a bill you are unable to pay.

Whatever your gross income over the year you then need to deduct anything related to work from that, which may include: room rent, heating and electricity expenses, telephone bills, paper and printer ink, play therapy materials, leaflets, purchase of large items such as a laptop or printer, new toys or furniture for the room, any training you attend and expenses related to that training. Do not forget clinical supervision, insurance, bank charges, membership of regulating bodies and marketing. Deduct any staffing costs and payment to the accountant. If you are not including travel costs (fuel and parking, train etc.) in your fees then these should also be deducted. You need to retain all receipts, invoices and records for 5 years after you have filed your tax return. It is worth noting that banks often offer deals for new businesses, such as no charges over the first 12–24 months whilst you are a fledgling business. I suggest booking a meeting with a small business advisor for some guidance.

Play therapy kit

There is plenty of guidance regarding which toys to have in your therapy room. Axline (1969) and Landreth (2012) both provide lists and I would advocate including items from key toy categories: sensory toys (bubbles, playdough), role play toys (dressing up, masks, doctor's kit), art and craft materials, a sand tray with small figures and other small items, dolls and baby bottles. In my experience children will find a way to express themselves using whatever you have. Not having a dolls' house will not stop your clients playing out something which happened in their home. Not having slime will not stop a child finding a way to explore unpredictability or having a sensory experience. I have seen a basic deck of cards used in many ways: to symbolise the fragility of home, for a game of chance demonstrating how they feel about their mother's love for them and theirs for her, as well as an ice-breaker or relationship builder, representing something familiar and safe.

When travelling to various clients or venues you will need to consider carefully what to include in your mobile kit. You will be limited in what you can carry or fit in your car. Consider how much time you have to spend setting up. Some therapists use stacking wheelie boxes, one containing the sand, one with the small figures, another with art materials, and so on.

When working with young children or those with developmental learning needs, ensure your kit does not contain choking hazards and that you use edible paint, homemade playdough, etc. It is also important to be aware of allergies and consider removing items such as shaving foam for a child with severe eczema. Wash your toys frequently and have a toy cleaning policy. If you have children with certain illnesses (i.e. those with cancer having chemotherapy) you will have to be extra careful.

Maintaining CPD

It is important to maintain high standards of play therapy practice (in line with BAPT Core Competence 15, see Appendix 1) by keeping up with the latest research and extending your skills. When working for yourself you are not automatically enrolled on training courses and will have to search and research training for yourself. You need to give yourself a training budget each year and prioritise your learning needs.

The BAPT conference is a great place to start. Each year the wealth of knowledge which is provided from such experienced therapists never fails to inspire me. I always come away feeling so invigorated. I find the mix of main lectures and experiential workshops are just the right balance to get the most out of me, as well as me feeling I have got the most out of it! And, of course, it is always great to catch up with my fellow play therapists.

The BAPT website lists some short courses as does the noticeboard in the BAPT magazine. Recommendations at networking groups or searching what is on offer at local universities are other places to check out. Supervision is a requirement of your membership and is part of your CPD (please refer to Chapter 3 by Platteuw on supervision).

There are thousands of books and articles to read on all sorts of subjects related to our profession and it is important to carry on reading throughout your career. Social media can be another great source for finding information or asking specific questions. There are numerous groups and pages to join which provide links to articles and documents as well as providing the opportunity to tap in to knowledge from other therapists using the sites. Of course, you should check references and critically evaluate sources of information.

Further training courses which many therapists choose to attend are filial therapy, supervision training, Child Parent Relationship Therapy (see Chapter 20 by Cowper), Theraplay, EMDR (see Chapter 18 by May), animal assisted play therapy and play therapy in the outdoors. You can also think about specific areas of need such as depression, anxiety, eating disorders, bereavement, physical disability, sensory processing difficulties, etc.

Ongoing support and self-care

Working alone can be isolating. It is important to keep in contact with others working in the same or similar field. This is another reason supervision is so vital. Check if there is a support group local to you, if not think about setting one up. Hold meetings in your place of work as part of a team or attend staff meetings.

We all know that there are cases that 'get to us' more than others. We read a lot of case histories which can describe horrendous abuse, awful situations and chronic suffering. This can take its toll on our own emotional state. I am sure we have all woken at night once in our career worrying about a child, because we care deeply about our clients. Therefore, it is important to create a good work/life balance. Think about how many cases you can manage at a time. We will inevitably experience life changes across our careers which will affect our capacity to manage cases. When I returned to work after having each of my children I knew I could only manage a few cases at first. I was lucky that I could leave the babies with my own mother and only work two half days to begin with.

Planning holiday breaks is vital for your self-care even if you are not actually going away. Other ways of looking after ourselves include mindfulness, relaxation techniques and exercise. It is important to be able to recognise when we are feeling overwhelmed by work and need extra support. We can explore feelings in supervision but sometimes we will need more than this. The personal therapy required on BAPT training courses helps us explore existing issues and opens us up to the benefits of therapy for ourselves (see also Chapter 2 by McCann) and the ability to recognise when it may be needed again.

Summary

This chapter has covered:

- Identifying potential suitable locations for practice – the benefits and challenges of working in family homes, within schools and renting a space
- Establishing yourself as a therapist
- Legal and ethical considerations including contracting play therapy services, confidentiality, record-keeping and data protection

- Financial matters including keeping accounts, insurance, paying tax and setting fees
- Play therapy kit – play materials and health and safety considerations within the play room
- Maintaining CPD for professional body membership
- Sources of support – the challenges of working alone and self-care provision.

Useful websites

BAPT website: www.bapt.info/
GDPR: https://ico.org.uk/for-organisations/guide-to-the-general-data-protection-regulation-gdpr
Health and Safety Executive: www.hse.gov.uk/
National Institute for Health and Care Excellence Guidelines: www.nice.org.uk/guidance
Self-Assessment Tax: www.gov.uk/self-assessment-tax-returns/get-help
Working Together to Safeguard Children: www.gov.uk/government/uploads/system/uploads/attachment_data/file/592101/Working_Together_to_Safeguard_Children_20170213.pdf

References

Axline, V. (1969) *Play Therapy.* New York: Ballantine Books.
Bond, T. & Mitchels, B. (2014) *Confidentiality & Record Keeping in Counselling & Psychotherapy.* Legal Resources Counsellors & Psychotherapists. London: Sage with BACP.
Department for Education and Skills. (2017) *Working Together to Safeguard Children: A Guide to Inter-Agency Working to Safeguard and Promote the Welfare of Children.* Available at: www.gov.uk/topic/schools-colleges-childrens-services/safeguarding-children/latest [Accessed: 17/06/18]
French, L. & Klein, R. (2012) *Therapeutic Practice in Schools. Working with the Child Within: A Clinical Workbook for Counsellors, Psychotherapists and Art Therapists.* Hove: Routledge.
Landreth, G.L. (2012) *Play Therapy: The Art of the Relationship.* (3rd ed.) New York: Routledge.
Padmore, J. (2016) *The Mental Health Needs of Children and Young People: Guiding You to Key Issues and Practices in CAMHS.* Maidenhead: McGraw Hill.
Ragusea, S.A. (2008) *A Professional Living Will for Psychologists.* Available at: c.ymcdn.com/sites/www.flapsych.com/resource/resmgr/docs/final_version_will.pdf [Accessed: 15/04/18]

Part II

Being a play therapist

Chapter 6

Being an ethical play therapist

Linda St Louis

Chapter overview

Becoming and being an ethical play therapist is a continual process of development and this ethical component of play therapy is worthy of closer exploration and understanding. This chapter provides an overview of the British Association of Play Therapists (BAPT) ethical framework and, as a starting point, I will address ethical principles, personal qualities and skill competences. I will highlight the importance, use and application of the BAPT ethical framework through the use of brief vignettes and a case study. I will make particular reference to considerations when establishing the play therapy contract. This includes obtaining consent, working with parental responsibility, applying the principle of confidentiality, addressing issues of safeguarding and protection and working systemically with support agencies and the family network. I will conclude with a discussion on preparing for play therapy and the legal framework which governs practice and delivery of interventions.

Introduction

While undertaking research for this chapter, I was struck by the dearth of literature on working ethically with children and young people within the field of play therapy in the United Kingdom. The increasing recognition of play therapy as an effective modality in addressing the needs of troubled, abused and neglected children, augments the need for skilled, knowledgeable, qualified play therapists in the delivery of appropriate therapeutic interventions. These interventions take place within a range of settings such as schools, hospices, Child and Adolescent Mental Health Teams, adoption services and child sexual abuse services, amongst others. Given the vulnerable nature of these client groups being referred for play therapy, it is fundamental that the reputation of the profession is underpinned by clear ethical procedures which ensure the protection and safeguarding, not only of clients, but also of the play therapist.

Ethical principles in play therapy

Play therapy is a therapeutic intervention which seeks to promote emotional well-being for children experiencing emotional and behavioural difficulties. The presentation of varying needs within this population group requires play therapists to work and engage with differing levels of vulnerability, which necessitates sensitivity, protection and safeguarding. The therapeutic relationship which develops between the play therapist and the client, is one based on trust and respect. Within this relationship, clients may well experience a power imbalance which is often true of the child–adult relationship but can be mitigated and counteracted within the setting of the play therapy intervention.

BAPT's *Ethical Basis for Good Practice in Play Therapy* (2014) is based on the British Association for Counselling and Psychotherapy (BACP, 2010) ethical framework which promotes transparency and accountability when contracting and engaging in counselling interventions. It is important to note that the BAPT code of ethics is not static, but is reviewed periodically and adapted in response to new and emerging changes in legislation and national standards. The code of ethics which underpins play therapy provides standards for its members, and the general public, concerning ethical principles and standards of competence, as well as good practice and procedures in the management of complaints. The challenge we all face as play therapists is in knowing how to give meaning to an ethical code and its application in our work on a day-to-day basis, and addressing dilemmas which may arise over the course of an intervention (BAPT Core Competence 12, see Appendix 1). The function of the BAPT code of ethics is to enable and support the safe delivery of play therapy within guidelines which take into account all consenting parties – the child, parent and play therapist. A clear ethical framework demystifies play therapy practice and promotes high calibre professional conduct by laying down principles which can be used to hold the therapist to account and to keep all parties safe.

BAPT's eight *Ethical Principles in Play Therapy* inspire play therapists to achieve the highest ideals of the profession (for the full list of descriptors see Appendix 2). So how do we, as play therapists, begin to give meaning to key concepts through our engagement and interactions with our clients? Each of BAPT's Ethical Principles will be discussed in turn.

Responsibility

All play therapists are responsible for upholding standards as we continue to develop professionally and within our relationships with clients. Keeping abreast of current knowledge and research is imperative. Implementing this knowledge in the therapeutic relationship could involve appropriate boundary-setting, contracting for play therapy and managing ethical conflicts, all of which must keep the child at the centre of the intervention. For example, Leroy (aged 9) was referred to play therapy as a result of his parents' separation. He reflected his enjoyment of the sessions when being collected by his mother. In the review meeting, Leroy's mother mentioned her dislike of the way her son related to me. She was aggrieved by the fact Leroy would not speak with her in the manner that he spoke to me. I felt a responsibility to address this issue as parents so often feel as though they are excluded from play therapy. By working with Leroy's mother, informing her of the support that she could provide and suggesting the type of comments she could explore and make to Leroy, I helped her to feel validated, which assisted the parent–child relationship. This, in turn, enhanced the therapeutic relationship with Leroy.

Beneficence

The interventions we undertake with children are to promote the welfare of the child. From time to time we are required to review the decisions we make, not just with the child, but with the wider family too. Zoe (aged 5) was referred to play therapy following the death of her father. She had not known her mother and was raised by her paternal relations. Initially, I agreed to an intervention of play therapy followed by life story work, and this began with play-based assessments. However, Zoe's mother reappeared and commenced legal proceedings as she was seeking full residency of Zoe. My intervention had to be reviewed in light of this information, as the outcome of the court hearing was for me to undertake a joint intervention with Zoe and her mother instead, which would comprise of life story work when Zoe was ready to engage. The court placed a large part of the decision-making in my hands. The dilemma I experienced at the time involved a conflict of interest. How would I manage the relationship with Zoe, who I had come to know, while 'facilitating' a parent–child relationship, without any knowledge about the parenting ability of Zoe's mother? These dilemmas and competing needs: that of Zoe, her mother and of the court, were explored in clinical supervision as I felt I would be compromising the therapeutic relationship if I had to change the emphasis of my work. For this reason, the decision was made that the life story work would be undertaken by an independent agency. The role of supervision can be advantageous when grappling with ethical conflicts such as this. As I explored this situation in supervision, the interconnectedness of BAPT's ethical principles of 'respect for people's rights and dignity', 'fidelity', 'justice' and 'self-respect' were present in this one case. Clinical supervision provided a safe space whereby the case and issues could be dissected, and ethical principles illuminated, in order to produce an ethical response which was most beneficial to Zoe.

Non-maleficence

The children being referred for play therapy are vulnerable and may have experienced either emotional or physical harm, or both. As a play therapist, I am all too aware that my actions and judgements may impact the lives of others and that I must avoid augmenting that harm. We also have a responsibility to undertake self-care by remaining fit to practice when delivering interventions. Struggling to undertake a session while in ill-health is not beneficial for the play therapist or the client. The following example explores the notion of harm and keeping the child safe. Ijaz (aged 8) had been referred for play therapy due to behavioural changes as a result of witnessing domestic abuse towards his mother (PTSD was subsequently diagnosed). At the end of one session I noticed clay marks on his uniform and as I reached forward with my hand to brush his clothing he jumped backwards and covered his head, thinking I was about to hit him. I was quick to reassure Ijaz, reminding him that there would be no hurting in the play room and explaining my actions. This example reminds me of the unintentional harm that can occur in the play room as we enable the child to process past trauma. My learning was never to assume that it is safe to enter the personal space of the child and always to maintain physical boundaries.

Fidelity

The therapeutic relationship is based on trust. During the course of an intervention and depending on whether or not the child is known to Children's Social Care, I could have access to an overwhelming quantity of information, not just about the child but also the relationship the child has with their family members. Maintaining confidentiality is of the upmost importance. When working within a professional network, for example Team Around the Family meetings (TAF), the assumption is often made that all professionals share information about the family. Nishat, the mother of Ijaz, was also receiving play therapy at the same time as her son. This was a parallel intervention which explored the impact on the mother–child relationship following separation due to domestic abuse (St Louis, 2011). The true extent of the abuse perpetrated against Nishat was shared during our play therapy sessions, but never with the school or the psychiatrist who had previously been treating Ijaz. (It is worth noting that when my intervention commenced with Ijaz it was agreed that his psychiatrist would suspend her intervention with him, as he had been due to commence child psychotherapy). I was conscious that the school and the family support worker were keen to learn about my work with Nishat and Ijaz. There is much value in discussing with clients beforehand the information that is acceptable to share with professional networks. Just as we ask children what they would like us to tell their parents about play therapy at review meetings, I use the same approach when sharing information about adult clients. This process of being transparent was reassuring for Nishat as I experienced a willingness on her part to disclose further acts of violence perpetrated during her marriage. This was a gradual process which culminated in Nishat feeling valued and with increased self-worth as she re-discovered her voice. In this instance, ethical principles of 'respect for people's dignity and rights', 'justice' and 'responsibility' converged in the process of the intervention.

Justice

When providing play therapy, we seek to ensure fair and equal access to services for the benefit of clients. In the past I have been required to access interpreters where the first language of the parent is not English. It is important in situations such as this not to use children as interpreters. As I work in a multi-cultural community, care is taken to ensure that the play equipment reflects that community, for example dolls which are African, Chinese and Asian in appearance. Accessibility is another consideration which should not be overlooked, especially in light of the Equality Act 2010. In my place of work this involves ensuring that clients with reduced or limited mobility can gain comfortable access of the building and play room with the aid of lifts and ramps. Our training enables us to screen referrals to assess their appropriateness for play therapy, but we also need to be cognisant of our own needs and limitations while considering the most appropriate intervention for the child. Burton (aged 11) had been referred for play therapy following parental separation due to domestic abuse. I had accepted the case and began to network with agencies involved with the family. As more and more information was gathered, I realised that Burton's needs would not be met through play therapy as a number of mental health concerns became known. Maladaptive behaviours, which involved urinating on the floor, led me to make a more appropriate referral instead to a child psychiatrist within Child and Adolescent Mental Health Service (CAMHS).

Respect for people's rights and dignity

Respecting the rights of children in play therapy is central to the therapeutic relationship. Children learn how to become autonomous individuals and are helped to understand concepts such as 'confidentiality' and 'respect'. Children learn that they are fully accepted by the play therapist and, in the process, develop positive self-regard and acceptance of self. Self-acceptance is further enhanced through the process of assent and the active involvement of children signing their own play therapy agreement.

Lee (aged 7) warmed to play therapy and used some of his time to regress. I was assigned the role of mother and he would be the baby pretending to suck on a feeding bottle, pretending to cry and asking to be soothed. Once out of role he told me he did not want his mother to know about him being a baby and playing with a bottle, which I respected. The trust and respect within our relationship facilitated expression of an unmet need within Lee. My response enabled him to feel accepted and treated with dignity both within and outside of the play.

Respect for people's needs and relationships

The child in play therapy is dependent on others to meet their emotional, psychological and health and familial needs. We often work with parents who are resistant to play therapy, hence the need to explore ways of involving them. I was undertaking bereavement work in a children's hospice with David (aged 10) and his mother would often arrive late. Once I began to explore the reason for David's late arrival, his mother poured out her guilt about the demands of parenting and lack of contact with David and explained that she used the time travelling to and from play therapy to 'catch up' with David. What initially appeared to be resistance to play therapy, led to David's mother asking for help, examining her travel arrangements and linking to the community support services of the Hospice. David no longer arrived late to play therapy.

Self-respect

Respect of self comes with acceptance of self. Self-respect is further heightened for play therapists with the increase of knowledge through continuing professional development and access to clinical supervision (BAPT Core Competences 13 & 15, see Appendix 1). In my interactions with clients I aim to enable and build on their self-respect and self-worth too. It is not uncommon for parents accessing play therapy to carry with them the guilt of remaining in a violent relationship. Neither is it uncommon for child victims of violence to experience guilt as a result of calling the police for assistance. A key component in working with victims of domestic violence is to enable victims and children to understand the source of their guilt. The process of empowerment starts with helping victims to understand the reasons why they remained in abusive relationships, such as fear, guilt, isolation, lack of access to finances and to protect the children. It is important that this work is undertaken with the victim of violence and the child as a means of addressing the guilt that they experience. In the process, this enables parents to understand the impact of parenting from the position of guilt. Ethical principles therefore become more than a guide or reference tool as the personal and professional overlap ensures that ethical principles are absorbed into our relationships with children and professionals.

Personal qualities

Being an ethical play therapist requires the possession of key personal qualities (for list of these see Appendix 1).

> The effective deployment of skills and knowledge in play therapy are of the up-most importance to clients, the public, and the profession. ... The core competencies of play therapists are defined as a set of personal and professional qualities that are a pre-requisite of good practice.
>
> (BAPT, 2014:5)

The therapeutic relationship between the play therapist and child is one which is based on trust. Norton and Norton (2008) and Bond (2015) both emphasise the importance of trust between the client and therapist. Bond argues the importance of clients being able to trust their counsellors and he goes on to state: 'They trust their feelings of vulnerability to someone who is committed to using their knowledge and skills to act in the best interests of their clients' (Bond, 2015:7).

Ajagbawa and Associates (2014) state that the expectation is not that counsellors and therapists exhibit all ethical and personal qualities, but that they become aspirational and serve as a reference point to the standard that is expected in the profession. It is not the intention of BAPT's ethical framework to provide answers to all ethical dilemmas play therapists may encounter. It is the ethical principles, when combined with personal and professional qualities, which serve to guide and direct the play therapist in the decision-making process where ethical dilemmas exist. Indeed, in situations where ethical dilemmas are not reconciled, play therapists may need to seek further advice and direction from clinical supervisors and managers. Depending on the nature of the dilemma, on rare occasions this could result in a complaint being registered against the play therapist. In circumstances such as this, BAPT's ethical framework is applied to assess any contravention from the ethical code.

Working with ethical dilemmas in play therapy

As previously mentioned, BAPT's ethical framework is used to provide guidance when establishing play therapy interventions and applied when an area of practice may have been brought into question. Ethical transgressions can be far-ranging, from not obtaining consent, misrepresenting the child or family members in a report, being requested to change the contents of the report, or sharing a report with an agency where permission had not been sought from the family of the child. This would be considered a breach of client data. As in the case study which follows, a complaint by one parent resulted in the cessation of play therapy following a court judgement.

Case study: Simone

Simone (aged 9) was referred for play therapy due to the impact of witnessing domestic abuse and exposure to her parents' acrimonious separation, following legal action by her father to secure residency. Simone was an only child and contact with her father occurred fortnightly and involved overnight stays. Both parents shared parental responsibility.

The referral received from the Family Support Worker stated that Simone presented with low mood, would return from weekend contact feeling sad and she sometimes exhibited angry and verbal outbursts towards her mother. After each outburst, Simone would cry and an apology would follow. During the apology, Simone would share with her mother the derogatory comments about her mother that her father had made to her during contact. Mother was keen to seek help for her daughter.

After the initial meeting with her mother, I met with Simone, as yet undecided on the type of intervention I would deliver. I always like to meet the child, partly to assess their communication skills and playfulness. I invited her to use any of the toys in the room to tell me a story. She warmed to the activity and told a story of an eagle attacking small rodents on the land and birds in the sky. We spoke about the play and Simone told me that the eagle reminded her of her father and how he treated her mother. She spoke about feeling sad and her father not listening to her when she made attempts to defend her mother. Based on this initial meeting and case history, I made the decision to undertake a play therapy intervention. Consent was obtained from Simone's mother and a letter was sent to her father to inform him of my involvement, describing play therapy and offering an appointment for us to meet and discuss the work I would be undertaking. Father declined the opportunity to meet. On the day of Simone's first play therapy session, I learned from her mother that the father had made an application to court, challenging my decision to deliver play therapy because I had failed to obtain his consent. Just three play therapy sessions were delivered before bringing the intervention to an end. The judge ruled that parental consent should have been obtained from the father. A tearful session had to take place where I informed mother and Simone that it was impossible for me to continue in the light of the court decision.

Two weeks later, mother brought to my attention letters written by Simone about her father destroying her life, taking away her play therapy and how she was planning to kill herself. Mother pleaded for me to recommence play therapy. I explained that I could not and instead sought legal advice. I learned that the mother could return to court on a *Specific*

Issue Order (SIO).[1] The accounts written by Simone, which documented her feelings, were used as an appendix to a report I was required to submit to court. I argued for Simone's mental health needs to be considered as paramount in the proceedings. The outcome was positive and welcomed by Simone and her mother: the judge ruled in favour of Simone accessing mental health intervention which resulted in a referral to CAMHS.

A number of dilemmas and issues appear to co-exist in this case study which required balancing the rights of the child and access to therapy, alongside the court ruling which supported and upheld the wish of one parent for the discontinuation of play therapy. When considering the needs of children living with domestic abuse, the Adoption and Children Act 2002 (DES, 2002) extended the definition of 'harm' under the Children Act 1989, to 'impairment suffered from seeing or hearing the ill-treatment of another'. Children harmed as a result of domestic abuse are in need of protection and support. Discontinuing play therapy had impacted negatively on Simone's mental health and well-being. In applying BAPT's code of ethics to assess this particular court ruling, one could contend that Simone's rights had been denied, thereby contravening the principles of non-maleficence, and that she was in need of protection from harm. Jenkins (2015) states that a professional code of ethics presents a framework which counsellors and play therapists can utilise when responding to complex challenges in their practice. Bond (2015) argues further, saying that counsellors have a duty of care to their clients. Whilst the nature of play therapy enabled Simone to be more autonomous, the legal challenge brought by her father to end play therapy resulted in the removal of autonomy for Simone. It was my responsibility to convey a duty of care towards Simone, and to act in accordance with BAPT's code of ethics and with the Local Authority child protection procedures, to secure her right to access treatment.

Daniels and Jenkins (2010) describe the shifting and competing roles child counsellors may experience within their interventions. The play therapist is required to respond to emerging information which unfolds while engaged in the therapeutic relationship. In Simone's case, where circumstances evolved quickly, I was required to assess and consider the impact of new information on my intervention. My role shifted from that of play therapist to that of child protection officer and advocate. The decision to stop or continue play therapy had been removed from my jurisdiction by the court. In turn, this presented a number of ethical considerations. I had the *responsibility* to ensure that Simone's needs were met at a time when her mental health was fragile. I sought to act in the best interest of Simone by promoting her welfare and access to services – *beneficence*. The change to my role from play therapist to advocate was appropriate in order to safeguard and register child protection concerns – *non-maleficence*. A central question when situations such as this emerge is to contemplate what the best course of action is for the child. In doing so, I was able to ensure *respect for the rights and dignity of my client.* The intertwining personal qualities of empathy, critical reflection, knowledge, congruence and compassion, enabled the self-examination of my practice as I kept the child at the centre of the intervention in an attempt to obtain a positive outcome.

The legal framework and what you need to know

The BAPT code of ethics exists to ensure standards and competencies are upheld and that ethical issues are examined and addressed in accordance with current legislation pertaining to working with children. An absence of knowledge can leave many play therapists struggling within legal systems, leaving their practice open to negative scrutiny. It is a requirement when working directly with children that play therapists possess an understanding of the legislation which safeguards young people. It is important to note that in providing play therapy interventions in England and Wales, we work within the parameters of the legislative framework for the protection of children in England and Wales known as the Children Acts of 1989 and 2004 (DES, 1989, 2004), and in Scotland, the Children Scotland Act 1995 (The Scottish Government, 1995). The Data Protection Acts of 1989 and 2003 (ICO, 1989, 2003) ensure the safekeeping and protection of client records and The Mental Health Act 1983 (DoH, 2015) upholds the confidentiality of children under 16 if shown to be 'Gillick competent'.[2]

This is by no means an exhaustive list of legislation. For example, in my direct work with children and families living with domestic abuse, it has become necessary to access the Domestic Violence Crimes and Victims Act 2004 (MoJ, 2004) and, no doubt, other specialisms will access other areas of legislation. There is however key legislation with which all play therapists should be acquainted, irrespective of being employed by an organisation or working within private practice. The document *Working Together to Safeguard Children* (DES, 2017) clearly states that the overall protection of children rests with the local authorities. However, agencies with a non-statutory role are not exempt and are required to act accordingly in partnership with local authorities to promote the welfare and protection of children. As play therapists, we are responsible for ensuring that the implementation of our roles and responsibilities remains consistent with the statutory duties of our employer. For some play therapists working in private practice, there may be a feeling of detachment from the safeguarding responsibilities required within their role, but we are all obliged to be cognisant of legal frameworks, policies and legislation pertaining to play therapy which underpin our work. The case study of Simone presented earlier is an example of how the ethical framework and knowledge of legislation worked to ensure access to play therapy for a child who had been suicidal.

Maintaining ethical practice

To maintain ethical standards, Landreth (2012) states that every play therapist should be engaged in self-critique aided by the process of clinical supervision. The remainder of this chapter will therefore focus on the importance of clinical supervision, record and note-keeping and continuing professional development (BAPT Core Competences 13, 24 & 15 respectively, see Appendix 1).

Clinical supervision

The BAPT ethical framework stipulates that:

> All play therapists, including supervisors, are required to receive on-going, appropriate, formal and regular clinical supervision.

Aside from the learning process, supervision provides a safety net which protects the play therapist and the client throughout. Supervision ensures accountability and responsibility where ethical dilemmas can be expressed and explored. Schuck and Wood (2011) state:

> Supervision is a collaborative process in which the supervisor works with the supervisee to explore their work reflectively. The role of the supervisor is often viewed as a mix of educative, mentoring, holding the ethical position and ensuring the safety of the supervisee and the supervisee's client.
>
> (2011:15)

Furthermore, as a play therapist working in the field of violence and abuse, clinical supervision provides a safe place for me to process the abuse and hurt that many of my clients have experienced. I consider clinical supervision to be an act of self-care for the benefit of my clients (see also Chapter 3 by Platteuw for more on supervision issues).

Record and note-keeping

The issue of record and note-keeping is continually being examined, debated and reviewed. At the point of engagement with the family, play therapists are required to explain the process of play therapy before the first session takes place, as clearly defined in the ethical framework. This involves agreeing the frequency and duration of therapy sessions, the location and time, expectations concerning information about the child in their therapy sessions and what will and will not be shared. Collectively, this is the process involved in establishing the play therapy contract (BAPT Core Competence 19, see Appendix 1). It is at this stage that play therapists are required to inform families about the information which will be gathered and stored, either electronically or as paper files, along with the process to gain access to records if required. This invariably includes providing information about the complaints procedure (Wilson & Ryan, 2005; Bond & Mitchels, 2015). For play therapists employed by an organisation, policies concerning the storage and retrieval of client data should be in place and established. Play therapists working privately will need to institute appropriate systems in accordance with the Data Protection Act 1989 and the General Data Protection Regulation (GDPR) 2018 (ICO, 1989, 2018), which requires organisations and individuals processing personal information to register with the Information Commissioner's Office (ICO). Some organisations and individuals are exempt from registering and it is advisable that play therapists working privately establish their status and requirements.

It is the expectation of all BAPT full members to maintain appropriate notes without compromising client confidentiality. In recounting the case study about Simone, I was required to produce a retrospective report of my play therapy intervention which, together with Simone's letters, became a deciding factor in formulating the final decision by the judge. Play therapists can be called upon at any time by a court to make available a copy of their notes. Clear and concise recording of therapy sessions, when shared with clinical supervisors, adds an additional level of safety within the ethical framework, providing protection for play therapists in the event that a complaint or disagreement arises.

Continuing professional development

Training to become a play therapist does not end with acquiring a postgraduate qualification. The continuing professional development of the play therapist is an essential requirement for Full membership of the professional body: BAPT requires all registered play therapists to maintain CPD logbooks to evidence their learning and development. As a play therapist working in the field of family violence and abuse, developments have a direct impact on procedures and how I implement my interventions. I am required to remain up-to-date with training and new research, not just within the field of play therapy, but child development, trauma and attachment as well as bereavement. The skills of a play therapist should therefore include an ongoing understanding of the attachment relationships and the trauma which may have brought the child to therapy.

To conclude, the field of ethics in play therapy is wide-ranging and there are aspects which have only been touched on in this chapter, such as children's rights. However, I believe that strengthening our ethical approach as play therapists, working to maintain boundaries and safety for ourselves and our clients, will enhance the profession and underpin our interventions with a sense of purpose and commitment. Children referred for play therapy often present with a number of vulnerabilities, some of which can be complex. It is important, therefore, that as a play therapist I work within my knowledge and understanding while utilising clinical supervision to enhance that knowledge base. Working within BAPT's code of ethics enables me to develop an effective therapeutic intervention with children, while supporting me to negotiate complex challenges which can arise.

Summary

- The need for an ethical basis for play therapy was explained.
- BAPT's ethical framework was outlined and the application of the eight principles to practice was illustrated by means of a series of brief vignettes and a case study.
- The importance was stressed of remaining aware of the legislative framework underpinning play therapy.

Notes

1 SIOs can be made under Section 8 of the Children Act 1989 when a specific direction is required, where parents sharing parental responsibility are not able to agree.
2 A child who is 'Gillick competent' may consent to their interventions and treatment if they convey an informed and competent understanding of the issues involved (Quality Care Commission, 2015).

Further reading

These are some of the key Acts of Legislation referred to in this chapter, which are worth familiarising yourself with:

The Adoption and Children Act 2002. Available at: www.legislation.gov.uk/ukpga/2002/38/section/120

The Children Act 1989. Available at: www.legislation.gov.uk/ukpga/1989/41/contents

The Children Act 2004. Available at: www.legislation.gov.uk/ukpga/2004/31/contents

Children Scotland Act 1995. Available at: www.legislation.gov.uk/ukpga/1995/36/contents

The Data Protection Act 1989. Available at: https://ico.org.uk/for-organisations/guide-to-data-protection/key-definitions/

Equality Act 2010. Available at: www.gov.uk/guidance/equality-act-2010-guidance

General Data Protection Regulation 2018. Available at: https://ico.org.uk/for-organisations/guide-to-the-general-data-protection-regulation-gdpr/

The Mental Health Act 1983: Code of Practice. Available at: www.gov.uk/government/uploads/system/uploads/attachment_data/file/435512/MHA_Code_of_Practice.PDF

Working Together to Safeguard Children: A Guide to Inter-Agency Working to Safe-guard and Promote the Welfare of Children 2017. Available at: www.gov.uk/govern ment/uploads/system/uploads/attachment_data/file/592101/Working_Together_to_ Safeguard_Children_20170213.pdf

References

Ajagbawa, O.H. & Associates. (2014) The role of ethics in career counselling in 21st century. *Journal of Humanities and Social Science.* 19 (5) pp. 12–22. Available at: www.iosrjournals.org/iosr-jhss/papers/Vol19-issue5/Version-5/C019551222.pdf [Accessed: 29/08/17].

Bond, T. (2015) *Standards and Ethics for Counselling in Action.* (4th ed.) London: Sage.

Bond, T. & Mitchels, B. (2015) *Confidentiality & Record Keeping in Counselling & Psychotherapy.* (2nd ed.) London: Sage.

British Association for Counselling & Psychotherapy. (2010) *Ethical Framework for Good Practice in Counselling & Psychotherapy.* Available at: www.itsgoodtotalk. org.uk/assets/docs/BACP-Ethical-Framework-for-Good-Practice-in-Counselling-and-Psychotherapy_1276615182.pdf [Accessed: 1/09/17].

British Association of Play Therapists. (2014) *Ethical Basis for Good Practice in Play Therapy.* Available at: www.bapt.info/play-therapy/ethical-basis-good-practice-play-therapy/ [Accessed: 1/09/17].

Daniels, D. & Jenkins, P. (2010) *Therapy with Children – Children's Rights, Confiden-tiality and the Law.* London: Sage.

Department for Education and Skills (DES). (1989) *The Children Act 1989.* Available at: www.legislation.gov.uk/ukpga/1989/41/contents [Accessed: 27/07/17].

Department for Education and Skills (DES). (2002) *The Adoption and Children Act 2002.* Available at: www.legislation.gov.uk/ukpga/2002/38/section/120 [Accessed: 27/07/17].

Department for Education and Skills (DES). (2004) *The Children Act 2004.* Available at: www.legislation.gov.uk/ukpga/2004/31/contents [Accessed: 21/09/17].

Department for Education and Skills (DES). (2017) *Working Together to Safeguard Children: A Guide to Inter-Agency Working to Safeguard and Promote the Welfare of Children.* Available at: www.gov.uk/government/uploads/system/uploads/attach ment_data/file/592101/Working_Together_to_Safeguard_Children_20170213.pdf [Accessed: 1/09/17].

Department of Health (DoH). (2015) *Mental Health Act 1983: Code of Practice.* Available at: www.gov.uk/government/uploads/system/uploads/attachment_data/ file/435512/MHA_Code_of_Practice.PDF [Accessed: 28/08/17].

Information Commissioners Office (ICO). (1989) *Data Protection Act 1989.* Available at: https://ico.org.uk/for-organisations/guide-to-data-protection/key-definitions/ [Accessed: 28/08/17].

Information Commissioner's Office (ICO). (2018) *General Data Protection Regulation 2018.* Available at: https://ico.org.uk/for-organisations/guide-to-the-general-data-protection-regulation-gdpr/ [Accessed: 16/05/18].

Jenkins, P. (2015) Ethics. In: Pattison, S., Robson, M. & Beynon, A. (eds.) *The Hand-book of Counselling Children and Young People.* London: Sage. pp. 278–293.

Landreth, G.L. (2012) *Play Therapy: The Art of the Relationship.* (3rd ed.) New York: Routledge.

Ministry of Justice (MoJ). (2004) *The Domestic Crimes and Victims Act 2004.* Available at: www.gov.uk/government/publications/the-domestic-violence-crime-and-victims-act-2004 [Accessed: 30/08/17].

Norton, C.C. & Norton, E.N. (2008) Experiential play therapy. In: Schaefer, C.E. & Kaduson, G.H. (eds.) *Contemporary Play Therapy: Theory, Research, and Practice.* New York: The Guilford Press. pp. 28–54.

Quality Care Commission. (2015) *Brief Guide: Capacity and Competence in under 18s.* Available at: www.cqc.org.uk/sites/default/files/20180228_briefguide-capacity _consent_under_18s_v2.pdf [Accessed: 25/08/17].

Schuck, C. & Wood, J. (2011) *Inspiring Creative Supervision.* London: Jessica Kingsley Publishers.

St Louis, L. (2011) Domestic abuse: Collateral damage – Collateral treatment. *British Journal of Play Therapy.* 7 pp. 42–57.

The Scottish Government. (1995) *Children Scotland Act 1995.* Available at: www. legislation.gov.uk/ukpga/1995/36/contents [Accessed: 18/05/18].

Wilson, K. & Ryan, V. (2005) *Play Therapy: A Non-Directive Approach for Children and Adolescents.* Oxford: Elsevier.

Chapter 7

Being a playful therapist

Karen McInnes

Chapter overview

In this chapter I will explore the role of play and the importance of playfulness for children's development. I will outline how current knowledge and research regarding these constructs informs therapeutic work with children and young people. I will draw on recent research into perceptions of play and enabling playfulness, as well as discuss how this might be utilised in order to become a playful therapist.

Introduction

Much has been written over many years about the role of play in children's development (Ray, 2011) and the dangers for children's social and emotional wellbeing if they do not have access to play and playful opportunities (Gray, 2011). Due to its long history, and having been studied from a range of perspectives, there is a wealth of literature concerned with play. However, there is limited discussion of play itself within the play therapy field, although there are some notable exceptions (e.g. Landreth, 2012; McMahon, 2009). Despite this, the British Association of Play Therapists (BAPT) includes knowledge and understanding of play and development within its core competences (Competence 6, see Appendix 1). Play clearly underpins play therapy, as Landreth (2012: 11) states, 'play therapy presupposes the presence of some possible activity that would be considered play'. However, what is this activity which may be considered play and who makes the decision regarding what constitutes play? In this chapter I will discuss both these issues, drawing on a wide range of play literature from various disciplines to demonstrate that it is the playful relationship which provides the power to heal, not necessarily the activity of play.

Play theory

Play is a universal activity shared by humans and animals and is commonly seen as a mechanism for making sense of life and facilitating development

(Chown, 2015; Henricks, 2015). Consequently, play has been studied and written about by scholars from different theoretical disciplines and is highly valued by children and those adults who work with them. There are many theories proposed as to why children play and its function. Early theories were philosophical in nature: the surplus energy theory of play proposed by Spencer (1820–1903) stated that play was a product of superfluous energy left over after all other basic needs had been met, whereas the relaxation theory of play by Lazarus (1824–1903) took an opposing view, that play was an activity which occurred after work in order to relax and build up further energy. The recapitulation theory of play by Hall (1846–1924) argued that through playing children acted out evolutionary stages of humans, whilst the pre-exercise theory by Groos (1861–1946) explained play as an opportunity to practice adult activities and prepare for adult life.

Early educational and developmental theorists such as Froebel (1782–1852) and Pestalozzi (1746–1827) both emphasised the importance of playful activity for learning. Parten (1932) proposed a developmental approach to children's social play which is still used in studies today. Slightly more recently, Piaget's theory of play (1951), which originated from his work on intellectual development, provided a concept of play which was seen as part of the process of assimilation, with children being able to make sense of what was already known through play. Vygotsky (1976) also saw play in relation to intellectual development, however he emphasised pretend play and the importance of language and social interaction in play. He proposed that through these means self-regulation could develop. From a socio-cultural and anthropological viewpoint, play is thought to reflect the cultural meanings of the society in which it occurs (Goncu & Gaskins, 2007).

Play theory, contributing to the development of play therapy, comes from the work of Freud (1856–1939) who postulated a strong relationship between play and creativity. He also proposed that during imaginative play children would re-enact traumatic events and this would provide them with a means to gain control over such events. Erikson (1963) also valued play, and playfulness, as means to overcoming traumatic events and provided a developmental framework for play and self-esteem. Anna Freud (1965) furthered her father's work in developing the concept of the 'therapeutic' environment enabling the relationship between therapist and child. This combination of the facilitating environment as well as the relationship allowed children to play out their unconscious conflicts and talk about their conscious feelings and thoughts. Melanie Klein (1960) compared children's play with free association, with play being indicative of conflict which was communicated from the unconscious mind. She saw the therapist's role as one of interpretation of play behaviour to ensure the easing of conflict. Winnicott (1971) saw strong links between play and creativity and believed that children needed to play and discover themselves. He introduced the idea of the 'playful space' and proposed that play was a form of communication which took place in the playful space between two people, initially mother and child, but, in a therapeutic environment, this would be the playful space between therapist and child. Axline (1969), the pioneer of non-directive play therapy, believed that children had the power to heal themselves through play, given the right therapeutic environment. Whilst the role of the therapist was crucial in enabling this, the notion of instruction or interpretation by the adult was rejected.

Whilst it is clear that the above psychological and psychoanalytic theories underpin the development of play therapy and its practice, other theoretical positions can be seen to contribute. Huizinga (1872–1945) took a philosophical stance relating to the centrality of play for human existence which would be embraced by play therapists; likewise, the anthropological view of play reflecting the cultural meanings of society would find sympathy within play therapy practice. In addition, play therapists should have knowledge of play and its development, and so need to draw on the theoretical insights of those such as Piaget, Vygotsky and Parten. Many play therapists work in schools or other educational settings, so comprehending the contributions of these play theories to educational practice brings shared understanding with educational practitioners.

What is play?

Play theory enables us to have some understanding of the development and functions of play, but does not necessarily bring us any closer to defining what might be considered play. Many note the difficulty and complexity in attempting to define play (e.g. Chown, 2015) whilst others say it is an impossibility (e.g. Moyles, 1989). However, it is important to have a definition of what play is for research purposes and to enable conversations about children's play activities. Similar to theories of play, notions of what play is depend on theoretical background and discipline. Play may be viewed as a natural and spontaneous activity, although this is less than helpful when trying to define it. Theorists such as Piaget (1951) defined play according to categories of practice play, symbolic play and games with rules, whilst Vygotsky (1976) only viewed imaginative play as play. Educationalists define play as a vehicle for learning, however this is problematic as too often we see play being hijacked to serve the needs of the curriculum (Pyle & Danniels, 2017).

Within the play therapy literature, play is viewed as children's language and a mode of communication (Axline, 1969; Landreth, 2012; West, 1996). Landreth utilises the language analogy to state 'toys are used like words by the children, and play is their language' (p. 12). This is useful but does not help us address the question: what is this activity we call play? Play as communication entails a process not an activity. Another approach to defining play is through the use of criteria which focus on behaviours and dispositions of play. The first definition of play using criteria was proposed by Neumann (1971). She suggested three criteria: locus of control (freedom to choose), intrinsic motivation (self-motivation to engage and stay with an activity) and internal reality (reality made for and by the child). Krasnor and Pepler (1980) proposed criteria approaches using different criteria such as: internal motivation, non-literality (displaying pretence), positive affect (having fun) and flexibility (rules by the players not outsiders). Using these criteria would enable an onlooker to determine whether an activity was play. Whilst this rather rigid and formalised way of using criteria might not appeal, much of the play therapy literature makes reference to such criteria, with play being described as freely chosen, personally directed, intrinsically motivated, engaging the child, enjoyable, not goal directed and involving flexibility (Chown, 2015; Landreth, 2012; McMahon, 2009; West, 1996). What is clear is that many of these criteria might not always appear to fit, for example, is play in therapy always enjoyable? More importantly, many of these criteria are not observable but rely on the felt experience of the player, the child.

Children's views of play

There is limited research on children's views of play (Howard & McInnes, 2013), however it has been shown that children use cues to differentiate play from non-play activities (Howard, 2002). Children mainly use the cues of adult presence, choice and location to make this differentiation and we have demonstrated that these cues are different to the cues adults use (McInnes & Birdsey, 2014). A lack of adult presence often enables children to have a sense of freedom, control and participation. Choice in an activity enables children to feel motivated, enthusiastic and in control and further research has shown that it does not necessarily need to be free choice that children are provided with but adaptable choice which they negotiate (King & Howard, 2016). Finally, having space and a lack of constraint in terms of the location enables children to move and be physical which aids concentration and enables involvement. Further research we have conducted, related to the role of the adult, shows that when adults understand play and can enter play on children's terms, children are less likely to use the cue of adult presence – the adult role and adult playfulness is critical (McInnes et al., 2011, 2013).

In our experimental studies (McInnes et al., 2009, 2010) some of these cues children use to differentiate play and non-play activities have been manipulated to create playful (on the floor, adult proximal, choice) and non-playful (at a table, adult present, lack of choice) practice conditions. When children have then been allocated to one of the practice conditions and undertaken problem-solving tasks in a four-stage procedure: pre-test, practice, post-test and delayed post-test, they demonstrate enhanced performance in problem-solving tasks, and greater wellbeing when in the playful practice condition (Howard & McInnes, 2012). They are also more relaxed, move more freely and are more motivated as shown by behaviours such as leaning towards the task and smiling. They are more flexible in their thinking, trying out different ways to solve the problem, and they are more involved in the activity.

This way of thinking is bringing us closer to being able to address the question regarding what might be considered play: it is what the child considers to be play and adults need to observe and listen to children to determine this. This recent research, and the conclusions stemming from it, accords with non-directive play therapy practice. In the playroom, play is free from adult interference and when the adult is invited into the play then the adult's role is defined by the child and the adult acts accordingly (Chown, 2015). Children are free to choose but, like King and Howard's (2016) proposition, it is negotiated choice as the play therapist sets limits in the playroom which enables the child to feel safe, experience responsibility and further the therapeutic relationship (Axline, 1969; Landreth, 2012). Children also have freedom to move in the playroom, they have a space although the location is always the same (Ray, 2011; West, 1996).

Playfulness

There is a distinction in the literature between 'play' and 'playfulness' despite these words often being used interchangeably and, as various commentators observe, the play act itself may not be that important for children's development and wellbeing. Rather, being able to take a playful approach or attitude to any activity may be the critical factor (Bundy, 1993; Howard & McInnes, 2013). Analysing the cues children use to determine play activities has shown that children act in ways that can be construed as playful (McInnes et al., 2009, 2010). There are two views of playfulness in the literature: one that it is a personality trait of the individual and the other that it is an attitude or approach to an activity. There is a wealth of literature viewing playfulness as a personality trait. For example, Lieberman's (1977) research identified five core traits making up playfulness: cognitive, social and physical spontaneity, sense of humour and manifest joy. Lieberman's work led her to view playfulness alongside a particular cognitive style involving creativity, imagination and divergent thinking.

Playfulness as an attitude or approach to an activity links to internal affective qualities of being such as: enthusiasm, motivation, willingness to engage, freedom to choose and freedom to try out new ideas (Moyles, 1989) and these are the behaviours viewed in the playful practice condition in our experimental studies discussed above (McInnes et al., 2009, 2010). The literature viewing playfulness as a style or an approach to an activity is also vast and it crosses academic and practice disciplines. In relation to play therapy, Erikson (1963) discussed how a playful approach to living was the essence of the spirit of play. As mentioned previously, the idea of a playful approach was extended by Winnicott (1971) when he identified the playful space which occurs between the playful client and playful therapist as they work together. Literature on this view of playfulness comes from the field of occupational therapy and the work of Bundy (1993) who stated that, 'playfulness is so important that ultimately we may find a person's approach to an activity is more important than any play or leisure activity in itself' (p. 217).

This view of playfulness also links with the work of Csikszentmihalyi (1990) and his concept of 'flow states'. He studied the experience of adults engaged in activities which gave them few extrinsic rewards but from which they derived deep pleasure and involvement. These adults identified being lost in the activity, having no sense of time and having feelings of happiness and pleasure. This links with Bundy's proposition that the activity itself is not that important, as Csikszentmihalyi's participants were engaged in all sorts of activities, many of them not play activities. It also resonates with the psychoanalytic work of Winnicott (1971) when he states that the content of a child's activity does not matter and what counts is the 'near withdrawal state' (p. 69) of the individual as they become immersed in their activity.

Playful play therapy

Based on the above discussion it can be argued that playfulness is the most important aspect of play therapy, rather than the act of play itself. McMahon (2009) itemises the essentials for play as being: safe boundaries, autonomy and an absence of serious consequences. The first two essentials are necessary prerequisites for children to feel playful based on our research into children's cue use in relation to play: having space and freedom to move without adult interference contribute to safe boundaries as children can be themselves in a safe space, whilst having choice accords with having autonomy. Furthermore, we have argued that playfulness is at the heart of the relationship between adult and child (McInnes & Yuen, 2017). Chown (2015) argues that playfulness is a key aspect of early experiences between primary caregiver and child and that where there is playfulness there is attunement, affection and affirmation. Winnicott (1971) has also argued for the centrality of playfulness within therapeutic encounters and describes the necessity of communicating within the playful space between therapist and child.

This takes us back to the foundations of play therapy practice and the work of Rogers (1951) and humanistic theory. His person-centred therapy placed the person and therapeutic relationship at the heart of the therapy. He saw therapy as a philosophy in which growth and fulfilment of the person was the goal, achieved by enabling the person to feel loved. Attempting to ensure the client feels loved is dependent upon the therapist's ability to convey empathy (entering into the feelings of the client), unconditional positive regard (valuing and respecting the client regardless of the client's behaviours, feelings or attitude) and congruence or genuineness (freeing the client to be themselves) (Rogers, 1951). The ability to convey these three core conditions underpins the quality of the therapeutic relationship. These factors also ensure that the child is listened to, that the child's play is understood on the child's terms and accepted – the basis for ensuring that the child is enabled to be playful. This is also the basis of Axline's (1969) principles which underpin non-directive play therapy practice.

The playful practitioner

Enabling playfulness in children requires play therapists to be playful practitioners and, as all play therapists know, this is not necessarily easy. Being a playful play therapist requires much of the play therapist. Playful play therapists need to:

• Have knowledge of play: what it is and its functions. As we have seen, literature on play definitions and theory is immense and covers a variety of disciplines. It can be argued that play therapists should have knowledge of this vast field to ensure complete and deep understanding of play which will impact on their practice (Ray, 2011). In an educational context, we have demonstrated that when practitioners understand play this influences their practice, which, in turn, has a positive impact on children's views of play: they see more opportunities to be playful (McInnes et al., 2011). A deeper understanding of play will also enable play therapists to develop their understanding of how other practitioners view and utilise play and this will facilitate inter-disciplinary understanding and working relationships in the context of play.
• Understand the development of play. This is one of the BAPT competences and as Ray (2011) states, therapists should have an extensive knowledge of the development of play within the context of typical child development. This then enables them to make sense of the child's play within their current context. It also informs discussions play therapists may have with parents and other professionals involved with the child.
• Understand the cues the child uses to determine whether or not an activity is play. This is important to understand as working with the cues the child uses to determine play activities will also enable child playfulness. Understanding and facilitating the cues children use falls within the remit of essential play therapy practice: enabling autonomy, negotiating choice and providing a safe space with clear limits of acceptable behaviour.
• Listen and observe the child whilst playing. Landreth (2012) describes this as the therapist taking 'an active role' (p. 110). This does not mean the therapist has to be physically active but that the therapist is active

emotionally. This requires active listening and observing, being alert to the non-verbal and verbal messages the child is communicating. This is the essence of the communicative relationship between child and therapist.

- Be playful in the playful space between child and therapist (Winnicott, 1971). Playful communication may be silent, non-verbal or verbal but involves conveying enthusiasm and motivation for, and with, the child, a willingness to engage with the child and their ideas in whatever manner the child desires, and providing them with the freedom to choose and try out new ideas. It is about being playfully minded (Yarnal & Qian, 2011). This entails us being psychologically upbeat: happy, optimistic, cheerful, enthusiastic, mischievous and creative. Embodying these cognitive attributes enables the same attributes in others as well as being important for our own and other's emotional health.

- Embrace Rogers' (1951) core conditions of empathic understanding, unconditional positive regard and congruence or genuineness, and provide them continually in their practice. These three conditions provided by the therapist create an environment which facilitates change in the child (Ray, 2011).

- Recognise and nurture one's own playfulness by reflecting on our characteristics which signify a playful approach to life and relationships such as being optimistic towards life and having a positive demeanour; being enthusiastic towards situations and others and being appropriately mischievous and creative; celebrating our playfulness and considering what we might need to develop further; and reflecting on the barriers to playfulness and utilising supervision and personal therapy to address those issues which might inhibit playfulness – this is important as otherwise our playfulness is not genuine but becomes 'constructed playfulness' (Chown, 2015) to which children are alert.

Case study: a playful encounter

Tom, aged 8 years

Tom was referred to play therapy due to his history of disruptive and aggressive behaviour in school resulting in his expulsion from a primary school at the age of 7 years. He lived at home with his mother who was seriously ill and had experienced multiple hospital admissions. At these times Tom was looked after by a variety of different family members including his aunt and adult siblings. At the time of attending therapy he was in school part-time, as he was unable to cope with a full school day. He had no friends either inside or outside of the school environment.

Session 10

Tom was sitting on the floor and said he wanted to paint. He took a pile of white paper for himself and gave the therapist a pile of paper as well. There was no verbalisation as he handed the paper across, just a quick glance to ensure he had her attention. He then took one set of paints to share and made sure both he and the therapist had a paintbrush. Again, no words were said just a quick glance and handing over the brush. He then said, 'Now we are going to make splash art' and smiled. He dipped his paintbrush in the water then into the paint. He then used his finger to flick the end of the paintbrush and flicked paint on the paper. He turned to the therapist and said, 'You can do this too' and nodded his head, beckoning her to join in. Both Tom and the therapist used lots of colours and splashed paint over multiple pieces of paper. Tom was lost in the activity, but a smile escaped from time to time indicating his enjoyment. He then stated that 'we have made lots of messy pictures' whilst sitting back satisfied and smiling. He then proceeded to fold the pieces of paper or placed them on top of one another, ensuring that the paint became completely mixed and oozed out of the sides of the paper. The therapist reflected, 'You seem to like making a mess' and he replied with a big grin, 'Yes'. The therapist then wondered aloud, 'I wonder why you like making a mess?' Tom replied, 'I can do what I want'. He proceeded to make more messy pictures and then said, 'If you don't like a picture you can screw it up into a tiny ball like this' and tightly scrunched up the wet ball of paper in his fist. He continued with this activity with the therapist playing alongside him. As the session came to an end Tom conveyed a sense of calm, stillness and completeness.

The case study above describes a playful encounter in the playroom. Many adults would not necessarily consider the activity play or playful. It did not overtly involve pretence, a pre-requisite for many definitions of play, and it was not exuberant and full of laughter, a view many have of playful activities. However, for Tom, this was a playful activity which enabled him to feel playful and have a sense of wellbeing. Drawing on Piagetian developmental theory the play could be construed as that of a much younger child. The repetitive and sensorimotor nature of the activity belonged to a child younger than three years of age, and indeed, many of Tom's behaviours belonged to this developmental age. However, there were symbolic aspects to the play in the way he made and contained his mess, reflecting the messy nature of his life. In terms of children's cues, Tom had negotiated choice (King & Howard, 2016) and there were limits to his activity. It occurred on the floor which gave him freedom to move and generated freedom of ideas. It was also free of adult interference, the therapist responded to the nonverbal invitation to join in.

The therapist was an active listener and observer. There was very little language, but the therapist was alert to the nonverbal signs being conveyed: glances, smiles, body posture – his emotional presence. The communication between Tom and the therapist was playful. The therapist was playfully minded, conveying enthusiasm and motivation for, and with, the child, engaging with the child willingly and responding to and participating with their ideas in whatever manner Tom desired. The therapist clearly embraced the core conditions of person-centred therapy being empathic, accepting all aspects of Tom's play and being genuinely playful as she was able to participate in the 'messiness' of the play.

Landreth (2012) stated that 'play therapy presupposes the presence of some possible activity that would be considered play' (p. 11). However, from the above discussion it would appear that more important than what *adults* consider this activity to be, is whether or not the *child* considers it to be play. If the cues are in place for a child to consider an activity to be play then the child will be playful, a far more important quality for their development and wellbeing. The cues children use to view play and be playful accord with the essentials of play therapy practice. In addition, play therapists need to nurture their own playfulness by reflecting on and celebrating their playful characteristics whilst considering and challenging the barriers to playfulness through supervision and, where appropriate, personal therapy. This will ensure that therapeutic encounters and the therapeutic relationship are playful and enable emotional growth and a deeper feeling of wellbeing for children.

Summary

- This chapter has provided an overview of play theories and how play is viewed. It has presented a view of play based on children's perspectives of play and using these to enable playfulness, a more important quality for wellbeing. It has argued for the need to embrace playfulness within the therapeutic relationship and that this enables the development of a playful therapist. Ultimately it makes the point that playfulness is the heart of the relationship which enables healing.
- What play is and why children play has been theorised from different perspectives and understanding these provides an holistic view of play.
- Listening to and observing children's views of play, which are often different to adults, enables an understanding of what activities children believe are play and enables playfulness.
- Playfulness is critical for children's development and wellbeing and is the heart of the therapeutic relationship between child and therapist.
- Nurturing one's own playfulness is necessary so that it is genuine and not constructed.

Further reading

Howard, J. & McInnes, K. (2013) *The Essence of Play*. London: Routledge.
This book is useful for further information on concepts and the discussion of play and playfulness.
Winnicott, D. W. (1971) *Playing and Reality*. Abingdon: Routledge Classics.
Although this is rather an old text it remains valuable for Winnicott's discussion of the playful space.

References

Axline, V. M. (1969) *Play Therapy*. (Revised ed.) New York: Ballantine Books.
Bundy, A. C. (1993) Assessment of play and leisure: Delineation of the problem. *The American Journal of Occupational Therapy*. 47(3) pp. 217–222.
Chown, A. (2015) *Play Therapy in the Outdoors: Taking Play Therapy Out of the Playroom and into Natural Environments*. London: Jessica Kingsley Publishers.
Csikszentmihalyi, M. (1990) *Flow: The Psychology of Optimal Experience*. New York: Harper Collins Publishers.
Erikson, E. H. (1963) *Childhood and Society*. New York: W. W. Norton & Co.
Freud, A. (1965) *Normality and Pathology in Childhood: Assessments of Development*. London: Karnac Books.
Goncu, A. & Gaskins, S. (eds.) (2007) *Play and Development: Evolutionary, Sociocultural and Functional Perspectives*. Philadelphia: Psychology Press.
Gray, P. (2011) The decline of play and the rise of psychopathology in children and adolescents. *American Journal of Play*. 3(4) pp. 443–463.
Henricks, T. S. (2015) *Play and the Human Condition*. Urbana: University of Illinois Press.
Howard, J. (2002) Eliciting young children's perceptions of play, work and learning using the activity apperception story procedure. *Early Child Development and Care*. 172 pp. 489–502.
Howard, J. & McInnes, K. (2012) The impact of children's perceptions of an activity as play rather than not play on emotional well-being. *Child: Care, Health and Development*. 39(5) pp. 737–742.
Howard, J. & McInnes, K. (2013) *The Essence of Play*. London: Routledge.
King, P. & Howard, J. (2016) Free choice or adaptable choice? Self-determination theory and play. *American Journal of Play*. 9(1) pp. 56–70.
Klein, M. (1960) *The Psychoanalysis of Children*. London: Grove Press Inc.
Krasnor, L. R. & Pepler, D. J. (1980) The study of children's play: Some suggested future directions. In: Rubin, K. H. (ed.) *New Directions for Child Development. Children's Play* (Vol. 9). San Francisco: Jossey-Bass Inc. Publishers. pp. 85–95.
Landreth, G. (2012) *Play Therapy: The Art of the Relationship*. (3rd ed.) London: Routledge.
Lieberman, J. N. (1977) *Playfulness: Its Relationship to Imagination and Creativity*. New York: Academic Press Inc.
McInnes, K. & Birdsey, N. (2014) Understanding play: The perceptions of children, adolescents, parents and teachers. In: Barnett, L. A. (ed.) *Play of Individuals and Societies*. E-book Oxford: Inter-disciplinary Press. pp. 105–116.

McInnes, K., Howard, J., Miles, G. & Crowley, K. (2009) Behavioural differences exhibited by children when practicing a task under formal and playful conditions. *Journal of Educational and Child Psychology*. 26(2) pp. 31–39.

McInnes, K., Howard, J., Miles, G. & Crowley, K. (2010) Differences in adult-child interactions during playful and formal practice conditions: An initial investigation. *Psychology of Education Review*. 34(1) pp. 14–20.

McInnes, K., Howard, J., Miles, G. & Crowley, K. (2011) Differences in practitioners' understanding of play and how this influences pedagogy and children's perceptions of play. *Early Years. An International Journal of Research and Development*. 31(2) pp. 121–133.

McInnes, K., Howard, J., Miles, G. & Crowley, K. (2013) The nature of adult-child interaction in the early years classroom: Implications for children's perceptions of play and subsequent learning behaviour. *European Early Childhood Education Research Journal*. 21(2) pp. 268–282.

McInnes, K. & Yuen, N. (2017) Play and playfulness: The foundation of development. In: Thomas, A. & McInnes, K. (eds.) *Teaching Early Years: Theory and Practice*. London: Sage. pp. 47–64.

McMahon, L. (2009) *The Handbook of Play Therapy and Therapeutic Play*. (2nd ed.) London: Routledge.

Moyles, J. R. (1989) *Just Playing?* Buckingham: Open University Press.

Neumann, E. A. (1971) *The Elements of Play*. New York: MSS Information Corporation.

Parten, M. B. (1932) Social participation among pre-school children. *Journal of Abnormal and Social Psychology*. 27 pp. 243–269.

Piaget, J. (1951) *Play, Dreams and Imitation in Childhood*. London: William Heinemann Ltd.

Pyle, A. & Danniels, E. (2017) A continuum of play-based learning: The role of the teacher in play-based pedagogy and the fear of hijacking play. *Early Education and Development*. 28(3) pp. 274–289.

Ray, D. C. (2011) *Advanced Play Therapy*. London: Routledge.

Rogers, C. (1951) *Client-Centred Therapy: Its Current Practice, Implications and Theory*. Boston: Houghton Mifflin.

Vygotsky, L. S. (1976) Play and its role in the mental development of the child. In: Bruner, J. S., Jolly, A. & Sylva, K. (eds.) *Play: Its Role in Development and Evolution*. New York: Basic Books Inc. pp. 537–554.

West, J. (1996) *Child Centred Play Therapy*. London: Hodder Education.

Winnicott, D. W. (1971) *Playing and Reality*. Abingdon: Routledge Classics.

Yarnal, C. & Qian, X. (2011) Older-adult playfulness: An innovative construct and measurement for healthy aging research. *American Journal of Play*. 4(1) pp. 52–79.

Chapter 8

Being an improvisational play therapist

Simon Kerr-Edwards

Chapter overview

In this chapter I will recognise how improvisation is an integral part of human interaction and how it has been developed as a concept and technique in the sphere of drama. I will show how researchers and practitioners have applied these ideas to the psychological and psychotherapeutic disciplines and will go on to develop my thoughts as to how aspects of improvisation can be applied equally and effectively to the practice skills needed in play therapy. I will argue that, through improvisation, a practitioner can develop the skill of spontaneity that allows them to bring their sense of self, to their work for therapeutic benefit.

What improvisation has to offer

Many of our interactions in daily life are improvised. We may have plans for events or relationships but what flows from those ideas are often spontaneous moments. The roots of this chapter began when I wrote about play therapists being 'more improvisational' when exploring the beginnings of play therapy interventions (Kerr-Edwards, 2012) and here I wanted to examine in greater detail what I meant by being improvisational and how this can be of benefit to the child and the therapeutic relationship. Although there is a plethora of literature in music, comedy and business about the importance of improvisation as a concept, it is the study of drama that generates much literature that is of most relevance. Frost and Yarrow (2007) refer to improvisation as an elemental part of all dramatic forms across cultures (western and non-western) and note that it has been the subject of suppression by authorities over time. They define it as a 'dynamic *principle* operating in many different spheres: an independent and transformative way of being, knowing and doing' (2007:17). This principle is valuable to the dramatic process, as Hahlo and Reynolds (2000:20) state that skills developed through improvisation will 'include creativity, co-operation, communication and concentration as well as the ability to listen, compromise, contribute and take initiative'. Furthermore, Hodgson and Richards (1974) believed this process can develop insight:

> Improvisation in drama aims to utilise the two elements from everyday life improvisation: the spontaneous response to the unfolding of an unexpected situation and the ingenuity called to deal with the situation, both of these to gain insight into problems presented.
>
> (1974:2)

Here they identify spontaneity as enabling us to react to something unexpected, as well as a means of leading us to problem-solving and the development of insight. This notion of spontaneity is further explored in the pioneering work of Spolin (1999), who devised games and exercises to expand the actor's spontaneous qualities. These involved physical tasks for using the whole body and sensory self, as well as developing character, emotion and acting skills. Such exercises were listening with the body, mirroring, physicalising and transforming objects, tug-of-war and jumping emotions. Furthermore, she believed that it was through spontaneity that 'we are re-formed into ourselves' (1999:4). Another important proponent in the development of improvisation was Johnstone (1979) who, when discussing narrative skills, considered how actors became inhibited when they focussed on the meaning of texts. He went on to say: 'Once you go on to ignore content, it becomes possible to understand what narrative is, because you can concentrate on structure' (1979:111). This proposes the idea that **how** something comes about (the process of construction) is as important or maybe more so than what is produced or what is 'meant' by what is produced.

These ideas from drama have provoked thinking in the literature of psychological therapies, especially in the field of dramatherapy. In his attempt to formulate a dramatherapy model, Landy (1986:105) saw improvisation (as well as role-play) as part of the therapeutic continuum and proposed that 'spontaneity is a midpoint between compulsive, inhibited styles of acting and impulsive, overinvolved styles'. Here he believes that the self and role are both separate yet merged, and that the actual world and the 'as if' world exist at the same time in therapy. Although he applies this to the client experience, I would argue that this is as crucial for the therapist experience. Our ability to experience in-play and out-of-play concurrently comes from a confident ability to move between the two.

The concept of improvisation has emerged in other psychotherapy and psychoanalytic texts such as when Pedder (1977), exploring the theories of Winnicott (1971), linked psychotherapy, play and theatre and highlighted the need for a safe space in which personal material can be explored. More recently, the work of Ringstrom (2012) focusses on how scripts, roles and sets and lines are part of the psychoanalyst's tool-kit that enables safety to be achieved. However, he goes on to identify that, 'Improvisation grasps how both implicitly and explicitly the minds of the analytic participants meet and co-author a quality of relational consciousness' (2012:449). Here he acknowledges that improvisation can reveal much about both sides of the therapeutic dyad and uses the unconscious of the therapist to the client's benefit. In addition, he identifies improvisational moments where the therapist and the client work off one another. These go beyond merely being spontaneous and highlight spontaneity as being essentially relational. Weiner (1994) also acknowledges how improvisation techniques can both support and enhance skills of the therapist as well as be used directly with families in therapy. He recognises the importance of play and story-making and goes on to show how other themes such as status, power and emotional expressiveness could be explored with families. Furthermore, he reflected on improvisation as part of clinical training:

> Since I view the effective therapist as creating a context of change via the use of self rather than by mere application of technique, improv can become a means by which therapists in training cultivate and expand their capacity to use the self fully.
>
> (Weiner, 1994:240–241)

How improvisation can be applied to the play therapist

Play therapy reflects the dichotomy of ritual and improvisation. It has its ritual elements: a prescribed time and duration to meet; a venue that is quiet and confidential; a play therapist who is keeper of the boundaries; a child, client or family who is the focus of the therapy. The toys also become the props of the ritual and can be used in a way that has a symbolic meaning. However, within the structures of therapy it is uncertain as to what is going to happen. There may be expectations but there is no script and it is not known what will take place during the hour. Furthermore, the symbolic expression may be personal to the experiences of that child and may only exist in the time and space of the therapy session and with that particular therapist. At its heart, play therapy is a considered, researched and taught modality of therapy that requires skill and practice in order for it to be successful. Undertaking the therapeutic journey with a child or family is not something that can be made up on the spot. Boundaries and expectations need to be clear and reiterated at the appropriate time in order for the play room to represent a safe and reliable container in which a trusting relationship can develop. But it is how each of us as individuals use our sense of self that develops the therapeutic alliance. As Landreth (2012:97) puts it, 'the difference between an effective play therapist and other adults, therefore, must come from within as the self of the therapist is made fully present and available to the child'. It is through exploring our improvisational self that we enable ourselves to be fully present in the relationship. When children are fully in relationship they can reflect on traumatic events or histories and gain some insight into them. This may lead to greater control of their inner selves and outer lives.

How play therapists behave (or improvise) will be crucial in allowing themselves to become 'fully present and available'. As Music (2017:145) says: 'Play is rarely rigid and planned, it is generally spontaneous and has elements of uncertainty and surprise'. This improvisation appears to be needed both in the play and also in the therapeutic relationship building. When we train as play therapists we may learn and practise how to talk about what play therapy is with the child and their parent. There are certain sayings or scripts that sound good to each of us and to which others have responded positively in the past. These may be said by rote to begin with and we may find ourselves being reliant for direction from our clinical supervisor or course tutor when in training. However, as our experience grows we may expand what we say and how we say it, depending on the cues we receive from children. We learn to set boundaries in the sessions (such as not to damage the toys), how to identify when a boundary needs reiterating and what to say if the need arises to state a boundary. However, what if we set the boundary and the child does not comply, what then? How can we react to this in a way that maintains the boundary and enables the child to remain connected with us? This may require a variety of responses according to the situation. In addition, we may add reflective, curious or empathic comments to the play, but these will be predominantly made-up or improvised by following cues from the child. On occasion, we may be asked to act out scenarios that require us to show a character or characteristics that the child wants expressed and to this we respond with our own spontaneous comments and ideas, in addition to what the child directs. Here we are allowing our self to the fore and this is where the 'co-creating' in therapy happens. If we are too inhibited, the child may not be able to connect with us. Too impulsive and we may take the play in a direction the child does not want. I believe it is through developing improvisational skills that we can better prepare our selves (and our unconscious) to being open to the complexities of the play therapy relationship. What is required of us is challenging, as Kronengold (2012:184) says: 'We may engage in play that can appear at turns intense, meandering, meaningful and downright goofy'. Here he argues that it is our understanding of the qualities of play that is vital in the supporting of the child's expression. Is play therapy a spontaneous and improvised discipline as much as a taught and researched modality?

So, how does the play therapy practitioner consider his own ability to improvise and how do these ideas impact on the therapeutic relationship? I suggest the following headings to enable me to structure my thoughts on the application of the processes of improvisation to play therapy.

The right amount of preparation

Improvisation is more than just about turning up and participating. It is a skill that has a theoretical base with time, attention and reflection needed when put into practice. An understanding of what is required is needed for the improvisation to flourish. Similarly, in play therapy there is an understanding that a thorough grounding in theory and time spent training and focussing on skills is needed for the therapist to be successful. To prepare for a piece of therapy, we gain referral information on the background of the child. We must not forget that this information may be subjective and incomplete. We may only have patchy information on which to formulate a plan. What is known enables the therapist to assimilate the child's personal circumstances with what they themselves know from theory and practice. However, an over reliance on the information gleaned pre-session may inadvertently distract the therapist from what is happening in the therapy room when the therapy begins. Here, clinical supervision is required to help reflect on what has been read, how this fits with understanding and theories and the therapist's previous experiences, as well as what it is he experiences in the room with the child. But ultimately it is the therapist's self that is taken into therapy sessions and not our books, referral form or supervisor, and we must rely on how we have absorbed and interpreted previous knowledge and understandings to be able to respond to what is presented to us. We must be aware of what has happened in the child's life but also recognise what preconceptions we may have of what we expect to happen in the therapy. If we anticipate seeing certain behaviours, then maybe we may see them or even steer the play in that direction and inadvertently miss other themes the child may express. Our attempt to over-prepare may be an attempt to manage anxious feelings and, although this is understandable, it may leave us inhibited in our approach.

Joining together to begin

At the start of any improvisational activity, a joining together is needed, which requires some discussion and agreement on what expectations and boundaries are needed for creating physical and emotional safety. This is the same for the start of the therapeutic process. How we come together in a therapeutic relationship and co-construct the therapeutic space can set the tone for what is to follow and can determine whether children engage in the process. Remember therapy belongs to those in the room as well as 'voices' that may appear from outside (parents, teachers, etc.). As most children are referred by someone else, it is vital to ensure that the child feels the process of therapy is hers to shape and benefit from and that she is the principal agent for what is about to happen. Being explicit about the therapeutic process is part of the therapeutic process.

Accepting what is on offer

Improvisation is about seeing and accepting what is on offer, even if this is sometimes ambiguous or confusing. What is not on offer cannot be responded to, so being content with what there is opens us up to appreciate it more. This is similar in play therapy, trusting that the child will offer up chances for relationship (no matter what her difficulties may be) and despite any possible indications to the contrary. We may wish the child in play therapy to be different – the child might be contained or uncontained and we may be challenged by this and wish it to be different. But paradoxically, our acceptance of how the child is, becomes a powerful tool for change. Children need to be seen for the shapes they are rather than the shapes they are not. The therapist needs to chime with what is presented, work with that and avoid being distracted by other preconceived notions.

Accepting that which you do not know

Not knowing what is going to happen next is an important part of improvisation. The idea of going into stressful situations with this element of 'not-knowing' can be a challenge to the therapist that may raise anxious feelings of failure. Yet not being clear about what will happen next may encourage our spontaneity and ability to focus in each moment with the child. When play therapy students begin, the 'not-knowing' part of them is understandably great and they may have mixed feelings about this. Sometimes, to manage these circumstances, what they believe they need is certainty and order. Although partly true, this might be hard to achieve when, as a student, there is so much to learn all at once. As experience is gained, insights are developed and practitioners will grow into knowing what to expect, as patterns in play and relating with children begin to emerge. These experiences will be understood and reinforced by knowledge of theory but still may at times appear novel or unique. Although this lack of 'knowing' can spur on our curiosity to know more, we may also remain 'in the dark' and we need to be comfortable with this position. We do not always know the outcome of the therapeutic journey but do know that insights will appear along the way and the adventure itself will be enlightening.

Deepening our observation

Any improvisational process requires us to see what is before us in order for us to respond. If we are to accept the offer of an idea we must be able to see the invitation as it arises. However, what we see before us may not be clear and may not be all that is going on, as some invitations to join may be disguised or inferred. Our tendency may be to categorise, assess or intellectualise the play, staying removed from it, rather than involving ourselves in it as it happens and experiencing the nuances as they occur. This deepening may require us to notice the 'small' things that may be the key to gaining insight about 'big' things. This could be a glance or a fleeting gesture. At this time, we need our intellectual and emotional 'eyesight' to co-operate with each other in both participating *and* observing what is going on. We also need to look within ourselves and our own internal responses and impulses need to be engaged. Some internal thoughts may be given back to the child ('Wow, you've got some big feelings about that') and others might need taking to supervision ('Wow, I've got big feelings about that') to reflect on them there.

There is also a caveat to observing the child closely. I cannot recall how many times I have been invited into playing 'hide and seek' with a child in therapy, but it has been many. This may require me to cover my eyes (and sometimes ears too) and when this happens I reflect to myself that too much 'seeing' of the child might be experienced as intrusive or overwhelming and therefore the game can reset this balance. The child may need to 'reveal' herself in her own time.

Turning up our listening

The basic tenet of any improvisation is to listen to what is happening with another. To know where we are in relation to another, we send out signals and listen to what responses return to us and, although this is largely through words, we use other communicative senses too. Listening is a foundation for any therapeutic modality and is often discussed and practised. However, there is more than one level of listening going on: we listen to the **content** (what is said), we listen to the **meaning** (what is meant by what is said) and also to the **process** (what does this say about how we are together?). All three of these processes happen simultaneously and we need to be able to consider all equally.

These layers of listening also interact with the internal voice or 'internal supervisor' (Casement, 1985), a voice or dialogue that we have within ourselves as practitioners that enables us to step back and see how we (child and therapist) are together. This enables us to listen to and monitor our spontaneous responses so that, when for example we act out a narrative with the child, we are using a level of emotional expression that fits in with what is required of us (and not what we may unconsciously wish).

Listening to our body

Aural listening is not the only listening that needs to be attended to. Improvisation has often focussed on using the entirety of what the physiological and emotional body can offer. Our perceptions through all our senses are our primary way of interacting with the world. Therefore, our sensory awareness is fundamental to our interactions as therapists in the therapeutic space. Our body might have vital signs (or as a medic might say, 'vital-signs') that can illuminate what is happening in the therapy room. Being too hot or cold, energetic or sleepy, fearful or relaxed, hungry or satisfied, may indicate something about the therapeutic relationship. Furthermore, how we sit, where we position ourselves and how we move about the room are all questions to consider. We can often work with children who have sensory processing issues, proprioception difficulties or hypervigilance, so our own connection with our sensory awareness and vigilance needs to be heightened to uncover as much as we can. For instance, sometimes distractions outside of the room may matter more to the therapist (fear of interruption or intrusion) than to the child (who is used to a busy classroom).

Taking opportunities and getting it wrong

An improvisation requires one person to take up opportunities given by another. This is saying 'yes' to another's idea. However, we may also have to say 'no' and set a boundary. This is an important balancing act but without being permissive there will be little progress. Things can go well and the relationship deepens or it may go awry and an interruption to the relationship may occur. Either way invitations must be considered on their merits. The decision-making of 'yes' or 'no' is crucial in developing the therapeutic relationship. There will be opportunities offered by the child but we always run the risk of us either not picking them up correctly or responding in an unhelpful way. The above themes of *listening* and *observing* are the precursors to taking up of these opportunities for relationship. Generally, if these are performing well we will pick up on the overt and covert invitations from the child to deepen our relationship with them. However, it is likely that we cannot always pick up the cues that are given and may at times respond in ways the child does not want or find useful. This is plainly called 'getting it wrong'.

I want to emphasise that 'getting it wrong' is an important part of the process of making a relationship and, if we do not occasionally get it wrong, how can we understand what is right? Sometimes the messages we are given by the child are mixed and we may easily respond to them in an unhelpful way or to the wrong part of them. In fact, I would reiterate that getting it wrong is essential to getting it right and we need to have a confidence in our failures. This allows us to work at repairing any ruptures in the relationship. We may be asked to be the 'shouting' teacher in a role-play, only to be told that we are not 'shouting' enough. Responding or trying something may not work so, if rejected, then let us be open to this, apologise and try something different. There will be times when we feel that all we try is rejected or fails and this may be part of the therapeutic journey. We may be tested to see how much failure we can take.

Children who have been referred to therapy can often bring with them strong notions of success and failure and may see the requirement for therapy as proof they have got it wrong or have failed.

Being playful whilst acknowledging despair

There is a willingness for engagement and connection with self-and-other, and in an improvisation this begins with a wish to participate or to play. It is easy to see how this playfulness could develop into something comedic or be perceived as fun. However, improvisation is something much broader and deeper and can encompass an array of feelings from euphoria to despair and is not confined to making someone laugh.

Playfulness is a basic skill in a play therapist's tool-kit as it is a means of showing that we strive to speak the language of the child. This playfulness requires spontaneity and may be considered as having a 'light' quality. There may be concerns that we become uninhibited in our playfulness. To avoid this, we need to accept that we may be facing and encompassing a range of feelings that are profound and moving, not only in the child but also in ourselves. This means the play therapist needs to be spontaneous with what they hear and see, even when encountering narratives of grief, shame and failure. We may have been told distressing experiences before but this is the first time with this child and in this moment. My understanding of playfulness is the ability to bring another, lighter perspective to emotional expressions, recognising and accepting them as creative and engaging experiences that come and go rather than ones that need to be hidden and reviled. (See also Chapter 7 by McInnes on the skill of playfulness.)

Stepping back

Reflecting back on an improvisation is part of the process. It can require a constant checking out and adapting as it unfolds. This is apposite for the play therapist who can be both in the play and separate from it. We may participate in play with a child but we also observe the play, the child, ourselves and the burgeoning relationship. The therapist may ask for a time out in immersive narratives or role-plays to ask for clarification or guidance. There may be a concern that this would break any flow or intensity, but in fact this may deepen the narrative as the therapist is showing how he wants it to be right for the child. This technique can also monitor our levels of engagement and whether we are at the correct level of involvement for the child.

Being persistent and trusting the process

When you try something in an improvisation and it does not work, it requires persistence, trial and error. An action may not work to begin with;

we may not connect and it may not produce interactions that are coherent or useful. This could be akin to the making and maintaining of therapeutic relationships with children. There will be some children who readily identify with the therapeutic process and those who are challenged by it. Sometimes it is hard to know where the work is going and of what benefit it is. At these times, we need to persist and trust that the process of therapy can garner positive outcomes. Remaining persistent could be related to our own resilience and how we, the practitioners, can take a setback and keep on working in an open, receptive and responsive manner.

Play therapy, like improvisation, is a meaningful journey to take both in itself and for what might happen as a result. The structure and process of the therapy need to be trusted as a worthwhile endeavour, despite times when there seems to be little effect or result. Because we engage with a child's powerful and complex emotions, which can often challenge but also support their wellbeing, we need to be the repositories of hope and belief that things can be different.

The study and practising of improvisational techniques has a great deal of relevance to our building of our relational skills as play therapists. Core competences, such as building therapeutic relationships, using a range of creative media and effective communication (BAPT Core Competences, 17, 26 and 27, see Appendix 1), can all be furthered through the exploration of improvisational and spontaneous skills. Furthermore, our internal selves as seen through personal qualities such as self-awareness, self-responsibility, congruence and critical reflection (BAPT Core Competence 11, see Appendix 1) can also be enhanced through the exploration of the improviser inside us. Improvisation's emphasis on process as much as content is a valuable lesson for practitioners to remember. If this becomes out of balance and meaning becomes dominant, then we ignore the valuable steps of how we arrived there. No two pieces of therapy are ever the same. Challenges to the therapeutic relationship are constantly experienced by the therapeutic dyad and being improvisational is a means of considering how we respond to these challenges. My belief is that improvisation is an essential play therapy practice skill about which we need to be more explicit. We are often required to be spontaneous but it is often either taken for granted or treated with caution, as if it, or we, might become out of control. By not thinking about it, are we at risk of not understanding our unconscious reactions to children? Surely it is by nurturing or developing our own improvisational nature that we allow a stronger and more moderated sense of self to be present in the play room. An improvisational ability is a way of summoning our tried and tested therapy skills into the 'here and now' as a means of deepening our unique therapeutic relationship with a child. Being improvisational can allow us to expand our responsiveness to the child, recognise our mistakes or mis-attunements and try to refocus our energy on the needs of the child. We often focus on the meanings and resonance of expressions in our therapeutic relationship with the child in therapy, but **how** we relate together, and **how** the therapist responds to the challenges a child sets, seems just as important. Our ability to engage the conscious and unconscious processes of both child and therapist, through spontaneous and improvisation skills, allows for the creation of a unique therapeutic journey that enables the child to become, as Spolin (1999:4) says, 're-formed' through the process. We often regard play as the language of the child but is it not in fact improvisation?

Summary

- Much of human interaction is improvisational.
- Improvisation is a principle in drama to explore how participants can be spontaneous in their reactions to others.
- Improvisation focusses on the process of relationship along with the meaning of it.
- Play is largely improvisational with no script and with emerging themes.
- Therapists can utilise their improvisational principles and abilities to meet the challenges of making therapeutic relationships.
- Play therapists are ideally positioned to use improvisational skills.
- Being improvisational can be learned with practice and application and can contribute to the core competences of a play therapist.
- An improvisational ability allows the self of the therapist be used for therapeutic benefit.

Further reading

Bergen, M., Cox, M. & Detmar, J. (2002) *Improvise This.* New York: Hyperion.
This takes improvisational ideas into the business sector.
Grimes, R.L. (2006) *Rite Out of Place.* New York: Oxford University Press.
A text about ritual and how it can take place outside a religious context.
Johnston, C. (2006) *The Improvisation Game.* London: Nick Hern Books.
This book looks at improvisational techniques and talks to leading proponents in the arts.
Madson, P.R. (2005) *Improv Wisdom.* New York: Bell Tower.
Here Madson proposes 13 maxims for all improvisers.
McNiff, S. (2015) *Imagination in Action.* Boston: Shambhala.
A book that examines the minutiae of the creative process.
Nachmanovitch, S. (1990) *Free Play.* New York: Jeremy P. Tarcher/Putnam.
Another text that delves into the creativity of play.

References

Casement, P. (1985) *On Learning from the Patient.* London: Tavistock Publications.
Frost, A. & Yarrow, R. (2007) *Improvisation in Drama.* (2nd ed.) Basingstoke: Palgrave Macmillan.

Hahlo, R. & Reynolds, P. (2000) *Dramatic Events*. London: Faber and Faber.

Hodgson, J. & Richards, E. (1974) *Improvisation*. (Revised ed.) London: Eyre Methuen.

Johnstone, K. (1979) *Impro*. London: Faber and Faber.

Kerr-Edwards, S. (2012) Let's start at the beginning. *British Journal of Play Therapy*. 8 pp. 12–20.

Kronengold, H. (2012) The adventures of Captain Pineapple. *International Journal of Play Therapy*. 21(3) pp. 167–185.

Landreth, G. (2012) *Play Therapy: The Art of the Relationship*. (3rd ed.) Hove: Routledge.

Landy, R. (1986) *Drama Therapy*. Springfield: Charles C. Thomas.

Music, G. (2017) *Nurturing Natures*. (2nd ed.) Abingdon: Routledge.

Pedder, J. (1977) The role of space and location in psychotherapy, play and theatre. *International Review of Psycho-Analysis*. 2(2) pp. 215–223.

Ringstrom, P. (2012) Principles of improvisation: A model of therapeutic play in relational psychoanalysis. In: Aron, L. & Harris, A. (eds.) *Relational Psychoanalysis, Volume 5, Evolution of Process*. Hove: Routledge. pp. 447–478.

Spolin, V. (1999) *Improvisation for the Theatre*. (3rd ed.) Evanston: Northwestern University Press.

Weiner, D.J. (1994) *Rehearsals for Growth*. London: W.W. Norton & Company.

Winnicott, D.W. (1971) *Playing and Reality*. London: Tavistock Publications.

Chapter 9

Containing feelings and setting limits in play therapy

Working with aggression

Peter Ayling

Chapter overview

This chapter will explore the role of the play therapist in responding to children's emotions within play therapy. I begin by discussing how theories of emotional development and new understanding from neuroscience can inform play therapy practice. In particular, I will focus on responding to aggression within both children's play and the therapeutic relationship. I will consider the role of limit-setting in supporting emotional development and end with a brief reflection on the importance of therapist self-awareness, as a core aspect of effective therapy.

Play therapy and emotional regulation

Child-centred play therapy pays particular attention to the emotional processes of children within their play interaction. Axline (1989:69) established the centrality of emotions as a therapeutic focus within her principles of play therapy, through her emphasis on empathic reflection: 'the therapist is alert to recognise the feelings the child is expressing and reflects those feelings back to him in such a manner that he gains insight into his behaviour'. Indeed, this early emphasis on empathy has become a fundamental aspect of play therapy practice, reflected in the British Association of Play Therapists' core competences for practice (Core Competences 5, 11, 26. See Appendix 1). Landreth (2012) emphasises the significance of the therapist's ability to offer acceptance of the child's emotions, whilst providing safe limits for their behaviour. This acceptance without judgement is at the heart of Rogers' (1951) original core conditions for person-centred practice.

A number of change mechanisms have been identified within play therapy (Russ, 2004), including catharsis, defined as the release of deep emotion; the provision of a corrective emotional experience with the therapist; and promoting the mastery of feelings and behaviour through rehearsal within play. These processes emphasise the role of the therapist in labelling and containing emotions, thereby supporting cognitive development and neurological re-structuring (Drewes & Schaefer, 2014). The therapist's role is to facilitate the expression of emotions, but also to help the child identify and differentiate their feelings. Fonagy et al. (2004) has proposed the broader concept of 'mentalisation' to describe the process by which children come to understand their thoughts and feelings, through the minds and narrative feedback of the adults around them. Within the play therapy relationship, the therapist consciously utilises both emotional and cognitive processes within the play, building the child's emotional understanding and supporting their overall executive functioning (Kestly, 2014).

Schore (2016) highlights the importance of the child's growing ability to identify and regulate their emotions as a vital aspect of healthy psychological development, one particularly important for managing negative emotions, due to the powerful physiological arousal of such feelings. This regulatory ability develops within the context of the primary caregiving relationship, and mostly through the nonverbal and sensory interaction of parent and child (Stern, 1985). Gaskill (2014) describes the role that 'mirror neurons' within our brains play in supporting a sense of inter-subjective sharing within both the parent–child and therapeutic relation-ships. This shared connection is communicated largely through 'vitality matching' (Patton & Benedict, 2016), whereby the therapist conveys the intensity of the child's feeling through their tone and facial expression, whilst also marking their experience as sufficiently different to convey mastery and self-management, promoting 'co-regulation' of emotional states (Schore, 2016).

Case study: Reuben

Reuben is a 10-year-old boy in a kinship placement with his maternal aunt. These excerpts of play are from his fourth and fifth play therapy sessions with me:

Week 4: Reuben is using the Incredible Hulk figure to fight a large army of soldiers.

REUBEN: *(Excited, aggressive tone)* They are all firing at the Hulk but he is smashing them down *(knocks the soldiers down with Hulk's powerful hands)* Ha, they can't hurt him!

THERAPIST: *(Matching excited tone and gestures)* The Hulk is fighting them all, and he feels strong and powerful. They cannot hurt him!

REUBEN: *(Determined, powerful tone)* Smash! *(Hulk slams into the soldiers again, stamping up and down on them)* Hulk is smashing them all up, but they can't touch him.

THERAPIST: *(Trying to match the strength of this tone)* Hulk is stamping all over them but they can't get him. No one hurts the Hulk.

REUBEN: *(Pointing to bruises on his arms and legs)* I fell off a shed roof, but it didn't hurt. Nothing hurts me – if you hurt me I get stronger *(Excited, proud, strong)*

THERAPIST: *(Reflecting his strong confident tone)* You feel so strong, it's like nothing can hurt you … it makes you feel stronger … But I would be frightened if I was climbing on a roof. Those cuts look really sore to me. *(Shifting to worried, but animated tone to match shift in content)*

REUBEN: *(Less powerful, more questioning tone)* Don't you like being hurt? I don't care about getting hurt.

THERAPIST: *(Conveying uncertainty, confusion)* It's confusing, even when things hurt, you don't mind, you even like it … so hard to know how to feel. I don't like being hurt – it makes me sad.

Week 5: The following week Reuben came into the session and immediately showed me his finger, where he had a tiny, almost indiscernible cut.

REUBEN: *(Vulnerable, childlike tone)* I hurt myself – I cut my finger.

THERAPIST: Oh, you hurt yourself this week and you are showing me. It really hurt and you noticed it … I think we need to take care of this hurt. Shall we find a plaster? *(We go to the first aid box to dress his finger. I stroke it gently with cotton wool)* We need to look after your finger because it hurts. You really felt it. *(Gentle, singsong, rhythmic tone to convey calm concern)*

Here, Reuben is exploring a number of emotional themes within his play, including aggression, but also tentative expressions of vulnerability and nurture-seeking. My tone matches Reuben's, but my facial expressions and posture convey interest, concern and acceptance, rather than aggression. Through my acceptance of these ambivalent emotions, Reuben is able to begin to identify and name his feelings more easily and to express his needs, both within the therapeutic relationship and then within his play.

For some traumatised children, play therapy can be a threatening experience, leading them to avoid engaging with the therapist. Perry (2007) stresses the importance of establishing a primarily sensory connection with such children, to support co-regulation of their stress reactions and help calm their defences. Barfield et al. (2012) emphasise providing patterned, sensory experiences, to help the child to soothe their arousal. Play therapy utilises a range of ways to provide this through rhythm, music, movement and touch.

Case study: Tyrone

When I began working with 11-year-old Tyrone, he refused to speak and hid away in a den, separated from me by blankets and chairs. After a difficult 30 minutes, he began to tap out a rhythm on the floor, pushing his hand through the blanket and into view, while the rest of him remained hidden. I sat nearby on the floor and joined in tentatively, until we gradually began to beat out a rhythm together. Over several weeks, we developed elaborate tunes together on the drums and, at his suggestion, began singing nursery rhymes and songs. By this point, Tyrone had emerged to sit opposite, smiling and looking straight at me. He was now ready to explore the playroom.

Badenoch (2008) describes how this process of co-regulating emotions at a sensory level with the child supports the development of more complex neurological pathways within their mid-brain and limbic system, which can help the child begin to exercise greater levels of control over their subsequent responses. For Tyrone, this experience of regulation enabled him to begin to think about and represent his experiences and feelings through symbolic play.

Understanding and responding to aggressive play

Ray (2011) describes aggression as a developmentally ordinary aspect of children's development, emerging around 18 months of age, often associated with frustration about wish fulfilment or interaction with others. Research suggests that aggressive behaviour usually peaks relatively early in childhood (Doherty & Hughes, 2014), as pre-school children begin to develop cognitive skills to support their social interaction. There appears to be a correlation between poor emotional regulation skills in early childhood and the incidence of aggression in later childhood (Röll et al., 2012).

Crenshaw and Mordock (2005) suggest that the development of more entrenched aggression relates to difficulties with a child's emerging sense of autonomy, leading to feelings of shame and inferiority. Many children we meet have experienced adverse life experiences, which can profoundly affect their emerging sense of self, with consequences for their emotional and social development. As a result, aggressive or impulsive behaviour appears to be one common cause of referral to play therapy (Foulkrod & Davenport, 2010). Play therapists need to be able to respond to aggression expressed both directly towards them, in the form of limit-testing and challenging behaviour, and also indirectly, through aggressive themes represented within the child's symbolic and role play interaction.

O'Sullivan and Ryan (2009) identify the importance of helping the child become aware of a range of underlying feelings that might initially present as aggression. They stress the importance of accepting children's aggressive impulses as part of them, worthy of respect and recognition. We must seek to focus on the underlying intention within the child's play, rather than simply tracking the aggression (Norton & Norton, 2002). The task here is to connect with the meaning and energy behind the action, rather than to focus on the act itself.

A number of research studies have supported the efficacy of child-centred play therapy in reducing aggression (Ray et al., 2009; Schumann, 2010). Crenshaw and Mordock (2005) identify a wide range of play themes relating to aggression, including domineering and controlling play, representing experiences of trauma, abuse, separation and loss experiences, alongside attachment and nurture-themed play. I find it helpful to provide a range of materials that support emotional expression, including dressing-up materials, toys and symbols that represent conflict and aggression – for example, soldiers, police, superheroes, monsters and dinosaurs. However, children will make use of whatever materials are available, including sensory materials such as sand and clay, competitive games, small world toys and nurture play materials. Indeed, some of the most aggressive play I have witnessed has involved nurture materials, such as baby dolls, family figures and stuffed animals, as children have sought to represent the pain of early attachment relationships and release deeply held emotions through cathartic play.

A number of developments in contemporary inter-personal neurobiology also influence my practice. Siegel (2012) has shown how early traumatic experiences significantly impact the structures and integration of the developing brain, leading to children who become over-sensitised to potential triggers for danger in their environment, while simultaneously having reduced access to higher brain functions that support cognitive, problem-solving skills. Such children can re-create these experiences in visceral and compulsive ways within their play, and are more likely to present us with aggressive themes and behaviour within the playroom. At times, this will include cathartic play, involving the release of apparently extreme emotions (Drewes & Schaefer, 2014). I have found it important to pay particular attention to children's initial attempts at cathartic play, noting the duration and intensity of play themes and emotions, without restriction where possible. Such play may include intense expressions of anger, fear, revenge and sadness, which the therapist needs to accept without judgement or interference. However, for catharsis to be truly therapeutic, the play therapist will need to come alongside the child, matching their tone and pace to provide a narrative that accurately conveys understanding and acceptance, leading to a gradual reduction in the intensity of expression and an increase in the child's cognitive processing of their emotion (Drewes & Schaefer, 2014). At other times, children may engage in post-traumatic re-enactment, and may require a more structured, psycho-educational response from the play therapist to support resolution of their experience (Gil, 2011; see also chapters in this volume by May and Waycott & Carbis).

Porges' (2011) polyvagal theory identifies that our autonomic nervous system supports us to react to emerging threats within our environment. Chronic exposure to danger causes children's nervous systems to activate fight or flight responses at an unconscious, sub-cortical level. Importantly, Porges and Daniel suggest that real play can only occur when children are in a relaxed state, the 'social engagement' mode (2017:115). This occurs when the child's central nervous system experiences safety and the absence of threat, enabling the child to be open to social connections. Play therapy can create the conditions to promote this safe environment, by enabling children to explore their experiences in pretend mode (see Chapter 17 by Daniel for a detailed account of polyvagal theory in play therapy). Thus for some children, aggressive behaviours within their play may reflect the activation of their autonomic nervous systems as they seek to integrate past experience. The therapeutic task here is to support the child to explore and represent their experiences within the safety of their play. In this context, we are seeking to support the child to optimise their arousal, extending their 'window of tolerance' (Siegel, 2012:281) whilst benefitting from the security of the therapeutic relationship.

To facilitate this, the play therapist will again rely mostly on playful mirroring to communicate understanding and safety, both within the child's symbolic play and in response to the child's limit-testing behaviour with the therapist. Dion (2015) argues that, within their play, children represent their neurologically hardwired brainstem responses of either fight/flight, characterised by aggression and conflict themes in the play (hyper-arousal), or as freeze/avoidance, leading to helplessness/sleep/death themes within the play (hypo-arousal). Dion suggests that therapists will need to modify their responses to match the arousal of the child's nervous system accordingly. When responding to aggression, it is worth repeating that the therapist's tone and facial expression should match the child's closely, but that the mode of communication and the therapist's active response must be different, so that the child experiences acceptance and recognition, rather than a stimulus that might escalate their aggression.

Case study: Matthew

During the first 6 sessions in the playroom, 6-year-old Matthew, a looked-after child, repeatedly played out scenarios using various wild animals, dinosaurs and monsters. While the characters varied, each story was essentially the same, involving a boy who was constantly in danger from enemies. He introduced a mother figure who came to protect him but became a source of danger, abusing, imprisoning and eventually killing the child. As the therapist, I sought to contain and reflect the extreme emotional themes of this play, including fear and danger, hope for protection and betrayal.

Across 10 sessions, Matthew's play themes continued to reflect his ambivalence about family security and parental caregiving. As the therapist, I made reflections as if I were the child in the play, often relying on my tone and facial expressions to capture my sense of what the play conveyed. For example, 'I just don't know if I can trust that mummy dragon, sometimes she looks after me and sometimes she frightens me'. I also gave my own authentic responses to the play themes: 'I am so worried about this child. Who is going to take care of him?' After some time, Matthew introduced a new protective mother figure into his play, in the shape of a large polar bear, who protected the child consistently from week to week. While the sources of danger remained, there was a noticeable drop in the level of aggression within his play. Matthew also began to take notice of me directly in the session, commenting on my facial expressions and that I was a 'good grown up'. There was a sense in which he was actively becoming aware of the adults around him as a potential resource to help him. His carers reported gradual improvements in his responsiveness within the placement.

Matthew's aggressive play combined elements of traumatic re-enactment and catharsis. At times, it felt difficult to contain the sense of hopelessness and maternal aggression that seemed to represent his lived experience. However, by mirroring the emotional tone of the play, my presence offers safety and emotional acceptance to Matthew, as well as validation through the sharing of my own congruent feelings about the welfare of the children within the play. This seemed to help Matthew achieve some distance from his lived experience and he was able to sustain the play, expressing a range of emotions, whilst developing a new, more hopeful play narrative. In this way, the traumatic aspects of the play were reduced and Matthew began to explore a wider range of feelings.

Limit-setting in play therapy

The provision of therapeutic limits within play therapy is a key mechanism to help the child to remain within their 'window of tolerance' by keeping the play environment safe and secure for both participants. Effective provision of therapeutic boundaries and limits is one of the core competences for BAPT accredited play therapists (Core Competence 22, Appendix 1).

Norton and Norton (2002) suggest that a period of limit-testing is to be expected in most play therapy interventions, as the child explores the trustworthiness of the therapist.

Play therapists often begin and end sessions with a phrase that seeks to convey the permissiveness and consistency of the playroom and relationship. For example, I might say 'Alyssa, this is our time in the playroom. You can do most of what you want to do in here, and if something is not OK, I will let you know'. However, even in this initial limit, practice varies and many therapists would prefer to emphasise permissiveness at this stage. Ray (2011) suggests that introducing limits too early within therapy can activate resistance for children with oppositional or aggressive traits. For me, conveying that the play space is permissive, but boundaries are present, feels authentic and allows children to begin to explore the therapeutic limits of the experience directly.

Landreth (2012) devised what has become a widely used technique for limit-setting within child-centred play therapy with his acronym 'ACT' (2012:273) – in which the child's feelings in the moment are **acknowledged**, the limit on a specific behaviour is clearly **communicated** and an alternative behaviour is identified (**targeted**). For example:

LAURA: *(Unexpectedly starting to throw Velcro balls at my face)* I can throw these really hard.

THERAPIST: You are feeling very strong and want to throw those really hard, but I am not for throwing at … you can throw them hard at that target *(directing her to the back of the door)* if you want to … *(watching her throw)* … You want to throw them as hard as you can.

Significantly, Landreth (2012) emphasises the importance of patience and persistence when setting limits, using this process a **minimum** of three times before escalating further. This sequence forms an important aspect of emotional containment within play therapy by supporting the child to identify their emotion, while also exercising some autonomy over their action. Within my own practice, I have come to value the process of limit-setting as providing an opportunity to work with the child's underlying anxiety – whether it be their need for control arising from a lack of trust, or their destructive impulses emerging from a distorted sense of self.

When children are struggling to accept a limit, I usually add an additional empathic statement at the end of the limit (Cochran et al., 2011). This might include re-stating the child's original feeling or, alternatively, naming a newly emerged emotion in response to the limit being set. By returning to a recognition of the child's emotion after the limit has been set, the sense of shared understanding and acceptance is heightened for most children – for example: 'You're disappointed that

I set that limit, feeling very cross about that'. It is not unusual to have to work hard to repeat and sustain limits for children, particularly in the initial stages of therapy, or as the intervention moves towards termination.

While I will seek to facilitate expressions of aggression within play sequences, it is important to manage direct expressions of aggression towards the room or myself, through careful setting of limits. For example:

Case study: Matthew (continued)

During my early sessions with Matthew, he also tested the limits of the playroom directly through his behaviour. During our play fighting, using foam bats and play swords, Matthew initially sought to inflict pain on me directly, hitting my knuckles and knees hard and invading my personal space. He mocked and belittled me, as well as subjecting me to frequent violent assault and extended death sequences within our play. It felt that he was expressing some profound feelings of rage towards adults in general. Within my responses, I sought to engage with his aggressive play and acknowledge his angry and destructive feelings, whilst setting limits to keep me safe:

'You are really enjoying this fight and feeling very strong … it feels horrible being cut up and killed'. (Reflecting the feeling with my face and tone).

He lunges for my knuckles with his sword – 'You feel so angry, and want to hurt me for real and show me how strong you are – I am not for hurting. You can hit my sword or hit my arm here with the foam bat' (I show him the length of my forearm as a limit) 'but I am not for hurting' (repeating the limit with a calm tone) 'feeling fed up that I won't fight for real' (final empathic reflection).

I needed to repeat this sequence a number of times with Matthew during the first weeks of our play together. Gradually, as he experienced my ability to set and keep limits and my concern for the safety and well-being of us both, his aggression reduced and he accepted the limits of the session more easily.

Some psychodynamic therapists emphasise the importance of providing resistance for children, to enable them to begin to experience a sense of agency and mastery as they push against therapeutic limits (Bellinson, 2009). I have met some children who have tried to beat me into submission, regardless of size, and others who seem floppy and listless, physically underdeveloped in their play. These children may require more than basic limit setting to support their development. McCarthy (2007) discusses the importance of the therapist being strong enough to offer both resistance and at times provocation, to facilitate the child's expression and release of pent up emotional energy. This will also be true for children who demonstrate dissociation or avoidance within their play (Dion, 2015). Levine (2017) discusses the importance of proprioception as a sixth sense, which supports the child's sense of physical self and presence within the world. Engaging energetically in push-pull games such as tug-o'-war or dodge ball with an active child or quietly engaging with the sensory experience of an avoidant or reluctant child to encourage movement and connection, as with Tyrone, are equally crucial aspects of play therapy practice. They support the child's sensory integration and developing sense of their own physical agency, requiring a flexibility in our approach to limit setting.

Both Landreth (2012) and Ray (2011) recognise that initial limits do not always work and that a further step in limit-setting may become necessary, where the child is provided with a choice relating to the limit. Returning to my example with Laura:

THERAPIST: Laura, it's so hard not to throw the balls at me and you are feeling cross about it, but I am not for throwing at … If you choose to throw the balls at me, then you will be choosing not to play with the balls any more today.

Such limits must continue to be offered with acceptance and warmth to the child. I have noted a tendency in many trainee therapists to escalate quickly to this stage of limit setting, driven perhaps by their own anxiety and need to retain control of the situation. There is a temptation to set an 'ultimate limit' of ending the session prematurely, in order to restore our own sense of control and efficacy. However, this really does need to be a last resort and I find I rarely need to do this if I can authentically connect with the child's feelings. Since the therapeutic relationship is the primary vehicle for change in play therapy, it is important to sustain the opportunity for relationship whenever possible.

Therapist's use of self

Offering acceptance in the face of children's aggression and at times overt hostility is challenging. It is important to maintain a deep awareness of our own defences and vulnerabilities, recognising that each of us will find particular issues or types of play challenging and we may need to work hard to maintain appropriate therapeutic limits. It is crucial for play therapists to be continually mindful of their own emotional responses within sessions and to be aware of personal experiences that might trigger transference reactions within the therapy relationship. Particularly when setting final limits for children, there is a danger that our own internal models of behaviour and parenting may intrude on our ability to offer unconditional acceptance and warmth. Additionally, we may have experienced interpersonal trauma, aggression or violence ourselves and will need to have resolved those experiences sufficiently to be able to tolerate exposure to potential triggers within the children's play.

BAPT trained therapists are expected to engage in personal therapy during their professional training and to make use of regular clinical supervision to enable them to reflect on their reactions to children within therapy (BAPT Core Competences 13 and 14, see Appendix 1 and see also other chapters in the volume by McCann and by Platteuw). Through supervision, I also realised I needed to work on my ability to offer resistance and to be an object against which children could push, without triggering punitive or rejecting responses within me. Cochran et al. (2011) remind us that children can also challenge us by being overly compliant or conformist, eager to please or seeking approval, and that we need to be conscious of how these strategies might impact us also.

Ray (2011) highlights the importance of maintaining our own emotional health and developing our ability to sustain empathy and acceptance in the face of aggression and limit-testing. This will require practice and using supervision to reflect on previous experiences that have proved challenging. There appears to be a high level of consistency amongst play therapists on the type of limits viewed as appropriate (Landreth & Wright, 1997), most specifically around limiting aggression towards the therapist and play materials, and managing dangerous or unacceptable behaviour. At a basic level, these limits support the ability of the therapist to maintain the therapeutic conditions for relationship. Norton and Norton (2002) distinguish between absolute limits, common to all therapy processes, and reactive limits, imposed by individual therapists in response to children's particular play to help maintain the therapeutic relationship. These limits will vary widely and are likely to reflect the character and life experiences of both child and adult to some extent. I recall in my early days of training, my own struggle with offering sufficient acceptance of children's highly messy play, particularly when it appeared to be a deliberate act of testing or defiance by the child. I needed to reflect on this experience within my own personal therapy and recognise the connection with the values of my own upbringing. This helped me to become aware of my responses within children's sessions and to begin to offer a greater level of acceptance, eventually taking pleasure in their – and my own – ability to create mess in the playroom.

Ryan and Courtney (2009) have argued for the active use of congruence by the therapist to support the child's understanding of the therapist's emotions and enhance the effectiveness of the relationship. This might involve talking about our own emotional processes and thoughts about the content of the play or the child's behaviour. For example, 'Oh I don't like having balls thrown in my face, it hurts', whilst also acknowledging the child's intent: 'You felt cross, you really wanted to hurt me when you threw that'. Such responses seek to provide the child with feedback about the therapist's experience, building their capacity for empathy and perspective taking, whilst also offering the experience of regulation and acceptance so necessary for play. I have found it particularly effective to also notice moments of heightened enjoyment in the play with the child and to recognise our shared relaxation and pleasure, as a key process for building trust and security in the therapeutic relationship. Dion (2015) also suggests that the therapist comment on their own bodily sensations and responses to support the child's growing awareness of their own physiological arousal, for example, 'I'm feeling hot and my heart is beating fast. I'm going to breathe deeply for a moment'.

As therapists, we need to remain open to challenge about our therapeutic practice and to utilise supervisory relationships to enhance our own self-awareness. Congruence and ongoing reflection are important tools in the process of providing an effective play therapy relationship that will ultimately support the emotional and cognitive development of the child and enable them to understand and manage their feelings more effectively.

Summary

- While children usually develop cognitive and social skills to support the regulation of aggression, adverse life experiences and relationships can undermine healthy development. Persistent aggression tends to be more common amongst these children.
- Play therapy promotes the development of both emotional regulation and neurological integration and can support the development of executive functioning to support new self-management skills.
- Play therapists seek to facilitate the expression of deep emotions, including aggression, within children's play, whilst managing to contain emotions within the therapeutic relationship.
- The use of therapeutic limits within play therapy is one means of promoting safety and creating optimal conditions for the processing of traumatic experiences through play.
- Play therapists must be aware of their own histories and emotional responses and make use of clinical supervision and personal therapy to understand and manage these responses.

Further reading

Crenshaw, D. & Mordock, J. (2005) *Handbook of Play Therapy with Aggressive Children*. Lanham, MD: Jason Aaronson.

A valuable resource integrating theoretical frameworks for understanding aggressive play alongside practical tools and techniques for working with children.

Dion, L. (2015) *Integrating Extremes: Aggression and Death in the Play Room.* New York: Aviva Publishing.

A brief, engaging attempt to integrate learning from neuroscience and trauma with children's fight, flight and freeze responses within their play.

Kestly, T. A. (2014) *The Interpersonal Neurobiology of Play: Brain Building Interventions for Emotional Wellbeing.* New York: W.W. Norton & Co.

Very helpful source for play therapists, which presents complex neuroscience and theories of trauma in a clear and applied way to play therapy processes.

References

Axline, V. (1989) *Play Therapy.* Edinburgh: Churchill Livingstone/Longman.

Badenoch, B. (2008) *Being a Brain-Wise Therapist: Practical Guide to Interpersonal Neurobiology.* New York: W.W. Norton & Co.

Barfield, S., Dobson, C., Gaskell, R. & Perry, B.D. (2012) The neuro-sequential model of therapeutics in a therapeutic preschool: Implications for work with children c with complex neuropsychiatric problems. *International Journal of Play Therapy.* 21(1) pp. 30–44.

Bellinson, J. (2009) You can't do that – Or can you? Historical and clinical perspectives on limit setting in child psychotherapy. *Journal of Infant, Child and Adolescent Psychotherapy.* 8(2) pp. 87–95.

Cochran, J.L., Cochran, N.H., Cholette, A. & Nordling, A.J. (2011) Limits and relationship in child-centred play therapy: Two case studies. *International Journal of Play Therapy.* 20(4) pp. 236–251.

Crenshaw, D. & Mordock, J. (2005) *Handbook of Play Therapy with Aggressive Children.* Lanham, MD: Jason Aaronson.

Dion, L. (2015) *Integrating Extremes: Aggression and Death in the Playroom.* New York: Aviva Publishing.

Doherty, J. & Hughes, M. (2014) *Child Development: Theory and Practice 0-11* (2nd ed.) Harlow: Pearson.

Drewes, A.A. & Schaefer, C.E. (2014) Catharsis. In: Schaefer, C.E. & Drewes, A.A. (eds.) *The Therapeutic Powers of Play.* (2nd ed.) Hoboken, NJ: John Wiley & Sons. pp. 71–83.

Fonagy, P., Gergely, G., Jurist, E.L. & Target, M. (2004) *Affect Regulation, Mentalization and the Development of the Self.* London: Karnac Books.

Foulkrod, K. & Davenport, B.R. (2010) An examination of empirically informed practice within case reports of play therapy with aggressive and oppositional children. *International Journal of Play Therapy.* 19(3) pp. 144–158

Gaskill, R. (2014) Empathy. In: Schaefer, C.E. & Drewes, A.A. (eds.) *The Therapeutic Powers of Play.* (2nd ed.) Hoboken, NJ: John Wiley & Sons. pp. 195–210.

Gil, E. (2011) *Helping Abused and Traumatized Children: Integrating Directive and Nondirective Approaches.* New York: Guilford Press.

Kestly, T.A. (2014) *The Interpersonal Neurobiology of Play: Brain building Interventions for Emotional Wellbeing.* New York: W.W Norton & Co.

Landreth, G.L. & Wright, C.S. (1997) Limit setting practices of play therapists in training and experienced play therapists. *International Journal of Play Therapy.* 6(1), pp. 41 62.

Landreth, G.L. (2012) *Play Therapy: The Art of the Relationship.* (3rd ed.) New York: Routledge.

Levine, P. (2017) Somatic experiencing. In: Daniel, S. & Trevarthen, C. (eds.) *Rhythms of Relating in Children's Therapies.* London: Jessica Kingsley Publishers. pp. 125–140.

McCarthy, D. (2007) *If You Turned into a Monster: Transformation through Play: A Body-Centred Approach to Play Therapy.* London: Jessica Kingsley Publishers.

Norton, C.C. & Norton, B.E. (2002) *Reaching Children through Play Therapy: An Experiential Approach.* (2nd ed.) Denver, CO: White Apple Books.

O'Sullivan, L. & Ryan, V. (2009) Therapeutic limits from an attachment perspective. *Clinical Child Psychology and Psychiatry.* 14(2) pp. 215–235.

Patton, S.C. & Benedict, H.E. (2016) Play therapy with children with attachment disorders. In: O'Connor, K.J., Schaefer, C.E. & Braverman, L.D. (eds.) *Handbook of Play Therapy* (2nd ed.) Hoboken, NJ: John Wiley & Sons. pp. 381–396.

Perry, B. (2007) *The Boy Who Was Raised as a Dog: And Other Stories from a Child Psychiatrist's Notebook – What Traumatized Children Can Teach Us about Life, Loss and Healing.* New York: Basic Books

Porges, S.W. (2011) *The Polyvagal Theory: Neurophysiological Foundations of Emotions, Attachment, Communication, and Self-regulation.* New York: W.W Norton & Co.

Porges, S.W. & Daniel, S. (2017) Play and the dynamics of treating paediatric medical trauma. In: Daniel, S. & Trevarthen, C. (eds.) *Rhythms of Relating in Children's Therapies.* London: Jessica Kingsley Publishers. pp. 113–124.

Ray, D.C., Blanco, P.J., Sullivan, J.M. & Holliman, R. (2009) An exploratory study of child-centered play therapy with aggressive children. *International Journal of Play Therapy.*18(3) pp. 162–175.

Ray, D.C. (2011) *Advanced Play Therapy: Essential Conditions, Knowledge and Skills for Child Practice.* New York: Routledge.

Röll, J., Koglin, U. & Petermann, F. (2012) Emotion regulation and childhood aggression: Longitudinal associations. *Child Psychiatry and Human Development.*43(6) pp. 909–923.

Rogers, C. (1951) *Client Centred Therapy.* London: Constable & Robinson.

Russ, S. (2004) *Play in Child Development and Psychotherapy: Toward Empirically Supported Practice.* Mahwah, NJ: Lawrence Erlbaum Associates.

Ryan, V. & Courtney, A. (2009) Therapists' use of congruence in non-directive play therapy and filial therapy. *International Journal of Play Therapy.* 18(2) pp. 114–128.

Schore, A.N. (2016) *Affect Regulation and the Origin of the Self: The Neurobiology of Emotional Development.* London: Routledge.

Schumann, B. (2010) Effectiveness of child centred play therapy for children referred for aggression. In: Baggerley, J., Ray, D.C. & Bratton, S.C. (eds.) *Child Centred*

Play Therapy Research: The Evidence Base for Effective Practice. Hoboken, NJ: John Wiley & Sons. pp. 194–208.

Siegel, J. (2012) *The Developing Mind: How Relationships and the Brain Interact to Shape Who We Are.* (2nd ed.) New York: Guilford Press.

Stern, D. (1985) *The Interpersonal World of the Infant.* New York: Basic Books.

Chapter 10

Time-limited play therapy

Jenny Reid

Chapter overview

Many play therapists currently work within tight constraints. Financial limitations, waiting lists and organisational policies often limit the number of therapy sessions that can be offered to each child, meaning that therapists are required to work within much more time-limited conditions than they would like, or than they experienced during training. Clinical and ethical decisions have to be made, both in terms of how to manage therapy under these conditions and whether it is advisable to undertake the work at all.

This chapter considers some of the ways in which I have adapted my own practice to work safely and effectively within strict time constraints, and some more general thoughts about offering time-limited play therapy. I will consider the advantages of short-term play therapy, as well as some potential dangers and contraindications to working in this way. I will also offer some alternatives to individual play therapy which might be usefully considered.

Advantages of short-term play therapy

Non-directive play therapy is a child-led approach which can provide a safe, effective and empowering way of supporting children, even within a very few sessions. If a child has a secure attachment style and a basic assumption that adults are trustworthy, this can form the basis for a trusting therapeutic relationship to develop quickly. The therapist can support the child to explore areas of distress and trauma, and to develop increased self esteem, within the safety of this relationship.

Until recently, much of my play therapy work took place within a cancer support centre, where children were offered between four and eight play therapy sessions. My clients there were primarily children who had suffered a recent bereavement or were living with the long-term illness of a family member. The majority of these children exhibited strong resilience factors: most came from loving and supportive families who were able to provide for their physical and emotional needs and who had proactively sought support for them during what they recognised would be a difficult period in their lives. For many of these children, six or eight sessions of play therapy, while far from ideal, could usefully allow them to feel heard and understood. They could begin to share and process their current distress and to develop new coping strategies, helping them to gain some sense of mastery over themselves and their experiences.

A skilled play therapist demonstrates the core conditions outlined by Carl Rogers in his Person-Centred model of therapy (Rogers, 2003). For many children, even a brief experience of this intense acceptance can be extremely powerful. Through the therapist's genuine acceptance of every aspect of them (unconditional positive regard), the child experiences themselves as acceptable, competent, valued and trusted. The therapist's use of empathy allows the child to feel heard and understood, recognising that their emotions are normal, acceptable, and manageable (Landreth, 2012). Just as adults can gain immense relief from realising that they are not alone in their distress, some children are able to internalise this experience in a short time, which can fundamentally alter their self-image.

In many respects, non-directive play therapy is ideally suited to situations where limited time is available. Play provides a direct connection with unconscious processes, bypassing verbal defences and allowing the client to access thoughts and feelings which may not have been brought into conscious awareness. The language of play is also one which is very familiar to children, allowing them to work directly on therapeutic issues without taking the time to learn 'adult' ways of describing their problems and strategies. The child-centred approach ensures that power and control remain with the client throughout; there is no need for them to develop a dependency on the therapist, which might then be ruptured before they are ready. The client is free to develop and adopt new coping strategies to replace those which have become problematic, but their emotional and behavioural defences are not undermined. Additionally, play therapists are skilled in working with endings and boundaries, which form a key part of the therapeutic process for many children. Many therapists use a chart or other pictorial representation to 'count down' the number of sessions remaining; others do this through verbal means. In either case, ample time is allowed to prepare the child or young person for the end of therapy, enabling them to process their feelings in relation to this ending.

Like all person-centred approaches, play therapy involves a fundamental trust in the client's ability to moderate and manage their own experience (Rogers, 2003). It is frequently observed that most children are able to pace themselves in therapy, introducing material only when they feel safe enough. As long as they are given clear information about the duration of the therapy, children will rarely overwhelm themselves with emotions which cannot be sufficiently unpicked and reworked within the time allowed.

In some cases, this means that children will choose not to bring their greatest distress to the playroom. Short-term interventions may focus on increasing the child's self-esteem and self-efficacy, developing solutions to immediate problems such as peer relationships or insomnia, or simply creating a refuge within a turbulent week. Of course, this can create considerable frustration for parents and carers, whose expectation is that the 'real problem' will be actively worked on. In time-limited play therapy, as in any therapeutic intervention, the expectations of adults around the child need to be taken into account, and this will be considered in more detail later.

Case study

Nine-year-old Alice was offered six play therapy sessions while her mother was terminally ill. She worked mostly in the sand tray, creating scenes of an island where animals could live in safety. These images often had a mandala-like quality, featuring concentric circles and increasingly decorated with sparkling 'treasures'. Alice spoke infrequently, appearing peaceful and relaxed, and her parents reported at the end of therapy that she seemed calmer and more able to soothe herself. My hypothesis was that she had internalised the sense of calm and safety which she created in the sand tray, and was able to draw on this when her home life became chaotic and unpredictable.

The end of therapy can also be a powerful trigger for change, and it is a truism among therapists, often described as 'doorknob syndrome', that clients will introduce new material when they know that work is about to finish. Clients may save their most dangerous disclosures for a time when the safety of ending means that they know they will not be pushed to explore these further.

Case study

Billy moved from his birth to his adoptive family at eight months, and came to play therapy at the age of five. His adoptive mother reported controlling, violent and sometimes dangerous behaviour, as well as signs of very low self-esteem. For most of his therapy sessions he acted out violent and dramatic scenes, exploring themes of punishment, power and revenge. After more than six months of work, he spent the last five minutes of his final session nurturing a baby doll, revealing a gentle, caring side which I had not seen during his previous play.

While it is important to have sufficient time to build a therapeutic relationship, significant therapeutic change can take place during the ending phase. Clients in long-term therapy can have something of a 'latency phase' in the middle, where the process settles into a comfortable routine. Time-limited therapy is necessarily more efficient in this regard, bringing the common themes of grief, loss, bereavement, need and insufficiency, anger and rejection into the foreground from the beginning.

Another potential benefit of time-limited work is that it reduces the likelihood of fostering a dependency on the therapist. This is consistent with the person-centred approach in which the child and family are viewed throughout as competent and self-sufficient. The therapist provides the optimum conditions for growth and change, but the real work is done by the child. The planned end of therapy indicates the therapist's confidence that the child can continue this self-guided work. Play therapy, in this context, is seen not as an ongoing support structure but as a gentle nudge in the right direction. A past supervisor suggested to me that I think of each period of therapy as a piece of work, rather than the whole work – meaning that I needed to let go of the idea that my intervention would 'save' a child or family. I had to learn to focus more on the positive in the child's life, and on the small changes which I could hope to effect through my intervention.

Contraindications

There are some situations where time-limited play therapy is not appropriate. All of the examples given so far assume that the child is in a place of safety, essentially able to self-regulate, and has carers who support the work that is taking place.

Children who are extremely dysregulated may not be able to keep themselves safe within the therapeutic process, or to hold back traumatic material which cannot be safely processed in the time allowed. For children with complex trauma, the painful memories may emerge despite the child's efforts, and a therapeutic ending might then be experienced as premature and rejecting, regardless of the way this was planned. A longer play therapy intervention might well be the ideal approach in these cases, as children can learn over time to gain mastery of their experiences and to re-process traumatic memories through sensory and narrative play in order to store them in more conscious areas of the brain (O'Connor et al., 2016). If longer-term work is not an option, therapists might consider more trauma-specific approaches to therapy, such as EMDR (Eye Movement Desensitisation Reprocessing), where the trauma can be addressed directly and consciously and contained within a clear structure (see Chapter 18 by May for more on EMDR).

Children with insecure or disorganised attachments (Ainsworth, 2015) are likely to take a lot longer to trust the therapist. Some children may still be able to make use of short-term therapy to self regulate and build resilience. Mooli Lahad (2013) recommends that long-term therapeutic interventions focus on rectifying the client's weaknesses, while short-term interventions amplify their strengths. It is my experience that a non-directive approach will often follow this approach naturally, particularly with anxious or highly-defended clients. Children often approach a new challenge such as that of the playroom by remaining 'in their comfort zone', applying the skills with which they feel most confident. This makes it easy for us, as therapists, to recognise and reinforce those skills through reflection and self-esteem-building statements (Landreth, 2012), increasing the child's confidence in their own self-efficacy.

However, some ambivalently attached children have a strong need to test boundaries during therapy, including testing the therapist's commitment and willingness to accept them. If therapy ends before the child has moved beyond this phase, they are likely to experience this as rejection, reinforcing their belief that they are unlovable or that adults are untrustworthy.

My experience of working with children who are extremely mistrustful is that boundaries need to be very clear, strong, and containing. For some children, this may mean that the relative freedom of non-directive play therapy is too frightening to be supportive in the short term, and that more directive techniques such as Theraplay[1] (Booth, 2010) or CBT (Fuggle et al., 2012) based approaches are more useful if long term work is not possible.

The question of whether to work with children who are not living safely is a dilemma facing any therapist, but I would argue that this applies particularly strongly to those offering only short-term interventions. There can be an argument that a longer-term piece of work could build the child's resilience and potentially work to change the systemic factors which are placing the child at risk, as well as providing the child with a model of an adult who is warm, available and trustworthy. However, short-term interventions cannot really offer any of these benefits, and so resources are likely to be better spent on practical interventions.

Special considerations

If time-limited work is to be undertaken, the play therapist may want to modify their approach somewhat. One practical adaptation which therapists might consider is to change the frequency of appointments. Traditionally, play therapy has been offered weekly, and most trainees on BAPT-accredited courses use this model. During my work at the cancer support centre, however, I found that most clients benefited from fortnightly sessions, allowing the therapy to extend over a longer period. Children grow emotionally and practice new behaviours between therapy sessions, and allowing longer for these changes to take root can be beneficial. Less frequent sessions are also less likely to create dependency, as contact with the therapist does not become part of the child's regular support structure. This in turn reduces the sense of loss and possible abandonment when therapy ends.

For children seen in private practice, where parents are paying directly for therapy, this option can also be made available. Offering fortnightly sessions reduces the financial impact on parents, which in turn may reduce stress in the household and help parents to feel positive about the therapist. It may also enable some families to budget for a longer intervention so that the number of sessions offered is actually increased. Of course, there are also some disadvantages, particularly in relation to very young children who may have difficulty retaining memories from one session to the next, or to very anxious children who are not able to maintain a sense of safety between appointments. An open discussion with parents about these dilemmas would form part of my initial meeting.

Work around boundaries, limit-setting and developing self control can be an important theme of play therapy under any circumstances (see also Chapter 9 by Ayling), but these become particularly crucial in short-term work. Providing clear, consistent boundaries reduces children's need to test the limits of the therapy room (Landreth, 2012). For some children, the permissiveness of play therapy can be unnerving, and a therapist might decide to hold tighter boundaries than usual in order to give a greater sense of security for short term work. For example, while some children enjoy and benefit from the opportunity to make mess in play therapy, others find this disorientating and are more able to relax when the rules are more similar to those they have experienced at home or school.

Working with families and systems

Play therapy is essentially a systemic approach, engaging parents and other caregivers to increase their understanding of, and ability to meet, the child's emotional needs, as reflected in BAPT Core Competence 7: Knowledge and practice of working with parents/carers (see Appendix 1). This is particularly important in short term interventions.

Children use 'social referencing' (Walden & Ogan, 1988) to determine whether or not an adult is trustworthy, so time spent building a trusting alliance with parents or carers can help to establish a trusting therapeutic relationship from the outset.

It is important to establish clear expectations, both in terms of the likely outcomes of therapy and the process itself. Parents are frequently heard in the waiting room telling children to 'have fun' or 'be good', and these suggestions can inhibit a child's free expression of the emotions which they most urgently need to process. Within our practice, we have a 'checklist' for parents re-uniting with their children after therapy which reminds them that the session may have been difficult, painful or thought-provoking. We encourage them to follow their child's lead in re-establishing contact in the way which feels right to them at the time – whether this means having a quiet cuddle and a biscuit, talking about the therapy session, or running around to discharge emotions and reconnect with their body.

Time spent discussing the aims and likely outcomes of therapy can be extremely valuable to both parents and therapists, and is an essential component of BAPT Core Competence 19: Planning and contracting for play therapy practice (see Appendix 1). To practice ethically, the therapist needs to recognise the limits of their ability to help the family and to provide realistic expectations. The therapist also demonstrates integrity in this way, enabling them to form a genuine and trusting relationship with the family. A child who displays difficult or worrying behaviours is likely to elicit a sense of urgency in the parents, who may find it very difficult to recognise small changes. A detailed initial assessment and a frank, congruent discussion of the limitations of therapy set the groundwork for a review which can highlight any improvements in the child's mood, behaviour and relationships. Therapists might want to draw on a solution focused (Ratner, 2012) or motivation interviewing (Herman et al., 2014) influenced approach with parents, drawing attention to positive changes in order to promote hope that these will continue. The therapist can also adopt an advocacy role, recommending specific changes through which parents, schools and others can better meet the child's needs in the longer term.

Managing parents' expectations can help to contain frustration, reduce their potential sense of anger with or betrayal by the therapist, and increase the likelihood that they will continue to seek support in the future, as well as reducing the likelihood that they will undermine the child's progress by criticising the therapeutic process. An extreme example of this, which can be beneficial in some situations, is to treat the entire intervention as an extended assessment. I have found this particularly helpful in situations where parents were concerned that there was 'something wrong' with their child. Framing the therapeutic work as an assessment of the child's needs and functioning can remove some of the urgency, reassure parents that their concerns are being taken seriously, and gently introduce the idea that change might take longer than they have anticipated. Any positive change is then viewed as a 'bonus' – the focus moves from the failures of therapy to 'cure' the child to the positive gains which have been made, for which the child might be allowed to take credit.

Case study

Chloe was a five-year-old girl whose parents were concerned about highly controlling behaviours, as well as some evidence of sensitivity in relation to clothing, food and other textures. They asked me to meet her with the hope of exploring the reasons for her behaviour, and possibly recommending a referral to the local NHS child development and neurodisability service. I met Chloe for eight sessions of non-directive play therapy, during which she explored her complex emotional response to mess and dirt and her ability to tolerate failure. Her parents requested feedback regarding my assessment of her functioning. During our review meeting,

however, they described improvements in her mood and overall functioning, particularly in school, leading them to conclude independently that
there was no need for any further intervention.

In some situations, a decision might be made to work entirely with the
parents. With young children in particular, having a parent present in the
room can help to establish a sense of safety more quickly, enabling the
child to address the issues which are most pressing and to take greater
risks than they might otherwise. With sufficient briefing, the parent is able
to observe the therapist's child-centred approach, reflections of the child's
feelings, and supportive limit-setting. Many consequently begin to adapt
their own responses both within and outside the sessions. The parent also
has the opportunity to experience the child's therapeutic play and to process this experience with the support of the therapist, and so can reach
a deeper understanding of their child's needs and behaviours than would
otherwise be possible.

Where resources, policies and the therapist's skills allow, filial therapy
(VanFleet, 2014) can be offered as an alternative to one-to-one play therapy. Landreth and Bratton's (2006) model of Child Parent Relationship
Therapy (CPRT) is particularly designed and validated by research as providing a relatively short-term, cost-effective way of engaging parents in
therapeutic play with their own children, creating the possibility of long-
term change. This approach takes advantage of peer support within
a group, and we have found in our practice that we are able to offer the
complete programme for approximately the same price as an eight-session
play therapy intervention with assessment and review meetings. (See Chapter 20 by Cowper for a more detailed discussion of the CPRT approach.)

Use of working hypotheses

Play therapists are accustomed to generating working hypotheses and using
these to inform practice (Wilson & Ryan, 2005). While this should be
a constant and conscious process in any therapeutic work, it is particularly
crucial in time-limited therapy for the therapist to remain alert and reflective,
revising their hypotheses continually to ensure that their decisions create the
optimum conditions for each child to make use of the therapeutic space.

As person-centred therapists, we endeavour to maintain the core conditions of empathy, congruence, and unconditional positive regard (Rogers,
2003), allowing these to inform all of our interactions with our clients.
Within this framework, however, we may relate to our clients on different
levels, or in different modes, depending on context. During assessments
and reviews, we are actively gathering information and might ask more
questions usual. In preparation for review, we are likely to take more of an
overview of the therapeutic process, perhaps remaining less than usual

within the metaphor of the child's play and offering more of our understanding. At the end of each session, and when setting other boundaries, we temporarily take control and direct the client towards acceptable behaviours.

In time-limited therapy, we can also call upon these 'alternative modes' to help to move the therapeutic process forwards and avoid becoming stuck. Gardner and Yasenik (2012) advocate a conscious decision-making process, the Dimensions Model, in which the therapist moves actively between conscious and unconscious, directive and non-directive modes of interaction with the child.

Early goal-setting with the client can be useful, and this process parallels the way in which we are likely to relate during the review process. It is important for both therapist and client to have a clear and, ideally, shared understanding of the purpose of the sessions. Part of my introduction is likely to include an overview of their situation and the presenting problems. I may then solicit their views, as in the following example:

> Your mum has asked me to meet you because you are still so sad about losing your nan, and you're finding it difficult to concentrate in school. She's also hoping that play therapy will help you to fall asleep more easily at night. I wonder whether those are the things that worry you as well, or whether there are other things that you would like to change through coming here?

This is an integral part of the BAPT Core Competences 18 (Assessment of need) and 19 (Planning and contracting for play therapy practice), as well as contributing to Engagement and facilitation of a therapeutic relationship (Core Competence 17, see Appendix 1).

Sharing additional information which I have been given by carers, as well as demonstrating a level of transparency which helps to build a trusting rapport, can help the child to feel at ease and allow them to access activities which feel safe and familiar. In short-term work, and where the child is able to tolerate this, it may be beneficial for the therapist to move more quickly into a more explicit mode of reflection which keeps the play firmly grounded in the child's daily experience.

In some situations, the therapist might also offer specific directive techniques. This deviation from the non-directive model requires considerable reflection, as it risks undermining the confidence which is placed in the child's own ability to determine the course of therapy and to find solutions. However, if a child is particularly anxious or finding it very difficult to engage in play, offering a brief directed exercise can provide a solution to a specific problem or a doorway to more creative expression. It would be unethical to allow a child to suffer through several sessions of very anxious and disjointed play in the knowledge that this is likely to form the majority of their experience of therapy.

Case study

Dinah was nine, and reported that she had felt tense and anxious since the death of her mother the previous year. Dinah had close and supportive relationships with her brother and step-father, who was now her sole carer. She sat opposite me on a chair, swinging her legs, and asked me to help her to sleep better. She spent the remainder of her first session in the chair, talking to me about her experiences at school and her close friendship with her brother. She occasionally glanced around the room at the toys and other materials available. I commented on this tentative interest, but she did not feel able to leave her chair.

In the second session, I offered Dinah the option of a guided visualisation exercise, which she enthusiastically agreed to try. She fixed her gaze on the wall while I talked her through a body-based relaxation, ending by focusing on her breathing, and then suggested that she picture herself walking along a path and into a garden. After the exercise was completed and I encouraged her to return her attention to the room, Dinah smiled. She spent the remainder of the session painting a picture.

Dinah repeated the visualisation exercise at the beginning of each of her remaining two sessions. The process took approximately ten minutes, after which she began to engage with the symbolic materials in the room to work through her anxieties. She made particular use of the paints and the sand tray, once depicting the 'worry tree' from her visualisation. This became an important symbol of her resilience.

I have also used Lahad's Six-Part Story Test (Lahad, 2013) both as an assessment framework, to add to my knowledge and hypotheses about a child, and as a therapeutic tool. I have found the structure and boundaries of the exercise invaluable in beginning to work symbolically with children and young people who are either unable to begin to engage with the sessions, or who are very 'stuck' in a rational verbal means of communication which prevents them from engaging emotionally with their therapeutic needs or from accessing new solutions. It can be particularly useful for older children and teenagers as it provides a bridge between the kind of structured work which they are used to doing at school and the imaginative freedom which can be so beneficial in therapy. Young people who might feel patronised or alienated by 'children's' toys are able to engage readily with pen and paper.

This exercise is introduced and processed using the therapist's usual skills. Empathy is demonstrated towards the child or young person, reflecting their process in making the story and their feelings about what they have produced. Empathy can also be shown towards the characters in the story, and the therapist might want to express congruent feelings about the events which are portrayed. Many children in my experience then move on to play in other ways or to draw and paint spontaneous pictures of their own.

A non-directive therapist does not usually provide information, as therapists are careful not to be seen as 'experts' by the child but to help the child to uncover their own expertise. In short-term work, however, a small amount of information-giving can greatly enhance the client's immediate and longer term wellbeing. Psychoeducation can fulfil a number of functions, providing information about the working of the brain and effect of emotions on the body, exploring social clues, and offering guidance around emotional safety and wellbeing.

Part of the role of a play therapist is to advocate for children and ensure that their needs are heard. It is vital that we continue to campaign for better services, and to highlight the need for adequate mental health support for children and young people. At the same time, I believe that even short play therapy interventions can be very effective for a large number of children, and that it is our responsibility to provide children with the best service we are able within the resources available.

Summary

This chapter has explored:

- Advantages of non-directive play therapy as a short term intervention
- Considerations of when play therapy might not be appropriate for short-term work
- Modifying the play therapy approach for short-term interventions
- Involving families and systems to support time-limited play therapy
- Use of working hypotheses to ensure that play therapists work ethically and effectively in the short term.

Note

1 Theraplay is a registered service mark of The Theraplay Institute, Evanston, IL, USA.

Further reading

Gardner, K. & Yasenik, L. (2012) *Play Therapy Dimensions Model: A Decision-Making Guide for Integrative Play Therapists*. London: Jessica Kingsley Publishers.
Gardner and Yasenik provide a robust model for therapists to analyse and amend their interactions during play therapy, allowing children to take the maximum therapeutic benefit at any moment.
Landreth, G.L. (2012) *Play Therapy: The Art of the Relationship* (3rd ed.). London: Routledge.
Garry Landreth's faith in the power of the therapeutic relationship and the ability of children to find their own way, provides a valuable anchor against the anxiety and competing priorities which can cause us to doubt our gentle approach.

References

Ainsworth, M.D.S. (2015) *Patterns of Attachment* (Psychology Press & Routledge Classic Editions). London: Routledge.

Booth, P.B. & Jernberg, A.M. (2010) *Theraplay: Helping Parents and Children Build Better Relationships through Attachment-Based Play.* San Francisco: Wiley.

Fuggle, P., Dunsmuir, S. & Curry, V. (2012) *CBT with Children, Young People and Families.* Los Angeles: Sage Publications.

Gardner, K. & Yasenik, L. (2012) *Play Therapy Dimensions Model: A Decision-Making Guide for Integrative Play Therapists.* London: Jessica Kingsley Publishers.

Herman, K.C., Reinke, W.M., Frey, A. & Shepard, S. (2014) *Motivational Interviewing in Schools: Strategies for Engaging Parents, Teachers and Students.* New York: Springer Publishing.

Lahad, M. (2013) *The Basic Ph Model of Coping and Resiliency: Theory, Research and Cross-Cultural Application.* London: Jessica Kingsley Publishers.

Landreth, G.L. (2012) *Play Therapy: The Art of the Relationship* (3rd ed.). London: Routledge.

Landreth, G.L. & Bratton, S.C. (2006) *Child Parent Relationship Therapy (CPRT): A 10-Session Filial Therapy Model.* London: Routledge.

O'Connor, K.J., Schaefer, C.E. & Braverman, L.D. (2016) *Handbook of Play Therapy* (2nd ed.). London: Wiley.

Ratner, H. (2012) *Solution Focused Brief Therapy.* London: Routledge.

Rogers, C. (2003) *Client Centred Therapy: Its Current Practice, Implications and Theory.* London: Robinson.

VanFleet, R. (2014) *Filial Therapy: Strengthening Parent-Child Relationships through Play* (3rd ed.). Sarasota: Professional Resource Press.

Walden, T.A. & Ogan, T.A. (1988) The development of social referencing. *Child Development.* 59 (5). pp. 1230–1240.

Wilson, K. & Ryan, V. (2005) *Play Therapy: A Non-Directive Approach for Children and Adolescents* (2nd ed.). London: Elsevier.

Part III

Play therapy in practice

Chapter 11

Play therapy within a CAMHS setting

Ruth Lazarus and Carrie Waldron

Chapter overview

This chapter will discuss the work of play therapists working in multidisciplinary Child and Adolescent Mental Health Services (CAMHS) teams and the challenges they face. We will consider how play therapists seem to offer something unique within CAMHS, in helping children and adolescents process the unconscious, sensory or bodily experience of trauma. This includes work with those who have experienced this pre-verbally, including developmental, attachment-related trauma. We will discuss the types of referral within CAMHS that tend to be referred to play therapists and argue that we are successful at engaging and maintaining engagement with these children, when other 'talking therapies' might fail. We present two case studies to illustrate play therapy practice within this context.

Who are we and what do we do?

By nature, Child and Adolescent Mental Health Service (CAMHS) teams are multidisciplinary (Dogra, 2017). CAMHS teams tend to include Psychology, Psychiatry, Nursing, Therapies including Systemic, Creative Art and Psychotherapy, Primary Mental Health Workers and Participation Workers, who directly represent young people's views. Historically such teams have been thought of as providing a comprehensive approach to understanding children and adolescent mental health needs (Padmore, 2015). They also consist of highly qualified practitioners who can offer specialist ways of working. Within individual teams, this allows for each professional modality to contribute their distinct knowledge base to individual cases, whilst finding collaboration and shared understanding between them. As a result, there can be lively debate about what the 'right' thing to do in each case might be.

The National Institute for Health and Care Excellence (NICE) (www.nice.org.uk) set out clinical pathways to steer decisions about treatment plans within CAMHS teams. Fonagy et al. (2014) have summarised the existing evidence in child and adolescent mental health treatment, to inform clinical decision-making and funding choices. In so doing, they present play therapists with a challenge to embed ourselves as a profession within the statutory context. Although there is international recognition of the benefits of play therapy to treat child and adolescent mental health, (Baggerly, Ray & Bratton, 2010; Lin & Bratton, 2015) as a profession, play therapy is not yet recognised as having a sufficiently robust research evidence base to feature in the NICE Guidelines. Notwithstanding, play therapy seems to be alive and well in many CAMHS teams across the United Kingdom. From our experience, and from the views expressed by children and young people within CAMHS participation groups, there is a growing preference for using creative ways of supporting children and for a less 'clinical' approach.

However, play therapy provision within CAMHS teams remains inconsistent, and play therapy in the UK remains an evolving profession, without the recognition that other treatment modalities have already established. Establishing this for the first time requires tenacity, resilience and support from the play therapy community. There are also more practical challenges such as negotiating appropriate child-centred spaces, working in noise- and mess-friendly buildings and being able to offer the consistency and length of treatment necessary for effective therapeutic play interventions (Lin & Bratton, 2015).

As CAMHS practitioners, we are expected to assume both generic and specialist roles (Dogra, 2017; Padmore, 2015). Generic work includes completing initial assessments and follow up, case co-ordination for children and adolescents awaiting specialist intervention, completing risk assessments and management plans, creating and reviewing care plans and completing outcome measures. We also engage in liaison and consultation with the professional network and schools, contributing to multidisciplinary discussion, team meetings and in-house training. CAMHS practitioners are also expected to fulfil roles related to being on duty, such as screening and triaging new referrals, responding to crises on open cases, consulting with other professionals and family members on new referrals and contributing to assessments following admission to Accident and Emergency departments, due to mental health needs such as suicidal ideation, self-harm or substance misuse. Our specialist work includes assessing for and providing therapeutic interventions, managing the waiting list for those interventions, in addition to the generic tasks of each case. Training as a play therapist prepared us for the specialist work, however learning about the tasks associated with the generic CAMHS work was acquired 'on the job' by shadowing more experienced colleagues and reflective learning in supervision.

Within CAMHS nationally, outcome measures are an integral aspect of the work, promoting efficacy and effectiveness (Padmore, 2015). Some of the measures most commonly used are: Strengths and Difficulties Questionnnaire (SDQ), Goodman, 2001), Child Outcome Rating Scales (CORS), Miller et al., 2003) and Child Experience of Service Questionnaire (CHI-ESQ), Brown et al., 2014). Within our own CAMHS team, we have also developed a specific evaluation tool called 'Bullseye' that aims to generate conversation and reflection about the clinical sessions a child or adolescent experiences in the service. In terms of evaluating specialist play therapy interventions these current measures present a challenge, as they do not naturally fit with a child-centred approach, although the conversations they evoke can elicit information which otherwise might not be available to play therapists. Within our specific CAMHS teams there have been attempts to develop some ideas about a more child-centred evaluation tool. For example, Jäger has developed a model of play based evaluations (Jäger, 2013) that has been met with much enthusiasm and regard by play therapists nationally. Such evaluation of play therapy outcomes and effectiveness is one of the core competences of play therapy practice (Core Competence 31, see Appendix 1).

Play therapists can occupy a variety of posts within CAMHS. For example, some practitioners find themselves in a primary mental health worker post, within which they can practice play therapy. Others may be employed in a more direct play therapy or creative arts therapy post. As authors, we recognised that our own employment within CAMHS differs. Ruth began her employment in CAMHS as a primary mental health worker, based mainly in schools, before being employed in a substantive post as a play therapist in a Tier 3 generic team. Carrie was employed as a specialist CAMHS practitioner in a Tier 3 generic team, offering play therapy as her specialism. It is important to note that within the structure of CAMHS there is potential for development, both as a practitioner and for influencing others' practice more generally. For example, one of Ruth's roles at CAMHS is Chair of an arts and play therapy practice network that involves advising on standards of employment of creative arts therapies in the service and maintaining their professional registration requirements.

Over the period of our employment, we have reflected on how our roles have changed and this seems to reflect a wider cultural shift within CAMHS as a whole. In our generic Tier 3 teams, there seems to be a move away from specialism, towards an emphasis on shared generalist skills. We are now expected to spend more of our time fulfilling generic duties and this is prioritised over specialist work. There is also a move towards more symptom-specific care pathways with potentially shorter-term treatment. These trends can present dilemmas for us within our therapeutic roles. We recognise this to be a response to the ever-increasing demands on CAMHS services that has been well documented over the past few years, with high thresholds for accessing services and lengthy waiting lists in many areas (Campbell, 2016b; Matthews-King, 2017). Within the UK, a recent Care Quality Commission (CQC, 2017) review identifies how fragmented CAMHS services have become. Arguably, the demands have further increased due to a greater awareness of mental health and willingness to seek help more generally in society. These challenges mean that children and adolescents may experience long waits, sometimes of over a year, for specialist services such as play therapy.

The following clinical example illustrates a child's journey through the CAMHS system and with a play therapist in particular.

Claudia: meetings at the Sweet Lemon café

Referral information

Claudia was 7 years old when we first met for a CAMHS 'Choice' appointment (initial assessment) with her father and step-mother. It was the winter and Claudia arrived wrapped in multiple layers of clothing. I wondered what she was protecting herself from apart from the weather. The GP made the referral due to concerns about anxiety with obsessive compulsive behaviours in the context of a 'very difficult start to life' including an acrimonious 'legal tug of war between the separated parents for care of their children'. The referral had been considered by colleagues at triage and accepted as in need of initial assessment. The average wait time for play therapy, post initial assessment, was around 8 months due to the demands on capacity and an emphasis on more generic work, as described earlier.

During the initial assessment, I learned that Children's Services had placed Claudia and her twin brother Stephen with their father 18 months previously. The children had been abandoned at school by their mother and cared for by their childminder for 4 months before moving to the care of their father and step-mother. A number of older half-siblings had remained living with their mother. There had been no contact between the children, their mother or maternal relations since placement. There were significant mental health difficulties on both sides of the family.

The concerns about Claudia were reported as her extreme levels of anxiety, fears of illness and rejection, a sense of worthlessness, preoccupation with her clothing including constantly changing her clothes, touching her genital area and complaining of discomfort, with no physical cause identified. Claudia and Stephen were said to be sexually inappropriate with each other and also very rivalrous. Dad later shared that Stephen had recently disclosed sexual abuse by his half-brother, whilst living with their mother. They believed that Claudia had not been sexually abused, but that her twin was acting out what was done to him in their sexualised play. A social worker had become involved; the children were placed on a family support plan. I advised Claudia, her father and step-mother that I would talk to the multi-disciplinary team (MDT) about how best we might help.

I discussed my initial assessment with the MDT and we agreed that play therapy would be the most appropriate therapeutic approach for Claudia. There is growing recognition that play therapy is a developmentally appropriate intervention for children. Play is recognised as the primary means of communicating and expressing feelings, experiences and inner conflicts (Landreth, 2012). Naderi et al. (2010) have supported the value of play therapy in addressing anxiety and hyperactivity disorders, while Gaskill and Perry (2014) propose that play therapy can help children to develop emotional self-regulation and promote the integration of traumatic experience.

I spoke to Claudia's parents about the proposed care plan and confirmed my assessment and plan in writing to them and the GP. When I had capacity to start, I arranged to visit Claudia at home to introduce the work. We agreed to start with six play therapy sessions and then review.

Play therapy process

At the first session, Claudia would not take off her coat but immediately engaged in play. She used animal puppets to tell stories of being under threat (including animals who attacked others in the same pack and gobbled each other up), destruction and revenge. Claudia played hard throughout the session and introduced me to the truly catastrophic nature of the threats, telling me 'it was as if the sky was falling down'. In the second session Claudia introduced a role play of running a restaurant which she called the Sweet Lemon Café. This became a regular meeting place in our play until the conclusion of therapy: somewhere we were able to explore multiple themes together.

In the early sessions, I was directed to play a customer, bringing my two children to the café. Claudia instructed me on how I should play the role. The children were described as unwell, not eating or sleeping well, having bad dreams, screaming in their sleep. They saw their daddy at weekends and had babysitters that needed to be properly checked. By session five, Claudia had developed some trust in our relationship and confidence to play the mum role herself. Claudia played herself as a caring mum, telling me there was another customer in the restaurant who was hitting and hurting her children. My attempts, within the play, to stop this were ineffective: Claudia repeated over and over the various ways the children were being mistreated which, she wanted me to know, could not be stopped. I was to witness the various ways children are harmed by their parents and carers. Claudia played all her own roles as someone who was exceptionally good, skilled and perfect in all they did.

After six sessions I held a review with Claudia and her parents, making time to speak to the parents alone. Claudia continued to show high anxiety in school, was selectively mute and not making academic progress. We agreed to continue sessions with reviews scheduled after every eight sessions. In addition to therapy reviews, I attended and contributed to the multi-disciplinary family support meetings called by Children's Services.

Claudia gradually began to shed the layers of clothing in the playroom, becoming fully engaged in choosing to dress up for roles at the Sweet Lemon Café. During the second sequence of eight sessions I was introduced to Spike. Claudia told me Spike was a monster who lived in her brain and told her to do terrible things: if she didn't, he would kill her. Spike was said to suck the blood of elephants and other animals. She could only control him if she was quiet and kept to herself. Night times in particular were difficult: Claudia was scared of Spike when trying to sleep.

As Claudia increasingly gave Spike a voice in the play room, she gained confidence. Claudia's parents were at first frightened by Spike and questioned if this was an indicator of psychosis. I encouraged them to think of Spike as a means for Claudia to communicate and externalise un-expressed feelings of rage and distress and for them to listen, accept and contain her expressions. As they were able to do this, Claudia's confidence continued to grow. After 9 months of weekly play therapy sessions (around 30 sessions) Claudia was consistently described as emotionally calm and settled, making academic progress and we agreed to end therapy.

Following an 8 month gap, I was asked to recommence sessions with Claudia. The children had become subject to child protection plans due to concerns of emotional neglect. I attended child protection case conference (CPCC) reviews, while continuing to hold therapy reviews. Claudia continued to make good progress, using sessions fully, managing school, making academic progress, joining the school council and attending a school trip to France. Claudia had one remaining goal, to ask her mother 'why she had left them'. Claudia asked me to help her talk to her mum and we arranged a final meeting in order that Claudia could do this. This was our last session together.

Reflection

There appear to be two key factors that enabled Claudia's therapeutic change. Firstly, the ability to explore traumatic experiences safely through role-play, allowing her symbolic distance (Gil, 2011). Claudia's introduction of Spike within her play seemed particularly important in this respect, providing a direct embodied expression for her feelings. The second factor was my ability to work with both Claudia and the systems around her, responding to changing needs throughout her CAMHS journey. Ryan (2004) suggests that for children who are looked-after by the local authority who may have attachment difficulties or have experienced abuse, consultation with the professional and familial network is an integral part of therapy practice. This is recognised within the BAPT core competences, which emphasise the therapist's ability to work with the professional system around the child (Core Competence 28, see Appendix 1).

So ... who do we see and why?

Referrals can come to us through different routes. Sometimes we will be asked to complete an initial 'Choice' assessment, as we have the appropriate skills and understanding for that particular referral. In these cases, we often continue working with the child, adolescent and family for the specialist therapeutic work. At other times, cases are discussed with us at the multi-disciplinary team meeting (MDT), following the initial assessment or a previous intervention.

Over time, we have developed our colleagues' understanding of the sorts of referrals that would be appropriate for play therapy interventions, by building close working relationships with other professional groups and through attending multi-disciplinary meetings which decide appropriate care pathways or involve complex case reflective discussions. We have also given presentations on play therapy cases in team meetings and provided training to wider professional networks. Within our teams, we seem to have developed a reputation for being able to build relationships with 'difficult to engage' populations, both in terms of children and adolescents and their family systems. We have also noticed some patterns regarding the types of referrals made to us and why.

Children and adolescents referred for assessments for neuro-developmental disorders such as Attention Deficit Hyperactivity Disorder, or Autism Spectrum Condition

Of this group, some are referred immediately for play therapy interventions without further neuro-developmental assessment, because issues of trauma, attachment or other interpersonal and environmental factors play a larger part in their presentation. Alternatively, some are referred after the neuro-developmental assessment has been completed, and they have either fulfilled the diagnostic criteria, or not. There is growing evidence in the literature to support play therapy practice with children and adolescents who have fulfilled the diagnostic criteria for a neuro-developmental disorder (Naderi et al., 2010; Bratton et al., 2005). Furthermore, Gaskill and Perry (2014) argue that, increasingly, neuro-developmental disorders are identified within children who have also experienced maltreatment or neglect, making it problematic to accurately assess the underlying origin of the child's difficulty. We find that these children are often able to make use of the non-directive therapeutic space that we provide.

Children and adolescents who have experienced attachment and/or developmental trauma or other traumatic events

This group comprises a large proportion of our longer-term caseload. Some of this group are identified early on in their journey through CAMHS while others have received other therapeutic modalities which have had limited success, before being referred for play therapy. There is also a strong literature base demonstrating the efficacy of play therapy in supporting children with attachment difficulties (Malchiodi & Crenshaw, 2014; Patton & Benedict, 2016). Gaskill and Perry (2014) suggest that early trauma and attachment disruptions adversely affect children's neurological development and may result in impulsive, globally dysregulated children. They argue that such children are less able to make use of cognitive-behavioural or cognitive-relational interventions but rather need to access other forms of treatment that support the neurological development of their lower brain networks. Play therapists can support such development through our use of child-led, rhythmic, patterned, sensory play activities, including music, singing, dance and shared play.

Children and adolescents who prefer non-verbal communication

This group includes younger aged children who are often referred automatically to us, given their natural preference for play. Also included are children and adolescents who present as selectively mute, traumatised and psychologically disassociated. Additionally, many adolescents find it difficult to verbalise their distress or emotional world in verbal conversation. Play therapy can offer a unique and deeply effective approach to working with the complexity of such cases (Fernandez & Sugay, 2016; Singhal & Mehrotra, 2014). The work meets the child or adolescent on an emotional, sensory and non-verbal level where trauma is often held and transforms this into a more explicit form that can then be explored in the metaphor. The metaphor allows symbolic distance for the child or adolescent, enabling them to make sense of their experience safely and at their own pace.

The following case study illustrates the use of play therapy with a child who fits within all three of these categories. She was referred to CAMHS for a neuro-developmental assessment, there were identified trauma and attachment difficulties and she preferred non-verbal communication.

Barefoot Hannah

Referral information

I first met Hannah and her Mum in the CAMHS waiting area three years ago. She was a slim, blonde-haired, blue-eyed 6-year-old, standing barefoot in a onesie. She refuses to wear anything else. And she refuses to wear shoes. Hannah scowled at me and refused to respond to my warm, open welcome. I felt like she was warning me to 'be careful!' and 'beware!' all at once. In the assessment, her mother seemed overwhelmed with how life was with Hannah. She described how Hannah behaved aggressively and impulsively and made frequent threats to hurt and kill others, including specifically named peers. There was huge concern with how Hannah chose to communicate these threats, as she would draw graphic pictures of harming and killing children in her class. Her mother spoke of Hannah's physical attacks at home and that these often seemed pre-meditated. At the same time, Hannah seemed to experience significant anxiety around her attachments, particularly with her mother. There was a distinct inter-dependence between Hannah and Mum. Hannah was unable to be without Mum, either physically or psychologically, and her mother described how she felt 'she couldn't breathe with Hannah.'

Hannah was also unable to manage any kind of change or challenge to her 'world order' and maintained a very concrete view of the world. Hannah struggled with some obsessive compulsions and behaviours. Mum shared how Hannah could be quick to make a judgement about other people and once she decided that she did not like you, there was no changing her mind. There were queries around Autism Spectrum Condition but Hannah had consistently refused to engage in any formal assessment, which had made it impossible to either identify this, or rule it out.

Hannah lived with her mother and elder sister, Jess. Hannah's mother and father had recently separated after many years of conflict that was compounded by their significantly different parenting styles. This conflict was not known to be violent at this time, although Hannah, later in therapy, disclosed direct physical and verbal abuse towards her. Hannah and Jess were having contact with their father but this seemed strained and the parental conflict seeped into their time together, causing further splits in the family. Her mother had ongoing mental and physical health difficulties.

Hannah had been through several professional services before we met each other; Educational Psychology, Paediatric Services and Children's Services. A theme ran through their reporting of Hannah – they found her overwhelming, just as her mother did. Hannah frightened people, from her peers to the professionals. No one understood how a girl of Hannah's age could present such a complex and extreme picture of violence and apparent remorselessness. Mum reported that the last paediatrician referred to Hannah as being 'beyond his experience'. His comment only served to compound her mother's experience of Hannah as being beyond help, and possibly even beyond her own love. Hannah had refused to engage with most of the professionals who had tried. She remained defensive and threatening and as a result, completely alone.

At this time, Hannah's school placement was in jeopardy, she was already on a reduced timetable and was struggling to manage even these few hours. Hannah was later permanently excluded from her mainstream school and due to her complexity of need and violent behaviour, was not placed in any other education setting for a further two years. Hannah remained at home, completely without educational input, for this whole period. Not surprisingly, this exacerbated the complex attachment difficulties that already existed.

Play therapy process

For some reason, Hannah decided to give me, and play therapy, a go. Mum was shocked. She had braced herself for Hannah to either refuse or attack another well-intentioned professional! However, Hannah engaged deeply in play therapy and consistent, powerful therapeutic play themes emerged very early on in her process. For a significant period of the therapy, Hannah placed me in role as a 'Blood Fairy', who was also a mother. Hannah seemed to be using me to share an experience of being mothered herself and possibly a fantasy of what a mother 'should be'. She asked me to role-play being a cruel and dismissive mother, but one whose baby cannot live without her. I often felt confused and detached in the roles she assigned for me, although the feelings I experienced in them were tangible. I wondered about her exploration of her own family 'blood lines' which she had little clear understanding about.

The following abstract is taken from my case note of one session and highlights how she used me to explore and make sense of the mother–baby dyad and experience:

> I am instructed to trust her (Hannah) with my baby girl, having to assure myself she will be safe. However, she maltreats my baby. I watch as she shakes her vigorously, makes her sick and is emotionally abusive and threatening towards her. Hannah sticks the dummy into the baby's mouth further and holds it in so she cannot cry or talk. Hannah wishes to deepen my experience of the baby, so instructs me to play the role of the baby directly. My baby cries annoy her and the more I cry the worse her treatment of me is. She then instructs me to tell my mother that "I love her (Hannah), please let me stay for a whole month, mummy".

Hannah's experiences of her attachment relationships, both with her mother and father, were confusing and ambivalent. Hannah was able to communicate her deep terrors about the world and project her vulnerability onto me in a profound, visceral way. She was also able to effectively communicate that she had learned to stay powerful in order that she stay safe; that attack was her best defence.

Another huge shift that occurred over the course of the therapy was Hannah's capacity to emotionally connect with me. For a long time, Hannah actively resisted any of my reflections about her emotional state. There was not a denial of the feelings that I wondered about in the play room, it was more like a total block to them. Similarly, Hannah seemed completely resistant to developing any form of relationship with me. For a long time she barely made eye contact with me and her face remained inexpressive. One day during supervision, I reflected on how I had noticed her teeth and realised this was because it was the first time she had smiled at me. She had needed to defend herself to the point of being emotionally numb. It seemed, through play therapy, this numbness was thawing.

Hannah's use of the therapeutic space enabled me to communicate out to the professional network around her, and more importantly to her mother, that Hannah was frightened, not frightening. This facilitated a new space, or rather supported her mother to get into a space within which she could take care of her vulnerable little girl. Due to limitations of the mother's emotional capacity, this space could only open up for brief periods, but it was enough.

To conclude the story, we continued to work together for a further year or so and Hannah made significant improvements. A placement was identified in a specialist school and Hannah returned to education. Although there were inevitable bumps in the road, Hannah thrived. For the first time I saw Hannah have a healthy degree of independence, self-esteem, ambition and hope for her future. Hannah tolerated wearing her school uniform (which included shoes!), and her violent behaviours gradually reduced at home. One of the most significant changes was her understanding of her own emotions and her ability to verbalise these to others. Hannah could allow herself to be vulnerable and trust in others to notice this. In the end, Hannah was also diagnosed with Autism Spectrum Condition, but with strong recognition of the trauma she had experienced and her significant attachment needs, which I was able to impress onto the assessment.

Reflection

Since my work with Hannah, I have often wondered what it was about me, or play therapy, that felt different to her. Was it that I could understand and accept Hannah's need to embody internal positions of vulnerability and attack simultaneously? Was it that she was able to remain in charge of her own process and the therapeutic relationship? For Hannah, this meant that she could remain in a defensive position as long as necessary, while allowing her therapeutic journey to begin. Play therapy, particularly non-directive play therapy, requires that the therapist does not assume knowledge of the child's internal world and certainly does not ask too many questions! (Landreth, 2012) We learn from the child, genuinely take their lead and deeply respect their need to remain in whatever conscious or unconscious internal position they need … and this enables the therapeutic work to occur and indeed, be effective. Maybe this is why play therapists can engage so well with these 'hard to reach' children, as we do not expect them to reach us?

Summary

- Play therapists are increasingly found as core members of multi-disciplinary CAMHS teams in the UK, working with a range of other creative therapists. Although they may be 'hidden' in other generic mental health roles ... so look out for them, they might be wearing a mask!

- CAMHS settings require play therapists to be flexible in their roles and demonstrate both generic and specialist skills. They also need to operate within organisational constraints including initial assessment and waiting list protocols.
- Play therapists in CAMHS teams face several challenges. Play therapy is not yet consistently recognised as a treatment pathway in CAMHS teams across the UK and many play therapists continue to fight for their worth. There are also practical challenges such as ensuring child-centred spaces and being able to offer the consistency and length of treatment necessary for effective play therapeutic interventions.
- However, once established within a CAMHS service, play therapists can attract referrals that are most responsive to this child-centred and non-verbal approach and enjoy great therapeutic success.

Further reading

Padmore, J. (2015) *The Mental Health Needs of Children and Young People: Guiding you to key issues and practices in CAMHS.* Maidenhead: McGraw Hill.
A good general introduction to key issues in working with young people's mental health.
Jäger, J. & Ryan, V. (2007) Evaluating clinical practice: Using play-based techniques to elicit children's views of therapy. *Clinical Child Psychology and Psychiatry.* 12 (3) pp.437–450.
This interesting article outlines some child-friendly methods for evaluating the effectiveness of clinical play therapy practice. Available at: http://journals.sagepub.com/doi/abs/10.1177/1359104507075937
Rye, N. (2008) Play therapy as a mental health intervention for children and adolescents. *The Journal of Family Health Care.* 18(1) pp.17–19.
A brief article which outlines some of the benefits of play therapy practice within mental health settings. Available at www.jfhc.co.uk/play-therapy-as-a-mental-health-intervention-for-children-and-adolescents

References

Baggerly, J.N., Ray, D.C. & Bratton, S.C. (2010) *Child-Centered Play Therapy Research: The Evidence Base for Effective Practice.* Hoboken, NJ: John Wiley & Sons.
Bratton, S., Ray, D., Rhine, T. & Jones, L. (2005) The efficacy of play therapy with children. A meta-analytic review of treatment outcomes. *Journal of Professional Psychology, Research and Practice.* 36 (4) pp. 376–390.
Brown, A., Ford, T., Deighton, J. & Wolpert, W. (2014) Satisfaction in child and adolescent mental health services. *Administration and Policy in Mental Health and Mental Health Services Research.* 41 (4), pp. 436–446.
Campbell, D. (20 October, 2016) Jeremy Hunt says child mental health services are NHS's biggest failing. *The Guardian.* Available at: www.theguardian.com/society/

2016/oct/20/jeremy-hunt-promises-better-mental-health-services-children-adoles cents [Accessed: 16. 01. 2018].

Care Quality Commission. (2017) *CQC Completes Initial Review of Mental Health Services for Children and Young People.* Press Release, 27 October. Available at: www.cqc.org.uk/news/releases/cqc-completes-initial-review-mental-health-services- children-young-people [Accessed: 19. 12. 2017].

Dogra, N. (2017) *A Multidisciplinary Handbook of Child and Adolescent Mental Health for Front-line Professionals.* (3rd ed.) London: Jessica Kingsley Publishers.

Fonagy, P., Cottrell, D., Phillips, J., Bevington, D., Glaser, D. & Allison, E. (2014) *What Works for Whom? A Critical Review of Treatments for Children and Adolescents.* (2nd ed.) London: Guilford Press.

Fernandez, K.T.G. & Sugay, C.O. (2016) Psychodynamic play therapy: A case of selective mutism. *International Journal of Play Therapy.* 25 (4) pp. 203–209.

Gaskill, R. & Perry, B. (2014) The neurobiological power of play using the neurodevelopmental model of therapeutics to guide play in the healing process. In: Malchiodi, A. & Crenshaw, D. (eds.) *Creative Arts and Play Therapy for Attachment Problems.* New York: Guilford Press. pp. 178–191.

Gil E. (2011) *Helping Abused and Traumatized Children: Integrating Directive and Nondirective Approaches.* New York: Guilford Press.

Goodman, R. (2001). Psychometric properties of the strengths and difficulties questionnaire. *Journal of the American Academy of Child and Adolescent Psychiatry,* 40 (11), 1337–1345.

Jäger, J. (2013) Facilitating children's views of therapy: An analysis of the use of play based techniques to evaluate clinical practice. *Journal of Clinical Psychology and Psychiatry.* 18 (3) pp. 411–428.

Landreth, G. (2012) *Play Therapy: The Art of the Relationship.* (3rd ed.) New York: Brunner-Routledge.

Lin, Y-W. & Bratton, S. (2015) A meta-analytic review of child-centered play therapy approaches. *Journal of Counseling and Development.* 93. pp. 45–58.

Malchiodi, A. & Crenshaw, D. (eds.) (2014) *Creative Arts and Play Therapy for Attachment Problems.* New York: Guilford Press.

Matthews-King, A. (10 November, 2017) NHS mental health services turn away 150 vulnerable children a day. *Independent.* Available at: www.independent.co.uk/news/health/ nhs-mental-health-services-children-turn-away-day-vulnerable-nspcc-study-a8047401. html [Accessed: 21. 01. 2018].

Miller, S. D., Duncan, B.L., Brown, J., Sparks, J., & Claud, D. (2003). The Outcome Rating Scale: A preliminary study of the reliability, validity, and feasibility of a brief visual analog measure. *Journal of Brief Therapy,* 2, pp. 91–100.

Naderi, F., Heidarie, A., Bouron, L. & Asgari, P. (2010) The efficacy of play therapy on ADHD, anxiety and social maturity in 8-12 years aged clientele children of Ahwaz metropolitan counseling clinics. *Journal of Applied Sciences.* 10 (3) pp. 189–195.

National Institute for Health and Care Excellence (NICE). Available at: www. nice.org.uk [Accessed: 28. 11. 17].

Padmore, J. (2015) *The Mental Health Needs of Children & Young People: Guiding you to key issues and practices in CAMHS.* Maidenhead: McGraw Hill.

Patton, S.C. & Benedict, H.E. (2016) Play therapy with children with attachment disorders. In O'Connor, K., Schaefer, C.E. & Braverman, L.D. (eds.) *A Handbook of Play Therapy* (2nd ed.) Hoboken, NJ: John Wiley & Sons, p. 381.

Ray, D., Armstrong, S., Balkin, R. & Jayne, K. (2015) Child-centred play therapy in the schools: Review and meta-analysis. *Psychology in the Schools.* 52 (2) pp. 107–123.

Ryan, V. (2004) Adapting non-directive play therapy for children with attachment disorders. *Clinical Child Psychology and Psychiatry.* 9 (1) pp. 75–87.

Singhal, M. & Mehrotra, S. (2014) The use of play for assessment and therapy: The case of a child with selective mutism. *International Journal of Play Therapy.* 3 (2) pp. 157–168. DOI: 10.1080/21594937.2014.886103

Chapter 12

Play therapy in schools

Sonia Murray

Chapter overview

Delivering play therapy in schools can be perceived as a natural and safe option, but there are a number of challenges that can affect the therapeutic process. This chapter aims to explore some of those challenges and to offer strategies to minimise the impact they may present. It will provide a tool kit for play therapists and assist in the planning, preparation and practice of play therapy within schools.

Introduction

In 1994, I was involved with one of the first schools within the UK to introduce play therapy as an intervention for its pupils. At that time, play therapy was in its infancy in the UK and there was little research to support us in developing procedures for play therapy practice in schools. Since those pioneering days, we have developed a greater understanding about the provision of therapeutic services within school. Harland et al. (2015) note that 62% of schools in the UK now offer some form of counselling services to their pupils, and play therapy has been recognised as one such intervention by the Department of Education (DfE, 2016a).

With a growing emphasis on supporting the mental health and wellbeing of children and young people, schools are increasingly expected to be first responders to children who are experiencing a range of difficulties. Schools are also key to initial identification of child protection issues and early developmental difficulties (Figley, 1995; DfE, 2016b). In an atmosphere where support services are limited and thresholds are high, schools are on the front line of providing initial helping interventions. Research indicates that when schools support their pupils'/students' emotional wellbeing and mental health, there is greater opportunity for both pupil and whole school attainment (Gutman & Vorhaus, 2012).

According to the British Association of Play Therapists, the benefits of undertaking play therapy in schools include:

- Therapy is delivered within a familiar and safe environment for both children and their parents/carers.
- Schools offer flexibility around the scheduling of the play therapy sessions to accommodate the daily timetable.
- Ease of access to staff perspectives on children in their care who can identify developmental and behavioural difficulties and changes early on.
- Facilitates effective communication between the therapist and school staff.

Preparing to deliver play therapy in school

For the play therapist, there are usually three routes to working in schools – as an employee, on a freelance basis or working for an outside agency. The play therapist will need to provide evidence of their identity and their qualifications, to demonstrate that they are part of a Professional Standards Authority (PSA) accredited register. As required for ethical practice (BAPT Core Competence 12, see Appendix 1), the play therapist will also ensure that they have professional indemnity insurance and public liability insurance and provide a current Disclosure and Barring Service (DBS) certificate to cover their practice within the school. It is worth recognising that the role can feel isolating at times, as there may only be one therapist in each school. Incorporating play therapy into the structures of a school takes time, and there is a need for information sharing, clear communication and developing effective relationships between the play therapist and school staff (BAPT Core Competence 28, see Appendix 1). For play therapy to gain respect and be valued within the school setting, the development of trust and confidence between all parties needs to be established.

It is important to convey a clear understanding of what play therapy is and how it works within a school setting. Using a written working contract, with identified lines of accountability and communication, supports a clear understanding of respective roles and expectations (BAPT Core Competence 19, see Appendix 1). The play therapist also needs to be aware of some of the contemporary demands in schools, including the diversity of the school population and range of academic ability, the role of the governing body and the pressures of the changing policy landscape in meeting Ofsted requirements.

A play therapist who does not have experience of working within a school should ideally spend time observing within their new school context, to gain a greater understanding of the working practices and procedures of the school staff. Schools are busy and complex environments and play therapy will only be one of many elements occurring within a school day. Whilst we know that play therapy is a proven effective approach in schools

(Ray et al., 2015), this needs to be understood within the context of it only being approximately 3% (1 hour) of the child's time in school per week (30 hours including lunchtimes).

Each school will also have its own values and ethos, developed by the staff, pupils, parents/carers, governors, and wider community. As stated by French (2012:55) 'Each school has its own culture and related priorities, which means that the emphasis placed on learning about and working towards emotional well-being can vary considerably'. It is important to understand the particular ethos of the school, as this will give an indication of the importance the school attaches to outcomes in relation to emotional health and wellbeing. The play therapist will need to market play therapy as an intervention that supports these values. As noted by Ray (2011:203) 'schools typically employ mental health professionals for the sole purpose of helping children progress academically'. A brief summary linking play therapy, emotional wellbeing and academic attainment, is an essential tool for all school play therapists.

Part of the play therapist's role is to make sure that all parties have a well-informed understanding of play therapy, realistic expectations about the play therapy process and an understanding of how it can benefit children academically. I provide specific training sessions about play therapy for the Senior Leadership teams and whole-school training sessions on the play therapy process, including explanations of any assessment tools used – for example Strengths & Difficulties Questionnaire (Goodman & Goodman, 2011).

The play therapist needs to stay informed about the school calendar and upcoming events such as exams or school trips. I recommend that the school identify a designated play therapy liaison staff member who may be the Head Teacher, SENCo, Pastoral Lead, Inclusion Manager etc. This person will require a full understanding of the play therapy process, from both an operational and strategic point of view. Their role can include identifying and overseeing referrals, acting as liaison point for updates regarding the referrals and plans for the academic term, scheduling progress reviews, and generally serving as a potential ally for play therapy with other staff members.

Developing an agreed communication plan with all parties is essential. Some suggested strategies are:

- Make contact with staff each play therapy day to check if the child is in school and there are no planned trips etc. that may restrict the child attending the session.
- If appropriate, agree with the parent/carer to contact you directly if their child is ill.
- Half-termly reviews with class staff, the designated play therapy liaison staff member, parents/carers and other agencies involved.

Maintaining confidentiality within school

I have found it important to establish an agreement on how to share information between staff, whilst in the presence of the children. In line with BAPT Core Competence 23 (see Appendix 1) the play therapist may need to model confidentiality for other staff members and support them to understand the limits of confidentiality when discussing the child's therapy. It may be worth agreeing a privately understood signal with school staff to indicate that things have been a bit difficult prior to collecting the child, or to convey that the child may still be processing some of the emotional aspects of the play therapy session on returning the child to class. It may also help to negotiate for some children to have a transitional activity with a staff member, rather than returning from play therapy directly into the learning environment.

School staff may try to discuss things with the play therapist in front of the child. I have found it useful to have a clear empathic script to help manage the situation without alienating the child and/or school staff. For example:

STAFF MEMBER: Jimmy's behaviour has been really challenging and I think it is the play therapy that is causing this, so I have decided that he shouldn't come today.

PLAY THERAPIST RESPONSE: I am sorry to hear that things are challenging at the moment. Thank you for letting me know. This sometimes happens. Do you remember that we discussed this possibility when we met to discuss the arrangements? When children explore their experiences and feelings, sometimes things spill over after the session. It is essential that the play therapy continues as arranged. However, let's book a time to meet to explore what is happening and perhaps plan a transitional activity to support his return to class.

Confidentiality can also be an issue for some children attending play therapy within a school environment. Children may see the play therapist collecting other children from their class. On the one hand, this can be comforting as the child knows that they are not the only one needing support, but it can also lead to issues about potentially not being perceived as special by the play therapist, or to questions about the other children. This may test the play therapist's boundaries around confidentiality. Over the years, this has presented itself in different ways to me and the play therapist will need to ponder what the underlying needs are behind the questions. Here are two examples:

Example 1:

CHILD: I was talking to Tyrone about play therapy and he has said you can tell me what he does in here.

Suggested response:

PLAY THERAPIST: I am guessing you are checking whether I will tell other people about what you are doing in play therapy. I agreed with you that I will not tell other people what you do here, so I cannot tell you about anybody else's play therapy.

Example 2:

CHILD: You can tell Tyrone what I do in here.

Suggested response:

PLAY THERAPIST: I am wondering if you are not sure whether you can trust that I will not tell other people about what you do here. I agreed with you that what you do in here stays between you and me.

Safeguarding children within school

Safeguarding is defined by the DfE (2016b:5) as 'protecting children from maltreatment; preventing impairment of children's health or development; ensuring that children grow up in circumstances consistent with the provision of safe and effective care; and taking action to enable all children to have the best outcomes'.

Child Protection covers the process of protecting individual children identified as either suffering, or likely to suffer, significant harm because of abuse or neglect. As a school play therapist, it is essential to know who the Designated Safeguarding Lead is within the school and to be fully aware of the school's specific child protection procedures. The play therapist has a professional duty of care to the children they are working with and it is essential to access regular updated safeguarding training (BAPT Core Competence 8, see Appendix 1). Current guidance is set out in *Working Together* (DfE, 2018) and *Information Sharing – Advice for Safeguarding Practitioner* (DfE, 2016b). Each play therapist will need to be aware of what is expected of their role in school as either an employee or a visitor, including what to say, what to report, and to whom. If the play therapist is freelance or employed by an agency, they will need to agree with the school how they will work within the school's particular procedures.

Child protection issues raise a number of ethical dilemmas. The play therapist needs to balance legal duties, safeguarding procedures and acting in the best interests of the child, whilst considering the management of risk. It is important to consider how their actions will impact the therapeutic relationships with the child, the parent/carer and with the school, particularly if there is a difference of opinion regarding the potential safety of the child. For example, there may be a difference of views as to whether the concerns merit referral to Children's Services. While this could potentially affect the therapist's relationship with the school management, the therapist must exercise their own professional judgement to ensure that safeguarding concerns are communicated clearly and adequately.

It is also important to communicate clearly their safeguarding role to all parties, including the child (within their level of understanding). When a child protection issue arises, it is advisable that the play therapist seeks guidance and support from their clinical supervisor and/or manager. If necessary, legal advice should be sought. In addition, the play therapist needs to carefully record the concern within agency procedures and report any actions taken.

If a child protection concern arises in the session, the play therapist needs to respond in a calm, considered way to ensure the child feels supported and understood, whilst explaining what will need to happen. As with other situations, it is important to prepare the child from the beginning.

For example – one child asked me if they could tell me a secret, which she had to keep. I gently reminded the child of our agreement at the start of the sessions that if the child told me of someone hurting them or others, then I could not keep this a secret and would need to tell the head teacher. However, if it was a secret about a surprise birthday party then I could keep it. With the child reminded of this information, they can choose to tell or not. The child on this occasion proceeded to inform me about being hit by her carer that morning and we were able to discuss how best to tell the headteacher together.

At other times, concerns emerge through the child's symbolic play and the child may state that this is happening to them. Again, the therapist needs to carefully manage the play and explain that they will need to speak to someone else as they have said that they are being hurt and they need to be kept safe. Children can naturally become very anxious about this and can try to withdraw the concern. In these circumstances, I need to reflect the child's feelings carefully, whilst explaining the importance of keeping the child safe and my duty to tell someone who will be able to help. It is essential not to make unrealistic promises or give false assurances, as potentially this can hamper the therapeutic relationship.

Expectations of play therapy

It is important to have an understanding of how play therapy is perceived by school staff and parents/carers. Some of these perceptions will be conscious and unconscious responses to therapy occurring in schools and/or to the therapist (French, 2012). Positive expectations can include a desire that the process will support their role as teacher, an expectation that it will enable the child to settle more to learning, feelings of relief that the child is absent from class for a period of time, and gratitude for providing help with the child. In contrast, staff may believe that play is for early years children only, not for older children, or believe that the child is missing out on valuable teaching time or will be viewed differently by their peers.

Staff may also have unrealistic expectations about the child's progress whilst in play therapy, believing that everything will be resolved after a few sessions. For example, one teacher said after six sessions, 'this play therapy is not working as the child's behaviour has not changed, in fact it has got worse, so it needs to stop.' Staff may even take the view that children are being rewarded for challenging behaviours.

On a more personal level, some staff might feel the therapeutic process could compromise their professional role. They may be feeling deskilled or overwhelmed, and may experience feelings of competitiveness or anxiety about the role of the therapist. The therapy process may evoke unconscious wishes for their own self as a child or for their own professional role. As Klein suggests (2012:64) 'this can engender jealousy of the therapist's relationship with the child and envy, whether conscious or unconscious, of her role.'

These responses are often internal defence strategies, such as projection, when we have thoughts or feelings that are uncomfortable so we project them onto another. For example, during a review meeting, a teacher interrupted me and said angrily, 'it is ok for you because you only have to focus on one child and you can give him what he needs. I have to split myself between 30 children and deliver the curriculum.' At their most extreme, these can include unconscious reactions that undermine the play therapy process, for example, by teachers asking the child to bring play materials out of the room for them, or insisting on prioritising class work rather than letting the child attend play therapy.

In these situations, the therapist may also experience counter-transference responses of their own about their skill as a play therapist. For example, if a teacher states there has been no change or the child's behaviour has got worse, the play therapist's own anxiety may be triggered and they may react by trying to justify the process or by becoming more directive within the playroom. It is essential for us as play therapists to develop a deep understanding of ourselves, and our own triggers, so that we can manage our counter-transference responses. BAPT Core Competence 14 (see Appendix 1) requires that play therapists undertake personal therapy as part of our training to help guard against defensiveness and enable us to remain open and aware of our responses within therapy.

It is important to seek to form strong relationships with the school staff supporting children in play therapy (BAPT Core Competence 28, see Appendix 1). These staff are living the journeys of these children, often with limited understanding of childhood trauma, attachment and loss and with limited support to process their own reactions to caring for the children in their school. Compassion fatigue (Figley, 1995) and blocked care

(Baylin & Hughes, 2016) are potential risks of providing care, particularly in ongoing stressful situations and without wellbeing support. Nurturing the staff–therapist relationship is essential to the ongoing effectiveness of the overall intervention. The play therapist will need to maintain the relationship through regular reviews and check-ins with the school staff, just as we would with parents/carers.

Parents/carers also have a range of expectations of play therapy. As Bromfield posits 'entrusting your child to any caretaker is hard. Entrusting your child to a therapist and to the vulnerability of treatment is even harder' (1992:46). Sometimes parents can feel particularly disconnected from the therapeutic process in school. It is essential to involve parents/carers for play therapy to be fully effective. Similarly to school staff, providing clear communication routes and regular reviews will help the parents to be engaged in the process (McGuire & McGuire, 2001).

For many children, awareness of their peers is an overriding factor that can impact their feelings about attending play therapy within school time. They may be reluctant to attend because they do not want to be seen as different and often do not know what to say to their peers about where they are going. Some may still feel a stigma about attending therapy, while others may view it positively, as they are able to miss particular lessons, and some just love play therapy and boast that they get to go.

Dual roles within school

Some children may believe that they have outgrown play, while others, accustomed to adults directing their actions, may see the play therapist as another teacher who is in charge (Klein, 2012). This viewpoint may be reinforced if the play therapist has a dual role in the school, such as teacher or behaviour coordinator, and can lead to confusion in therapy sessions. I resolved this issue within my own school by wearing a specific jumper that identified when I was in the therapeutic role. I informed the staff and children that when I was wearing this jumper I was working as a play therapist and would not respond to other school issues. I introduced this idea in a staff workshop at the beginning of the school year and it was also explained to each class at the start of term. The jumper worked as a visual prompt for children, as to whether or not I was available to speak to them about play therapy and was easy to refer to if children or adults forgot in the moment.

I would recommend that, if possible, play therapists avoid working with children if they also have a teaching role for that child within the school, as this can also cause confusion for the child. Often in the teaching role, there is a need to be directive and set boundaries to help manage the learning environment for all the children. This can be too great a contrast with the role of play therapist, which focuses solely on the child and provides fewer boundaries within sessions.

Managing the play space

Another significant aspect that needs special consideration is the allocation of the play therapy space, particularly when the therapist may be visiting a number of different schools each week. The venue for therapy needs to be negotiated with the designated play therapy liaison at the start. It is necessary to emphasise the security, privacy and consistency required for the space to promote safety for the child (BAPT Core Competence 29, see Appendix 1. See also Chapter 5 by Fullalove). Unfortunately, space is always a challenge in schools, however this is a priority and, in my view, a prerequisite before play therapy can begin. I always create a visual calendar with session times included for the designated play therapy liaison, the admin team (who may book the rooms), class staff, parents and the child. It is important to regularly re-confirm the arrangements with everyone, as this will make certain that it stays in the minds of busy staff.

I also explore the issue of interruptions with all staff. Interruptions disrupt the therapeutic process and disturb the sense of safety within the room.

For example – one occasion whilst working in a school, a member of staff entered the room to get some paper. The child's body jumped and then she froze, briefly dissociated (freeze stress response) before getting up and saying, 'I want to go now' (flight stress response). It took empathic responding, time and repeated experiences of non-interrupted sessions for the child to feel safe again within the therapeutic space. That one small interruption hampered the therapeutic process and took time to repair.

To gain an empathic understanding about the importance of this, I ask school staff to imagine they are having a massage or a facial and are lying back, relaxing when suddenly someone walks in and disturbs them. This helps them to consider the potential impact on the child and to respect the therapeutic space more easily.

Often, a space designated for play therapy may be used for multiple purposes and consideration needs to be given as to how to delineate the play therapy space. The play therapist may also need to consider how the child may have used the room previously or is currently using the room, in case it has particular negative connotations for them. In these circumstances, I use a large mat to provide a boundary for the space (Cattanach, 1994). Everything to do with play therapy takes place on the mat, but as soon as they step off the mat, the child is back in school's rules.

Case study: the play therapy process with Sam

Sam was a child who struggled to regulate his emotions and behavioural responses. He would often be resistant to following adults' instructions and found it difficult to manage the constraints of a class. He had limited internalised constraints and would often challenge the teacher's authority. Unfortunately, he had experienced inconsistent parenting, at times neglectful and punitive. He regarded people as inconsistent, unpredictable and unsupportive and this played out in the therapeutic relationship. Sam repeatedly challenged the boundaries of the playroom, to see if I was able to contain him and to safely maintain boundaries. He needed the different spaces in school to be clearly defined, and would repeatedly test my ability to maintain consistency for him. When I went to collect him, he would run up the corridor to the playroom in breach of the school walking rule. I would acknowledge his feeling of wanting to get to the playroom quickly, but explain that we were still within school's rules. I would then wait until he walked up the corridor. Through supervision, I explored whether it would be more appropriate for someone else to bring and collect him from the playroom, but, due to his significant need for predictability, we decided that it was best for me to collect him each time. This also allowed me to model for Sam how to modulate his impulses and feelings.

He also tested my consistency by standing with one foot either side of the door frame, one foot in the playroom and one foot in the school corridor and saying a swear word. I reminded him that he was in school's rules and swearing was not OK. He replied that he was in the playroom where he could choose to swear. I reflected that he was really checking out if I was going to stick to the rules and if I would do what I said. To further support Sam to demarcate the different boundaries in the different spaces, I would add as we left the playroom, 'you are now back in school's rules.'

Sam needed repeated experiences of my ability to be consistent and persistent with the boundaries before he was able to internalise a sense of trust in the therapist. Gradually, the need to test the boundaries lessened and at the end of the therapy he said 'you showed me that there are people who do what they say.'

Conclusions

Play therapy in schools can easily become immersed in the complexity of meeting a wide range of demands, but also provides a unique opportunity to work collaboratively as a team with school staff and parents/carers, to provide a holistic approach to individual children. The key to effective play therapy in schools is preparation and education. In addition, developing strong working relationships, with clear lines of communication and accountability, will support the effectiveness of play therapy and promote positive outcomes for children within the school.

Summary

*   Schools are complex and dynamic organisations but offer a unique practice context for play therapists.

- Identifying a designated play therapy liaison within the school will facilitate effective communication and support the integration of play therapy within the school.
- It is vital to explain the benefits of play therapy in supporting children's emotional and academic development to school staff and parents/carers.
- Providing training for the whole school team will help staff to better understand the importance of the therapeutic space and to respect therapeutic boundaries.
- Play therapists need to keep updated with national and school safeguarding procedures, and clearly explain this responsibility to children at the beginning of their work.
- Play therapists within schools may need to manage dual roles and need to develop strategies to preserve their therapeutic identity, alongside other roles within the school.

Further reading

Drewes, A. A. & Schaefer, C. E. (2010) *School Based Play Therapy* (2nd ed.). Hoboken, NJ: John Wiley & Sons. This book provides an overview of play therapy in schools and discusses how different types of play therapy can be used in a variety of school situations.

French, L. & Klein, R. (eds.) (2012) *Therapeutic Practice in Schools: Working with the Child within: A Clinical Workbook for Counsellors, Psychotherapists and Arts Therapists.* London: Routledge. This book offers a comprehensive guide to providing therapy within a school setting. It explores and expands on the complexities and dilemmas that may arise from providing school-based therapy.

Landreth, G. L. (2012) *Play Therapy: The Art of the Relationship* (3rd ed.). New York: Routledge. This book is a must for play therapists as it provides a thorough grounding in play therapy and will enhance the therapeutic practice within schools.

References

Baylin, J. & Hughes, D. A. (2016) *The Neurobiology of Attachment-Focused Therapy: Enhancing Connection & Trust in the Treatment of Children & Adolescents.* New York: W.W. Norton & Company.

Bromfield, R. (1992) *Playing for Real: The World of a Play Therapist.* New York: Dutton.

Cattanach, A. (1994) *Play Therapy: Where the Sky meets the Underworld.* London: Jessica Kingsley Publishers.

Department for Education (DfE). (2016a) *Counselling in Schools: A Blueprint for the Future – Departmental Advice for School Leaders and Counsellors.* London: DfE.

Department for Education (DfE). (2016b) *Keeping Children Safe in Education.* London: DfE. Available at: www.gov.uk/government/uploads/system/uploads/attachment_data/file/550511/Keeping_children_safe_in_education.pdf [Accessed: 01. 04. 2017].

Department of Education (DfE). (2018). *Working Together to Safeguard Children: A Guide to Inter-agency Working to Safeguard and Promote the Welfare of Children: Draft for Consultation*. London: HMSO. Available at: https://consult. education.gov.uk/child-protection-safeguarding-and-family-law/working-together-to-safeguard-children-revisions-t/supporting_documents/Working%20Together%20to%20Safeguard%20Children.pdf [Accessed: 03. 05. 2017].

Figley, C. R. (ed.) (1995) *Compassion Fatigue: Coping with Secondary Traumatic Stress Disorder in those who Treat the Traumatized*. New York: Brunner/Mazel.

French, L. (2012) The symbolic function of a school-based therapy service. In: French, L. & Klein, R. (eds.) *Therapeutic Practice in Schools: Working with the Child within: A Clinical Workbook for Counsellors, Psychotherapists and Arts Therapists*. London: Routledge. p. 53

Goodman, A. & Goodman, R. (2011) Population mean scores predict child mental disorder rates: Validating SDQ prevalence estimators in Britain. *Journal of Child Psychology and Psychiatry and Allied Disciplines*. 52 (1) pp. 100–108.

Gutman, L. & Vorhaus, J. (2012) *The Impact of Pupil Behaviour and Wellbeing on Educational Outcomes*. London: DfE.

Harland, J., Dawson, A., Rabiasz, A. & Sims, D. (2015) *NFER Teacher Voice Omnibus: Questions for the Department for Education – June 2015*. London: DfE.

Klein, R. (2012) Working in the primary school setting. In: French, L. & Klein, R. (eds.) *Therapeutic Practice in Schools: Working with the Child within: A Clinical Workbook for Counsellors, Psychotherapists and Arts Therapists*. London: Routledge. pp. 60–66

McGuire, D. & McGuire, D. E. (2001) *Linking Parents to Play Therapy: A Practical Guide with Applications, Interventions, and Case Studies*. Lillington: Edward Brothers.

Ray, D. C., Armstrong, S. A., Balkin, R. S. & Jayne, K. M. (2015) Child-centered play therapy in the schools: Review and meta-analysis. *Psychology in the Schools*. 52 (2) pp. 107–123.

Ray, D. C. (2011) *Advanced Play Therapy: Essential Conditions, Knowledge, and Skills for Child Practice*. New York: Routledge

Chapter 13

Narrative group play therapy in a school setting

Sharon Pearce

Chapter overview

In this chapter I will provide an overview of how group play therapy can work in practice, to support the normalisation of experiences, develop socialising techniques with peers and encourage emotional catharsis. I will present a case study of a school-based group of three children experiencing parental separation. Through 12 sessions of group play therapy, each child found ways to deal with their experiences and to negotiate new relationships with their families. All made significant gains during and after the group. I will discuss some of the challenges and practice considerations when setting up group play therapy interventions.

Introduction

My interest in running groups for children came after a series of requests from the children that I worked with which culminated in a heart-felt request from an 11-year old boy 'I wish there was a group for children like me.' The children were expressing their desire to seek support and acknowledgement of their feelings with their peers. I have worked with children in both structured groups and small play therapy groups. Play therapy with school age children is often undertaken individually and often away from school, yet my experience of working with children is that, in many cases, group intervention can be very helpful for school-age children. Alpert-Gillis et al. (1989) observed that the school location maximises the number of children who can participate, including children from low-income families who may otherwise be excluded. Further advantages of working in the school include the children being familiar with each other, thereby enhancing the process of group cohesion, and the school providing a dedicated room for therapy. Children whose parents would not be able to transport them to therapy are able to attend in school with parental support.

Research literature on groups

Sweeney and Homeyer (1999) argue that group play therapy is supportive for psychosocial problems while Panksepp et al. (2003) reported that group therapy reduced behavioural disorders in children, and Chinekesh et al. (2014) have found improvements to the socio-emotional competence and skills of group participants. Research has shown that schools who offer caring discipline, clear rules, boundaries and expectations act as a buffer for children facing stress in their lives, particularly effective for boys who have difficult temperaments or experiencing multiple stress events (Hetherington, 1999).

Children referred to this group were those identified by teachers as performing below expectations academically, socially and emotionally. However, it is essential that the group composition is not composed solely of children with a single characteristic, as this can decrease safety for all members of the group. The benefits of group play therapy for the school include improved educational and social behaviour, as well as improved personal confidence in the children. Whilst this is a potential driver for the school referral, it should not affect the therapist's judgement over who will benefit from group play therapy. As Ginott (1961:17) argues, the essential criteria for group membership is 'social hunger' or the desire for peer acceptance, which motivates the child to change.

Group play therapy provides a social setting in which children can explore effective ways to relate to their peers and test new insights within their group relationships (Ginott, cited in Sweeney & Homeyer, 1999). The group itself can be therapeutic, normalising participants' shared experiences and providing a potentially supportive network for children. Children may be more comfortable with other children who have gone through similar experiences, rather than with an adult therapist in individual therapy (Sweeney & Homeyer, 1999). Kolvin et al. (1981) list the advantages that flow from the dynamics of group therapy as including the instillation of hope for participants, providing an opportunity for shared experience, effective imparting of information, development of socialisation techniques, and developing group cohesiveness.

Assessment for group play therapy

Each of the three children in this group were struggling to deal with the impact of parental separation. I held an intake assessment meeting with each child's family to gain consent for their child's attendance, as well as clarifying their understanding of the reasons for referral to the group. Where conflict levels remained high, I met with some parents separately. After further background interviews with class teachers and consultation with the Safeguarding lead for the school, I assessed all three children as having sufficient pro-social peer skills to be able to participate in the group play therapy format (Aichinger & Holl, 2017).

Narrative play therapy

Narrative play therapy (Cattanach, 2007; Taylor de Faoite, 2011) is based on social construction theory and narrative therapy (White & Epston, 1990), in which the stories used by individuals and by others to describe experiences are explored, and new stories may emerge, based on the idea of partnership or co-construction of the narrative between the adult and children (Cattanach, 2008; Taylor de Faoite, 2011). This enables me to integrate a range of theoretical approaches within my play therapy practice (BAPT Core Competences 4 & 5, see Appendix 1). I use narrative play therapy to help the children adjust to the circumstances in which they now find themselves. The stories allow children to give expression to and question their own experience. Play is triggered by the exploration of the story and the materials provided are wide ranging to maximise the opportunity for narrative play.

The children make sense of their experiences through narrative integration, and process those events via the stories, memories, sensations and feelings that they integrate within the group narrative, while supporting the individual's brain development (Spiegel et al., 2006). A child can take on a role of choice, experiencing a different reality within the role, actively constructing their own knowledge, creating and strengthening their sense of identity as his or her world evolves. Maladaptive expressions of behaviour from the children reflect their lack of mastery in situations that they are unable to control, and through narrative play therapy, we seek to achieve mastery and adjustment of these situations (Taylor de Faoite, 2011).

Story-making

Classical storytelling includes a beginning, middle and end – in which the main character seeks to overcome the problem. The 6-Part Story Method is an idea devised by Alida Gersie (Gersie & King, 1990) and developed in Israel by Lahad and Ayalon (1993). It has six parts:

- the main character/s in their setting
- the main character faces a task
- an obstacle opposes the main character/s
- things that help the main character/s
- the turning point of the story or the main action
- how the story ends.

I adapted this model within a group play therapy format to allow the children to explore together and negotiate the obstacles that befell them in a dramatised format. This allowed for the construction of the whole environment in which the story was to develop. The story addresses relationships, possible obstacles and ways to overcome them and is thus helpful for the child in identifying possible resolution to their challenges.

By providing dramatic distance from their daily lives, the group's stories were the basis for engaging with painful events and sometimes-hostile families. Whilst acting a story, it is possible for children to consider alternative reasons for events and explore a variety of potential endings. By storytelling the therapist is using a therapeutic metaphor that is related to the child's experiences, whilst being different enough to establish safety (Cattanach, 2008; Taylor de Faoite, 2011). Working with narratives allows the children to explore painful past experiences, to express their emotions, and achieve some mastery over emotional events. By placing their experiences within an imaginary context, they are able to externalise their own life story whilst making their feelings more manageable and coherent (Butler et al., 2009).

Resources

Some key considerations for narrative group play therapy are the character of the play space, organisation and predictability, special play areas, and the need for flexible boundaries (Kestly, 2014). For groups to be successful they need to have a calm, safe, invitational and welcoming space, large enough for the children to be able to use the space provided and allowing for storage of required items. Resources for the children vary depending upon the nature of the group but will include at a minimum: art and craft materials as well as puppets and small figures, animals and people. A sand tray can also be considered if the decision is to use small figures for projective exploration. The children in this group used the art materials to create the external world of their story, including a castle, and then used puppets and small figures to represent various characters with whom they collectively interacted throughout their narrative.

The room provided by the school was set aside for play therapy, which meant that the play environment could be retained from session to session, providing the children with a sense of continuity and security. The room was allocated for children's therapy with an agreement from school that staff and children would not interrupt the sessions themselves (BAPT Core Competence 29, see Appendix 1).

Sessions

The number of sessions offered will affect a group's ability to process experiences. I have found that children need at least 10–12 sessions, as it allows them more time to process their experiences and achieve mutuality within a group (Corey, 2014). A school term offers an external mediating boundary for children and parents alike, and allows children to process their issues within the group more fully, than say within a 6-week timeframe. The duration of each session will be determined by the level of structure required for the group and the number of therapists available. The children in this group received twelve sessions lasting for an hour.

The aim of group play therapy is to balance the needs of the group members so that they can encourage each other in their growth. A 'mix of active versus passive or inhibited versus pro social or susceptible to peer's pressure versus resistant to pressure, can make the group a setting where they are more likely to learn from each other' (Kottman, 1999:70). In this environment, the therapist can remind the children of the rules and encourage them to resolve conflicts with one another. The leader has responsibility to ensure safety of the group but, within this, the wishes of each child can be reflected whilst encouraging them to find solutions amongst the group. The children in the group had to negotiate with each other in the session to agree upon a story and re-negotiate any alteration or development in the story-line together.

Group composition

Carl: Carl was a 10-year-old boy whose relationships with peers were causing concern: he regularly lashed out at other children in the class and on the playground. Despite being stronger than many of the other pupils, he saw himself as a victim, claiming that he had been provoked by name calling from other children. Academically, Carl was said by his teachers to be underachieving. At home, he was the younger of two siblings but at the time of referral to the group, his older sister was living with his father and his new wife. The breakdown of his parents' marriage was acrimonious. His mother had had two new relationships since the separation from his father. Carl had been close to his stepsiblings in the first relationship and had enjoyed the support of the second stepfather in his main passion of football. By contrast, Carl's relationship with his father was becoming difficult, worsened by his father's relentless criticism of Carl and his mother during their fortnightly contact visits.

David: David, aged 10, was the older of two boys born to young parents. David was the only child in the group to live in a split custody arrangement. When referred to the group he had developed a pattern of anti-social behaviour towards his peers, physically hitting other children in the playground and the classroom. Academically, he was struggling and his teachers described him as a sad and angry boy. He was acutely conscious of dividing his time, ensuring that he saw and maintained contact with all of them was his method of coping.

Edward: Edward, also aged 10, was the younger child of two children born to his parents, whose relationship ended when his father left to live with another woman. Whilst Edward lived with his mother and older sister, his father lived with his second wife and younger son on the same street. He was a small child, appeared anxious and fragile and had low self-esteem, particularly with his academic work. His lack of stature made him vulnerable to bullying by his peers. Edward had little understanding as to why his parents had separated and he attempted to bridge the gap by maintaining daily contact with his father and half-brother, of whom he was fond.

First story: sessions 2–6

During the first session, we spent time identifying the rules for the group, such as confidentiality and rules about not hurting each other. We discussed the story and the journey that the boys were to travel in the next session, before the story began in earnest. The three boys spent several sessions creating a castle, the environment surrounding it and creating characters for themselves. Carl had chosen to be a knight on horseback, David was a fierce lion, while Edward elected to be a Power Ranger. The story took several sessions to tell. They decided to journey to a magic castle. A lively discussion took place about the content and shape of the story. Finally, they agreed that it was about an evil king who lived in the castle and controlled the land. The boys, acting out their roles, decided to leave the village and try to attack the castle and defeat the king, ridding the land of his evil power. On the way to the castle they each encountered an obstacle that they had to overcome using the help of the others. In the first session, they set off but were stopped almost immediately by some large beasts. Carl challenged them to a knock out football match, which he won. The beasts were angry but David and Edward tied them up and they all escaped. Then two monsters attacked David and tried to pull him apart. Carl and Edward used their magic axes to chop off the monsters' heads and they fled in the direction of the castle. Just before they reached the castle, a flying dragon chased Edward away from the others. Carl and David told the dragon that there was gold in the castle that the dragon could have if it left Edward alone and helped them. The dragon agreed and joined them on their journey.

Second story: sessions 7–11

The story continued in the second half of the group. The boys and the dragon reached the castle but dinosaur guards protected it, the boys surprised the dinosaurs and killed them. The dragon tricked the evil king into coming outside and the boys killed him with a magic sword. Together they went through the castle until they found the treasure and divided it up between them. The castle started to collapse and the boys had to flee. They escaped on the dragon's back with the treasure. The dragon flew them home where they were welcomed as heroes because all the evil power in the land had vanished. Edward said he wanted to keep the dragon as a pet. Carl and David agreed that Edward could keep the dragon. The boys then unanimously agreed that they should destroy the castle and the surrounding environment.

Discussion of group process

During the sessions, the boys learned that they could co-operate and survive the threats facing them together as a team and as individuals. They learned to care for each other by being attuned to each other's needs (Aichinger & Holl, 2017). The process of normalisation within the group allowed the boys to care for each other and to give each other support, whereas previously they had felt isolated and angry. When Edward experienced bullying in school, Carl and David supported him in the group to manage his distress and suggested ways of managing the situation, which included letting his parents and teachers know. They also extended their support to him in the playground. My role as the group play therapy leader was to be a facilitator for their safe exploration on their journey together (Sweeney & Homeyer, 1999), allowing them to experience closeness to an adult without being hurt. Within the group, they could shed defences and remain protected. In turn, this allowed them to achieve emotional closeness in the group rather than just physical proximity to others (Ginott, 1999). Through the group process, the children became more connected and empathic towards each other and developed self-regulation where previously it was lacking. Further, through the repeated narration of their story-making, they were no longer flooded by emotions or old behavioural patterns and could move forward in their lives (Sweeney & Homeyer, 1999).

The co-operative setting of the group helped the children to normalise their experiences of their parents' separation (Yalom, 1975). The co-constructed story between the group and myself, with its elements of obstacles and dangers to be overcome, allowed the children to collectively explore their anxieties about parental separation. A feature of their story was their expression of cathartic anger (Ginott, 1961) towards 'authority', as represented by the King in the story and illustrated by the destruction of the castle, a structured, physical activity that they negotiated between them. This session marked the turning point for all three boys. In subsequent sessions, the boys explored ways of re-negotiating their relationships with their parents, establishing their own identity, and moving on to form significant peer relationships, an age-appropriate task of late latency aged children. Group play therapy is based on the assumption that children will modify behaviour in exchange for acceptance (Ginott, 1961). The group had progressed and were now engaged in concerns for their own future including their forthcoming transfer to secondary school.

Evaluation

Evaluating outcomes is an important aspect of play therapy practice (BAPT Core Competence 31, see Appendix 1). Play therapy interventions may be evaluated by an assessment of whether there are changes in the child's presenting circumstances. O'Connor (2000) makes the point that such adaptations are usually accompanied by changes in the child's wider eco-system. The children in the group responded quickly to the intervention. The evaluation tools included shields drawn by the children before and after the group sessions and interviews with their parents and school staff (Pearce, 2011). Collectively, they showed significant progress both in and out of the school environment, including academic and behavioural progress. According to school staff, Carl, who had been failing academically due to disengagement, achieved an excellent result in his SATS. David received a Merit award for improved behaviour in school, whilst Edward improved in confidence both at home and in school. The social and emotional competence gains that the children made following their sessions were confirmed on follow-up three months later.

Carl's review: Carl's review indicated that he had a more realistic understanding of his parents' separation and his place within his family. He focused on events in the present rather than being consumed by the past. He had shared with the group that he felt angry with his father and received their support. Carl went on to decide, in consultation with his mother, to end his visits to his father and shared this decision in the group. Carl's wishes, identified by his second shield assessment, were to be a family unit with his mother and sister again. He could accept the reality of his parents' divorce, no longer wishing for them to reunite. This occurred shortly after the group ended. He had also begun to separate himself from a difficult relationship with his father.

David's review: David was initially described by his teacher as a very sensitive boy, emotionally literate, often able to open topics for other students when they struggled to express their pain. Within the group, David had the opportunity to be listened to and drew support from the other boys in his struggle to cope with his parents' separation. As David developed through the group, he began the process of separating from his parents, becoming realistic in his wishes and enabling him to negotiate for more freedom from his parents and to concentrate on the age-appropriate task of developing his friendships and identity away from home.

Edward's review: Edward showed considerable development in his understanding of his situation. He had asked for, and been given, explanations for his parents' separation, which in turn enabled him to begin the process of moving on. Edward had been bullied at school: Carl and David offered him support in the group, helping to restore his self-esteem, and the joint support of both of his parents in the aftermath of the bullying incident, reassured him of his importance to them.

Considerations for planning group play therapy

As a single play therapist working with children, there were obvious advantages to seeing children in a group, as I could see more children in the time available. The school were aware of this and were therefore keen to support this approach. In my experience, a play therapy group may optimally contain up to four children with a single play therapist, providing all the criteria for participation in the group has been met.

Of crucial importance, Sweeney and Homeyer (1999) highlight both the ability to form empathic relationships between the children and the commonality of the issue between them to support both bonding and the eventual catharsis of the group approach. Where these conditions have been met, but the group demand was high, I have introduced a second play therapist to help provide safety and containment of all the children involved.

Groups are not a panacea for children's problems. They involve as much work in the planning and preparation, delivery, reflection and supervision stages as working individually with each child. The goals for group play therapy are to improve social functioning, increase trust, security and self-esteem, and enhance coping skills for emotion regulation through re-enactment, re-examination, redirection and reintegration (Smith & Smith, 1999). Groups work because they can help the participants instil hope, build new friendships and empower the children in the light of new learning and changes in their own self- perception (O'Rourke & Worzbyt, 1996). Successful groups help children to feel safe within the group via shared understanding of their situation. They allow safe expression of feelings and acceptance of different views, as well as allowing members to support each other in trying out new ways of being. They also allow group members to provide support to each other, in line with their age and abilities, and finally, to take these experiences and to apply them to their own personal situations. The key to their success is the emotional bonding and catharsis that takes place between the children as they learn from each other and share ways to take care of themselves in the face of adversity.

Perhaps the last word should go to the children. In an essay written for his teacher some months later, and shared with his consent, Carl wrote:

> The problems that many children experience when their parents' divorce has affected my life being pulled in all directions. I have one father and two sorts of step-fathers who I grew to be attached to only to be disappointed when my Mum's relationships ended. This has led me to be very angry and (with) no support and lack of understanding, I thought it was my fault. It is only now after counselling that I have discovered and expressed my feelings and have after discussions with family have sorted out my worries. I now intend to concentrate on my studies and on football. I want to be like my hero David Beckham.

Summary

- Planning is essential for any group: you will need sufficient time to plan, run and follow up from every session. You will need space to meet and resources to lead a group, as well as supervision.
- Intake assessments are vital to ensure the right group members. You will need to ensure that you have consent from the parents if you are seeing their children in school. Be aware that if you are co-working a group you also need time to plan the sessions together.
- As a play therapist, your primary consideration when assessing pupils for group therapy should be the needs of the children, not the school's need for discipline or behaviour management.
- Follow the school and local safeguarding procedures. All schools are required to have safeguarding policies and to abide by them. Ensure that you know the safeguarding lead within school, and that you understand the circumstances surrounding each child's referral, as part of your intake assessment. Be prepared to discuss any concerning information in supervision.
- A co-therapist is recommended for four or more children.
- Supervision is vital to pay attention to the group dynamics and process.
- The group should run, ideally, for 10–12 weeks in order to allow for children to process their feelings sufficiently and for you to work safely with them. Such a timescale allows for a beginning, a middle and an ending for the group.
- A suitable room should ideally be welcoming, safe, and available throughout the life of the group.

Further reading

Cattanach, A. (2007) *Narrative Approaches in Play with Children*. London: Jessica Kingsley Publishers. An essential text for play therapy students wishing to understand the power of narratives and social construction in play therapy.

Drewes, A., Carey, L. & Schaefer, C. (2001) *School Based Play Therapy*. New York: John Wiley & Sons. A helpful text for play therapists working in schools.

Yalom, I. D. (1975) *The Theory and Practice of Group Psychotherapy*. (2nd ed.) New York: Basic Books. A seminal text in the working with and understanding the process and dynamics of group psychotherapy.

References

Aichinger, A. & Holl, W. (2017) *Group Therapy with Children: Psychodrama with Children*. Cologne: Springer.

Alpert-Gillis, L. J., Pedro-Carroll, J. & Cowen, E. L. (1989) The children of divorce intervention program: Development, implementation, and evaluation of a program for young urban children. *Journal of Consulting and Clinical Psychology.* 57 (5) pp. 583–589.

Butler, S., Guterman, J. T. & Rudes, J. (2009) Using puppets with children in narrative therapy to externalize the problem. *Journal of Mental Health Counseling.* 31(3) pp. 225–233.

Cattanach, A. (2008) *Play Therapy with Abused Children.* (2nd ed.) London: Jessica Kingsley Publishers.

Chinekesh, A., Kamalian, M., Eltemasil, M., Chinekesh, S. & Alavil, M. (2014) The effect of group play therapy on social-emotional skills in pre-school children. *Global Journal of Health Science.* 6 (2) pp. 163–167.

Corey, G. (2014) *Theory and Practice of Group Counseling.* (9th ed.) Boston, MA: Cengage Learning.

Gersie, A. & King, N. (1990). *Story-Making in Education and Therapy.* London: Jessica Kingsley Publishers.

Ginott, H. (1961 reprinted 1994) *Group Psychotherapy with Children.* Lanhan, MD: Jason Aronson.

Ginott, H. (1999) Play group therapy: A theoretical framework. In Sweeney, D. S. & Homeyer, L. E. (eds.) *The Handbook of Group Play Therapy.* San Francisco, CA: Josey Bass. pp. 15–23.

Hetherington, E. M. (1999) The adjustment of children with divorced parents: A risk and resiliency perspective. *Journal of Child Psychiatry and Development.* 40 (1) pp. 129–140.

Kestly, T. A. B. (2014) *The Interpersonal Neurobiology of Play: Brain-building interventions for emotional well-being.* New York: W. W. Norton & Company.

Kolvin, I., Garside, R. F., Nicol, R. A., Macmillan, A., Wolstenholme, F. & Leitch, I. M. (1981) *Help Starts Here.* London: Tavistock Publications.

Kottman, T. (1999) Group applications of Adlerian play therapy. In Sweeney, D. S. & Homeyer, L. E. (eds.) *The Handbook of Group Play Therapy.* San Francisco, CA: Josey Bass. pp. 65–85.

Lahad, M. & Ayalon, O. (1993) *BASIC Ph - The Story of Coping Resources, Community Stress Prevention (Vol. II).* Kiryat Shmona, Israel: Community Stress Prevention Centre.

O'Connor, K. J. (2000) *The Play Therapy Primer: An Integration of Theories and Techniques.* New York: John Wiley & Sons.

O'Rourke, K. & Worzbyt, J. (1996) *Support Groups for Children.* New York: Brunner Routledge.

Panksepp, J., Burgdorf, J., Turner, C. & Gordon, N. (2003) Modeling ADHD-type arousal with unilateral frontal cortex damage in rats and beneficial effects of play therapy. *Brain and Cognition.* 52 (1) pp. 97–105.

Pearce, S. (2011) Narrative play therapy with children experiencing parental separation or divorce. In Taylor de Faoite, A. (ed.) *Narrative Play Therapy, Theory and Practice.* London: Jessica Kingsley Publishers. pp. 151–168.

Smith, D. M. & Smith, N. R. (1999) Relational activity play therapy group: A "Stopping off place" for children on their journey to maturity. In Sweeney, D. S. & Homeyer, L. E. (eds.) *The Handbook of Group Play Therapy.* San Francisco, CA: Josey Bass p. 234.

Sweeney, D. S. & Homeyer, L. E. (eds.) (1999) *The Handbook of Group Play Therapy.* San Francisco, CA: Josey Bass.

Taylor de Faoite, A. (ed.) (2011) *Narrative Play Therapy.* London: Jessica Kingsley Publishers.

White, M. & Epston, D. (1990) *Narrative Means to Therapeutic Ends.* New York: W. W. Norton & Company.

Yalom, I. D. (1975) *The Theory and Practice of Group Psychotherapy.* (2nd ed.) New York: Basic Books.

Chapter 14

Play therapy with children affected by sexual abuse

Developing awareness, safety and trust

Tim Woodhouse

Chapter overview

In this chapter, I will explore some of the elements of undertaking play therapy with children affected by sexual abuse. My focus is on the factors that promote a safe intervention for the child, within a legal framework. There is an opening discussion about the child's experiences prior to therapy, before going on to explore preliminary meetings and potential blocks to developing a therapeutic relationship. I go on to explore the definition and parameters of sexual abuse before considering the impact of the experience on the child and their family. The chapter concludes with a discussion of the care-giver response and the implications of video-recording the therapy sessions.

Considering the child's experiences

Four-year-old Bethany was in a pre-adoptive placement when she was referred for play therapy due to the mother's concerns that Bethany was oppositional, defiant and controlling with her (but not with the father). Bethany had been placed for adoption at birth at her mother's request, who had not felt able to be a parent. There were no concerns about the mother's background, mental health or behaviour before or during her pregnancy. The labour and birth were unremarkable. Bethany spent the next three and a half years in a short-term foster placement. She was a child of dual heritage; was bright, articulate and engaging. There were no obvious reasons for the delay in finding permanence for this child.

A therapist considering this referral might hypothesise that the antecedent to Bethany's behaviour may be an insecure attachment pattern born out of the trauma we all experience as we are arguably born into the pain of the world, fragmented and displaced. In addition, Bethany did not receive the comfort, familiar smell, heartbeat, skin contact and rhythm of her mother's biology, that is our introduction to being regulated by another and part of the four-year journey to becoming an integrated individual (Nijenhuis, 2004). Instead, she had to face the strangeness of unfamiliar carers with whom she would languish, but who would never fully claim her. She also had to overcome the grief and loss of a foster placement that had become her family and were her primary attachment figures. She may have harboured distress and disorientation in respect of her new geographical location, the significant differences in the make-up of the new family, or their parenting style, demeanour or attitude. She also had unmet identity issues. However, this child's history suggested she had been safe in the care of the local authority and had not experienced further disruption in her birth family.

The consideration of the possibility of sexual harm is not always at the forefront of most therapists' minds when accepting a referral for therapy. The type of therapy practiced, the age, background or gender of the therapist and of the person being referred, or the reason for the referral, may all be contributing factors that deflect us from the need to remain aware of the potential existence of this type of harm. When considering the experience of harm in others, we must also be mindful of the harm we, as therapists, have experienced. In order to be available to others, we need to ensure we have not become defended, dismissive, avoidant or over-focussed on particular issues. Therapists stay grounded by maintaining their open disposition through clinical supervision, personal therapy and adherence to the BAPT Core Competences (see Appendix 1).

Developing a sense of safety through preparation

Many therapists will collate the information they gather on the child, their history, background and familial relationships, as well as professional, educational, medical and social information, to develop a psychodynamic formulation to cultivate their hypotheses, before deciding on a therapeutic intervention plan (O'Connor & Ammen, 2012; Johnstone & Dallos, 2014). Often, the plan is merely a map to help the therapist keep an aide memoire of the child's chronological experiences, in order to keep in mind where change might occur, rather than for any directive script. The over-arching philosophy in non-directive play therapy is that the child can bring to therapy whatever issues they want or need to and is therefore free to direct the therapy around the issues that are the most troubling. Unfortunately, there are many reasons why children may be resistant to the notion of focussing on their experiences. These include threats, pressure or responsibility placed on them by their victimiser, a lack of safety, support, belief or emotional warmth from their safe carer, or ongoing contact with the person who harmed them. The assessment of the child's current situation may include challenging issues like ongoing contact, where there are contraindications, or there is evidence to suggest contact is not in the child's best interests.

At Tiptoes Child Therapy Services, our clinical practice is to start interventions with oversight of local authority files, paperwork, reports and court bundles before meeting parents, social workers, foster carers, teachers and others involved in the child's life. Once satisfied with the available information, we meet the child. Children are at an awful, unfair disadvantage in this process of becoming a client. Unlike adults, who typically choose to enter therapy, children usually do not. Children are often told, persuaded or cajoled (sometimes, not unlike their experience of harm) to go to therapy by their parents, carers, educators or others. Initial challenges in the therapeutic relationship are to overcome the power differential, lack of choice and anxiety the child is likely to be experiencing when meeting this unfamiliar adult.

Bethany was already communicating her feelings via her behaviours, which arguably stemmed from a state of anxiety. She may have had anxiety about my gender or confusion about understanding the process, feeling that she had no real choice whether this process proceeded or not. Anxiety reduction therefore is always a primary goal in any intervention. Anxiety is born out of a lack of safety (Norton & Norton, 2002) which, in turn, can be a result of a lack of trust in our primary care-givers to keep us safe. I start with the premise that children will feel safer at their home location rather than somewhere unknown, like a centre or clinic, even when the child has experienced abuse, neglect or even ongoing harm at their home location. When children have a negative and harmful experience, particularly a recurring one, this becomes a known or familiar experience and whilst undeniably anxiety-provoking, this familiar experience can be somewhat less scary than going to see a stranger in a new and unfamiliar place. Therefore, it is beneficial to have the first meeting with the children at their home. I usually take a brochure (Woodhouse, 2015), that gives the child a clear description of the therapist, centre/clinic and an understandable description of play therapy, which includes photographs and maps. This can become a reference and reminder for them in later years. The need for this type of concrete information was seen clearly during the investigation of North Wales Children's homes (Department of Health, 2000), where one of the recurring themes to emerge was adult survivors' confusion about which adults from the past had harmed them and which had not.

Meeting the child

Despite being seen in the company of her adoptive mother, Bethany was tense, prone to spurts of activity that seemed to have no purpose other than to move (run – flight), to talk (avoid – flight) and resistance to her mother's direction (control – safety). The messages from her mother were not received, Bethany did not appear to be connecting to her higher cortex, she could not process information such as communication, limits or even expressions of love (Fisher, 2017), she was not connecting to her parents and clearly did not feel safe or contained in her mother's presence. This is a difficult time for the parents or carers of scared children: they worry for their child, they worry about how they are seen to parent and worry about how best to respond to their child. My task was to take responsibility for the meeting. The building of trust is not just with the child but also with those people around the child. Anxiety breeds anxiety (Woodhouse, 2015) and if we do not help regulate the parent/carer, we cannot hope to regulate the child (BAPT Core Competence 7, see Appendix 1). During an initial meeting with the parents, and prior to meeting Bethany, we agreed an explanation about why she was coming to therapy and ascertained what her response was likely to be. Being forewarned enables the parent/carer to observe and be available to respond to the child, whilst allowing the therapist to be prepared to respond to the child's dialogue and their behavioural, emotional, or physiological responses. I named Bethany's feelings, whilst allowing her the possibility of correcting me: "It's sometimes really hard to meet new people when you don't know why they are here. I'm not a social worker come to move you and I'm not a grown-up who hurts children".

Bethany calmed, showed some signs of curiosity and eventually increased her proximity to her mother and myself, although she did not attempt to make physical contact with either of us. She remained wary, said little, but started to draw. Regardless of how we prepare the parent/carers, all too often the responses they make come from a place of discomfort, and so it was with Bethany's mother who stated, "Don't be rude Bethany, listen to Tim when he's talking to you". These curveballs require sensitive handling, as we neither want to alienate or shame the carer, nor side with them and ignore the impact of the violent (shame-inducing) communication on the child. My response aimed to make a repair on the parent's behalf and allow both mother and child to feel supported. I stated, "Sometimes children need to be doing something, like drawing, in order to listen, and I can see that Bethany is listening really hard, but she is also wanting to show us something really important". I still had not given a rationale to Bethany as to why I was going to be seeing her, nor sought from her why she thought I was here. Instead I said, "You concentrated really hard to draw that picture whilst listening to me. I'm wondering if you want to tell me about the picture you drew". This gave her permission to make the choice over whether or not she wanted to share her picture.

Bethany talked about her picture in the third person, stating, "A little girl is making a snowman. The mummy is nice and warm with hats and gloves and a scarf on, but the little girl is very cold, her mummy didn't make her warm". Bethany had said all that she wanted to say and would not be drawn to give further detail. We did not know which mummy she was referring to, or indeed, if "the little girl" to whom she referred was even her. We need to develop hypotheses about what this communication may mean. One possible hypothesis here could be that Bethany was referring to her physical needs not being met, either now or in the past, or that while some needs were met, the care she received had failed to assuage her sense of a lack of emotional or physical warmth. Further information came from the sense of how emotionally withdrawn Bethany's current adoptive mother presented. Whether overwhelmed in her own right, emotionally illiterate, or withdrawn for some other reason, the mother seemed unable or unwilling to connect with her daughter.

Using congruence

On preparing to leave, after my introductory visit, Bethany ran down the hall to catch me up, then flung her arms around me and pushed her face into my groin. Her body was tense, rigid as she held onto me, I felt locked-in, pinned and unable to move with ease. The experience was uncomfortable and neither of the parents commented or intervened, although they too looked awkward and shocked. As therapists we are 'feelings finders', looking for congruence or incongruence in the child's feeling and how it is expressed. If this is true, then so too are the children we work with. If we are incongruent when we have a feeling and try to disguise it, we are in danger of creating greater problems. The child may be confused about what we are feeling, or whether, like their abuser, we are trying to hide something. I recognised my discomfort, but felt that if I tried to disguise it as a demonstration of affection, then the child may be confused further. They may feel that something is wrong with them, distrust their reactions or think that I am dishonest and, therefore, untrustworthy. Of course, a therapist could give many possible responses at this point. If our chosen response is correct, then it is an insightful intervention, potentially liberating or cathartic. If it is wrong, then it is crucial we overtly apologise and make a clear repair.

In this instance, I chose to break the 'hug'. A hug is usually a greeting, a farewell, a sign of affection, or comfort where both participants gain an empathic response or support in a mutual, consensual and positive emotional experience. This experience however, did not feel affectionate, mutual, or beneficial to me – it felt sexual. The breaking of such a connection, even when that connection is clearly skewed, can be experienced as a rejection by the child, and so, I held her shoulders to bring us apart and I simultaneously crouched down, sliding my hands down to her arms as I went. This enabled us to maintain physical contact but to redirect it in a healthier manner, whilst I dropped to her eye level.

I stated, "It seems as though you are trying to tell me something really important huh?" (This was met by silence and a watchful gaze, and so I anticipated no further verbal response). I continued, "I'm not a grown-up who touches children's private parts or does sex things with children".

She sighed, and I could see and feel her previously rigid body relax and slump slightly. Before I let go, I stated, "You can talk to me or your parents as much or as little as you want about the things that make you feel worried or mixed up or tense or anything else, but I won't promise to keep what you say a secret as sometimes I need help from other grown-ups to keep children safe".

Bethany continued to be silent; she half smiled and returned to her parents as I stood and turned to leave. That night she disclosed the sexual abuse she had experienced at the hands of her foster mother to her new parents.

There will be debate here about whether my response was a directive or non-directive approach. I maintain that this was a non-directive response as it utilised 'congruence', one of the three main tenets of non-directive play therapy (Ryan & Courtney, 2009). I experienced a feeling as a result of a non-verbal communication instigated by the child and sought to demonstrate through my response that these feelings and experiences are permissible to talk about, think about or play about within the therapeutic space. To be vague or avoidant could confuse the child about the therapist's motivation, beliefs or potential behaviour. Sometimes the child believes that they will be re-victimised, that it is not an 'if' but a 'when' it will happen. Nothing we can say will take that belief away, the new experience of a safe adult–child relationship has to be lived. The naming of the child's fear can actually reduce the child's anxiety, helping them to feel 'safe-enough' to enter the therapeutic space with the therapist. There does, however, need to be a cautionary note: the emphasis of my reflection was on the type of adult **I am** and not on a leading statement that something had happened to the child (Bannister & Print, 1989; Ministry of Justice, 2011). The statement offers the child the potential to refute, clarify or challenge and thus leave the therapist room to repair or further reflect. At this moment, whatever the therapist has said or done is now potentially under the scrutiny of the judicial and legal arenas. Apart from her behaviour, there was no other information to suggest that Bethany had experienced or had been exposed to the risk of sexual harm.

Defining sexual abuse

The premise of being vigilant to the possibility of sexual abuse as part of the child's history is not about being 'abuse-over-focussed', but practical preparation for an event that is likely to happen at some point in the therapist's career, given the prevalence of child sexual abuse in the UK. Research findings suggest "1 in 20 children (4.8%) have experienced contact sexual abuse" (Radford et al., 2011:7.2) and that 18,915 sexual crimes against children under 16 were recorded in England and Wales in 2012/13 (Radford et al., 2011). The latest figures, as cited by Bentley et al. (2018:29), indicate "In

2016/17 there were 43,522 recorded sexual offences against children under 16 years old" and that "sexual activity involving a child under 13 has increased by 30.1% since 2015/16", showing a steep upward trend in the reporting of such offences. Statistically, the chance of a child having had some form of exposure to sexual harm is notable and the impact on the therapist can be as broad in severity as the sexual harm can be on the child.

In order for sexual harm to be seen, understood and accepted as a possibility by the therapist, a definition is needed to give parameters around what is abuse and what is ordinary, and healthy sexual development. Without a definition, it is sometimes difficult to see what has happened to others or ourselves as sexually abusive. Whilst on holiday in 2017, a conversation started between myself and two other men whom I had never previously met, with whom I shared our guide. The conversation went something like this:

MAN: When you say you work with children, you're a therapist right? Have they kind of gone off the rails and gotten into trouble with the law?

TIM: Sometimes children and young people I see get into trouble with the law, but really whatever their behaviour is, the behaviour really isn't the problem but it's the child's answer to the problem.

MAN: So what is the problem?

TIM: I work mostly, but not always, with children and young people who have experienced sexual harm.

MAN: Oh that's horrible, I mean that's awful, but you mean there are enough children that have that happen for you to only work with children who have been sexually abused?

TIM: *(Gives examples of the numbers of children seen at Sexual Assault Referral Centres and the statistics that are anything between 1/3 to 1/20).*

MAN: *(Looks at me and our thus far silent companion)* But that means two of us *(there were 8 people on this particular holiday)* have been abused, that's a bit far-fetched!

TIM: Yes, if you follow the greatest statistic, it even suggests one of us three has been abused doesn't it?

MAN: Well that's not likely is it? I've never had anything like that happen to me *(man's face screws up in disgust)*

TIM: Something has made you feel disgusted, huh?

MAN: Well, I've just thought of something. As a child we went to visit my cousin and on this one time he shoved his hand down my trousers and grabbed my penis, but that's not abuse is it?

TIM: I don't know because I wasn't there that time your cousin grabbed your penis, but maybe I can ask you some questions that might help you make sense of the experience?

MAN: Ok.

TIM: Was your cousin older, younger or about the same age as you?

MAN: Older by about 4 or 5 years.

TIM: Where were you when it took place?

MAN: It was outside, but we were on our own and no one else was around

TIM: How were you feeling when your cousin did that to you?

MAN: It was horrible *(face turns to disgust again)* He wouldn't stop even when I told him to get off!

TIM: What happened next?

MAN: I ran away.

TIM: You seem to be saying that your cousin was older, that he touched you in a place you didn't want him to touch, in private/secret, when there was no one else around, you didn't appear to like it, and your face screwed up in disgust, he didn't stop when you told him to and it only stopped when you ran away. Did you tell anyone?

MAN: No I didn't tell anyone! I can't believe he did that to me, I mean I never really saw him that much and not since I was a child … I can't believe I didn't see that! I'm going to tell him he shouldn't have done that!

MAN: So that's one in three.

TIM: No. You know that you are one out of three, but you don't know if you are the only one.

The notion that we do not know what has happened to us is not just seen in the random meeting of strangers, but also in our clinical practice. The first adolescent girl I saw was Tracey. I had read her files and reports and wondered how anybody could have survived such a globally abusive childhood. She had suffered the full spectrum of abuse and sexual abuse by family, friends and strangers, and I wondered how a child could survive such torture. While Tracey had known about her sexually abusive experiences, she had not known that these were wrong and illegal. She had believed that this was how families demonstrated love to each other and thus could not disclose it as sexual abuse, as to her, it was love.

Sexual harm is a term that covers the wide spectrum of harm from sexual abuse, rape, sexual assault to child sexual exploitation to sexually reactive behaviours and sexually harmful behaviours often referred to as SHB or HSB.

"Sexual abuse is defined as the involvement of dependent, developmentally immature children and adolescents in sexual activities they do not truly comprehend to which they are unable to give informed consent, or that violate the social taboos of family roles" (Schechter & Roberge, 1976:130). Sexual abuse can range from non-touch exposure to any form or format of pornography, voyeurism or indecent exposure, to being forced or manipulated into observing sex acts, to direct sexual assaults on the person by an individual or individuals. The draft document *Working Together to Safeguard Children* (HM Government, 2018:109) defines sexual abuse as: "forcing or enticing a child or young person to take part in sexual activities, not necessarily involving a high level of violence, whether or not the child is aware of what is happening". It goes on to state: "The activities may involve physical contact, including assault by penetration (for example, rape or oral sex) or non-penetrative acts such as masturbation, kissing, rubbing and touching outside of clothing" (ibid). They may also include non-contact activities and clarifies that "Sexual abuse is not solely perpetrated by adult males. Women can also commit acts of sexual abuse, as can other children" (HM Government, 2018:109).

Thus, like the work with Bethany, play therapists, male or female, must hold this knowledge within their awareness in the room, in order to be prepared to respond to any physical, verbal, emotional or play reaction relating to sexual harm that may manifest in the therapeutic relationship.

The impact of sexual abuse

The impact on the child depends on so many variable issues, that it is hard to gauge how each child or young person will respond to their experiences. Friedrich (cited in Gil, 1991:7) stated that the impact of sexual harm is on a continuum from "neutral to very negative" but concluded "it is important to recognise this variability because it reminds us again of the hopefulness that can be present even in traumatic events that the possibility for positive change always exists". Unlike physical abuse, child sexual abuse often leaves little physical evidence in terms of scars (Radford et al., 2011) due to the relatively quick healing capacity of the human body, especially in relation to the often-longer period it takes for the child or young person to disclose, which also reduces the chances of finding DNA evidence. Whilst physical damage, sexually transmitted infections and pregnancy are always possible, most offenders will not want to be caught as a result of the child's need for medical intervention. Twenty-five year-old Carmen for example, had been groomed and sexually abused from the age of 13. By age 15, she had been sold to a gang of men who sexually exploited her before selling her on to another group of men who continued to traffic her. Her abuse and grooming had been so robust that even facing this daily brutality she continued to return to her original abuser, a man whom she saw alternately or sometimes simultaneously as her lover, friend and father figure. The result was that she had very confused and mixed feelings about her involvement in the abuse, and thus was unable to remain consistent with her disclosures, staying loyal to the older male neighbour who had started this process. Psychological, cognitive and emotional impacts however, are often far less obvious with a range of states, traits and behaviours (actions) seen in the child's presentation and demeanour, specifically in reference to relationships. Thus, in therapy, children may often not see their abuse experiences as their reason for attending, they may not see it as abuse, they may not recall or even remember it. In addition, their understanding of any relationship, let alone a therapeutic relationship, may be distorted, requiring the therapist to be alert to the child's feelings towards them.

The closer the relationship, e.g. intra-familial, or more frequent the contact, e.g. school, pre-school, the greater the chance sexual harm has been repeated. Finkelhor (1995) argues this repetition is one of the conditions likely to cause developmental disruption while Beitchman et al. (1991) described how the frequency and duration of the abuse is associated with more severe outcomes. It is known that child physical, emotional or sexual abuse and neglect and domestic violence are causal factors in the mental and physical ill-health of children and adolescents (Richardson et al., 2002; DOH, 2004; Itzin, 2006). However, as Guelzow et al. (2002:57) eloquently stated, "a high level of parental (or carer) support lessens the impact of the child's sexual abuse and leads to a higher level of global self-worth".

Response by the parent/carer to the actual disclosure

How the family responds to an actual disclosure of sexual harm is important information that may enable therapists to gauge how supportive they will be to the child in any future intervention. For example, Caffaro (1995) argues that if the child's disclosure is denied by their family then the child may identify with their protectors' stance. This has clear implications for the therapist. If the child is not informed that the therapy is being provided, at least in part, because of their experience of sexual abuse, the danger is that the child will not know whether the therapist is aware of the abuse and may feel inhibited or shamed by their experience. We may compound this 'conspiracy of silence' by trying to avoid the subject and thus restrict what the child has permissions to explore.

Lusk and Waterman (1986) and Palmer (2001) describe a number of factors that impact on how a child makes sense of their experience of sexual harm. These include not just what the parent(s)/carer(s) do for the child, but also what they say to the child following their verbal disclosure, and how they respond to behavioural challenges arising as a result of sexual abuse. Bethany was believed by her pre-adoptive parents, who acted appropriately, contacting both the local safeguarding team and the police. However, her progress in therapy was also perpetually hampered by the mother's low-warmth and emotional detachment. The pain of the parent/carer's own experience can often result in counter-transference towards the child and lead service providers to question whether the child's needs are being met in placement. This is an important issue which should always be considered carefully.

Use of video-recording in clinical practice

Bethany was video-interviewed, using the Achieving Best Evidence (ABE) protocol for potential criminal proceedings (Ministry of Justice, 2011), during which she gave strong evidence of sexual abuse against her former foster mother. It emerged that the use of video-recording had been a part of her abuse experience. In addition, video was a necessary part of her complaint (ABE) experience and, later, became an integral component of her therapy. The idea of video-recording therapy sessions for many therapists is anathema (Landreth, 2012; O'Connor et al., 2016). However, the notion of safety is a complex one that is borne out of a number of factors. These include the therapist's self-belief in their safety as a person, as any self-doubt will most definitely be transmitted in one's body language, mirror neurones or transference to the child. Whilst positive self-belief inspires confidence, it must also be tempered with humility and acceptance of our own limitations. Safety is borne out of consistency, routine, predictability, presence and Rogers' core conditions (1957). Still though, doubt can remain. What makes a person safe?

I seek to create safety by not avoiding what we may assume to be unbearable for the child, but by proactively creating a transparency that is opposite to the conditions of the secrecy, grooming, pressure, manipulation and lies that allowed sexual abuse to thrive in the first place. This transparency is not easy, when we need to balance the growth of safety against maintaining the child's confidentiality, and this only becomes harder within criminal proceedings. The use of video gives a strong message to the child that you are looking out for the child's safety and your own wellbeing. The argument that it reminds the child of their abuse is only as valid as highlighting a bed, or a man (or woman), or a time, a season, a situation or any of the boundless number of sense-perception triggers that may remind the child of their abuse (Ogden et al., 2006; Ogden & Fisher, 2015; Fisher, 2017). All of these triggers are the triggers that need to be worked through, rather than avoiding them or trying to rescue children. Therapy is about enabling children to face their pain and their adversity by being emotionally held, socially regulated, having the opportunity for an act of triumph, the potential of transformation and to move on. When we can create safety around ourselves, we create safety around the child.

Summary

- It is important to consider a number of factors before working therapeutically with children who have experienced sexual harm, including planning to meet the child within their home and agreeing with parents how the purpose of therapy should be explained to the child.
- We need to consider how to create a safe space for the child and to reduce the child's initial anxiety by the use of child-centred skills and, in particular, using congruence to convey authenticity and transparency to the child.

- Issues of trust and safety within the therapeutic relationship are particularly significant for children who have experienced sexual abuse.
- The therapist will need to be mindful of the legal frameworks for working with children and young people affected by this type of harm and work within agreed procedures when dealing with disclosure of abuse or preparing for court.
- The therapist also needs to consider the involvement of parents/carers and wider systems within the therapeutic process.

Further reading

Daniels, D. & Jenkins, P. (2006) *Therapy with Children: Children's Rights, Confidentiality and the Law*. London: Sage. This is an accessible book that helps consider the issues of working therapeutically with children within a legal framework in the UK context.

Goodyear-Brown, P. (2011) *Handbook of Child Sexual Abuse: Identification, Assessment, and Treatment*. Hoboken, NJ: John Wiley and Sons. A good, relatively recent book that considers the major components of interventions in this field.

Horvath, M. A. H., Davidson, J. C., Grove-Hills, J., Gekoski, A. & Choak, C. (2014) *'It's a Lonely Journey': A Rapid Evidence Assessment on Child Sexual Abuse within the Family Environment*. London: Middlesex University. This research will help therapists understand the process that leads children from experiencing CSA within an intra-familial context and future vulnerability.

Levine, P. A. & Kline, M. (2006) *Trauma Through a Child's Eyes: Awakening the Ordinary Miracle of Healing*. Berkeley, CA: North Atlantic Books. A tool that helps therapists remain non-violent in their interventions.

Warrington, C., Beckett, H., Ackerley, E., Walker, M. & Allnock, D. (2017) *Making Noise: Children's Voices for Positive Change after Sexual Abuse. Children's Experiences of Help-Seeking and Support after Sexual Abuse in the Family Environment*. Luton, UK: University of Bedfordshire. This research is the child's voice on what has helped or hindered their recovery.

References

Bannister, A. & Print, B. (1989) A Model for Assessment Interviews in Suspected Cases of Child Sexual Abuse. *Occasional Paper Series Number 4*. London: NSPCC.

Beitchman, J., Zucker, K., Hood, J., Da Costa, G. & Akman, D. (1991) A review of the short-term effects of child sexual abuse. *Child Abuse and Neglect*. 15 pp. 537–556.

Bentley, H., Burrows, A., Clarke, L., Gillgan, A., Glen, J., Hafizi, M., Letendrie, F., Miller, P., O'Hagan, O., Patel, P., Peppiate, J., Stanley, K., Starr, E., Vasco, N. & Walker, J. (2018) *How Safe are our Children? The Most Comprehensive Overview of Child Protection in the UK: Every Childhood is Worth Fighting For*. London: NSPCC.

Caffaro, I. V. (1995) Identification and trauma: An integrative-developmental approach. *Journal of Family Violence*. 10 (1) pp. 23–40.

Department of Health. (2000) *Lost in Care: Report of the Tribunal of Inquiry into the Abuse of Children in Care in the Former County Council Areas of Gwynedd and Clwyd since 1974.* London: The Stationary Office.

Department of Health. (2004) *Choosing Health – Making Healthy Choices Easier.* White paper London: The Stationary Office.

Finkelhor, D. (1995) The victimisation of children: A developmental perspective. *American Journal of Orthopsychiatry.* 65 pp. 177–189.

Fisher, J. (2017) *Healing the Fragmented Selves of Trauma Survivors: Overcoming Internal Self-alienation.* New York: Routledge.

Gil, E. (1991) *The Healing Power of Play: Working with Abused Children.* New York: The Guilford Press.

Guelzow, J. W., Cornett, P. F. & Dougherty, T. M. (2002) Child sexual abuse: Victims perception of paternal support as a significant predictor of coping style and global self-worth. *Journal of Child Sexual Abuse.* 11 (4) pp. 53–72.

HM Government. (2018) *Working Together to Safeguard Children: A Guide to Inter-agency Working to Safeguard and Promote the Welfare of Children.* Draft for consultation. London: Department for Education.

Itzin, C. (2006) *Tackling the Health and Mental Health Effects of Domestic and Sexual Violence and Abuse.* London: DoH.

Johnstone, J. & Dallos, R. (2014) *Formulation in Psychology and Psychotherapy: Making Sense of People's Problems.* East Sussex, UK: Routledge.

Landreth, G. L. (2012) *Play Therapy: The Art of the Relationship.* (3rd ed.). Hove, UK: Routledge.

Lusk, R. & Waterman, J. (1986) Effects of sexual abuse on children. In: MacFarlane, K. & Waterman, J. (eds.). *Sexual Abuse of Young Children: Evaluation and Treatment.* New York: Guilford Press. pp. 299–311.

Ministry of Justice. (2011) *Achieving Best Evidence in Criminal Proceedings: Guidance on Interviewing Victims and Witnesses, and Guidance on Using Special Measures.* London: Ministry of Justice.

Nijenhuis, E. R. S. (2004) *Somatoform Dissociation: Phenomena, Measurement, and Theoretical Issues.* New York: W. W. Norton & Company.

Norton, C. C. & Norton, B. E. (2002) *Play Therapy: An Experiential Approach.* (2nd ed.). Denver, CO: White Apple Press.

Ogden, P., Minton, K. & Pain, C. (2006) *Trauma and the Body: A Sensorimotor Approach to Psychotherapy.* New York: W.W. Norton & Company.

Ogden, P. & Fisher, J. (2015) *Sensorimotor Psychotherapy: Interventions for Trauma and Attachment.* New York: W.W. Norton & Company.

O'Connor, K. & Ammen, S. (2012) *Play Therapy Treatment Planning and Interventions: The Ecosystemic Model and Workbook.* (2nd ed.). Cambridge, MA: Academic Press.

O'Connor, K. J., Schaefer, C. E. & Braverman, L. D. (eds.) (2016) *Handbook of Play Therapy.* (2nd ed.). Hoboken, NJ: Wiley.

Palmer, T. (2001) Pre-Trial therapy for children who have been sexually abused. In: Richardson, S. & Baron, H. (eds.). *Creative Responses to Child Sexual Abuse: Challenges and Dilemmas.* London: Jessica Kingsley Publishers. p. 152.

Radford, L., Corral, S., Bradley, C., Fisher, H., Bassett, C., Howat, N. & Collishaw, S. (2011) *Child Abuse and Neglect in the UK Today.* London: NSPCC.

Richardson, J., Coid, J., Petruckevitch, A., Shan Chung, W., Moorey, S. & Feder, G. (2002) Identifying domestic violence: Cross sectional study in primary care. *BMJ.* 324 pp. 1–6.

Rogers, R. (1957) The necessary and sufficient conditions of therapeutic personality change. *Journal of Consulting Psychology.* 21 pp. 95–103.

Ryan, V. & Courtney, A. (2009) Therapists' use of congruence in nondirective play therapy and filial therapy. *International Journal of Play Therapy.* 18 pp. 114–128.

Schechter, M. & Roberge, L. (1976) Child sexual abuse. In: Helfer, R. & Kempe, C. (eds.). *Child Abuse and Neglect: The Family and the Community.* Cambridge, MA: Ballinger. p. 130.

Woodhouse, T. (2015) Subcutaneous, subcortical, subconscious and subterranean; the most toxic boy in the world's search for mum. In: McCarthy, D. (ed.). *Deep Play - Exploring the Use of Depth in Psychotherapy with Children.* London: Jessica Kingsley Publishers. pp. 81–98.

Chapter 15

Working with bereavement and loss in play therapy

Chris Stone

Chapter overview

Following an introduction to how children might be affected by bereavement and loss, this chapter will consider theories of loss and their implication for play therapy practice. I will discuss a number of practice issues, including working with the child's wider system, the therapist's use of self, trusting the child's process, working flexibly, and evaluating therapy outcomes. I present three case examples. Names have been changed in case material to ensure confidentiality, and permission given.

Introduction

Death affects us all in different ways, but it does affect us all. A child or young person's bereavement experience, regardless of their age, can be just as painful and overwhelming as that of any adult (Wells, 2007). Their responses, however, differ.

Children's grief tends to be sporadic: they have a shorter 'sadness span' than adults, whose awareness and experience of loss is more persistent (Dyregrov, 2008). Adults will have already encountered a range of losses in their lives, and to some extent, developed strategies for managing such experiences (Di Ciacco, 2008). Most children have not. With limited ability to 'make sense' of the situation, what might otherwise seem like 'waves of grief' can be experienced by a child more like a 'tsunami' ...

Most families journey through their grieving process adequately, both collectively and individually, particularly if they have a reliable support network in place (Walsh & McGoldrick, 2004). The need for professional intervention is more likely where the child's needs are insufficiently met, e.g. in the case of the death of a partner or child, parents may be so engulfed by their personal grief that they are, understandably, not as emotionally available to the remaining children as they might otherwise be.

Individual experiences of grief vary and are influenced by such factors as the nature of the loss, the relationship with the deceased, previous experiences of loss and how they were dealt with, the age and developmental stage of the child, and other circumstances after the loss. Hence, know-ledge and understanding of child development is essential (BAPT Core Competences 1 & 2, see Appendix 1). Dyregrov (2008) describes the signifi-cant correlation between chronological age and level of cognition. For example, an infant can experience and display distress due to the absence of their primary carer. At the more concrete level of thinking, a young child will worry about who will feed/keep the person warm. The pre-school child's egocentricity may lead them to believe that the death is due to something they have said or done. The older child/adolescent has a greater sense of the long-term impact of such, realising death to be universal, per-sonal and irreversible. Therefore, children are likely to re-experience their grief repeatedly, in line with their developing understanding. This can be confusing for both the child and adults around them, particularly as their inability to verbalise/process emotions can erupt into 'negative' behaviour.

For the child, the sense of security in their world, which is fundamental to healthy emotional growth (Sories et al., 2015), has been snatched away and they may become anxious, regress behaviourally (e.g. separation-anxiety, bed-wetting), become withdrawn or act out their bewilderment and despair through anger. 'Sometimes the behaviour presented by grieving children is not linked to their bereavement at all and the child ends up labelled as bad, when in fact, they are just sad' (Smith, 1999:10). The spon-taneous 'Rap' song below appears to bear this out. One child in a group of 7-year-olds, began to tap her pencil rhythmically on the table, and the others joined in, adding words in what seemed to be an effortless way:

> Why, why, why did you die, die, die?
> I'm sitting here wanting to cry, cry, cry …
> I didn't have a chance to say 'Bye, Bye, Bye' …
> I would like to say 'Hi, Hi, Hi'.
> I think you are in the sky, sky, sky.
> When my teacher says I'm being bad, bad, bad,
> I am really feeling very sad, sad, sad.
> I am kicking the door madly, madly, madly …
> And I'm going to sleep sadly, sadly, sadly …
> I want to see you so badly, badly, badly …

As children's responses hinge greatly upon their perception of what has hap-pened to the deceased, the words used by adults are important (e.g. 'gone to sleep' might engender a fear of going to sleep themselves; 'gone away' can imply the possibility of them returning). Children can only manage to assimi-late the facts and tolerate the feelings gradually. Consequently, a child will often change the subject when the bereavement is being explained: 'Can I go out to play now?' Or appear uncaring about such: 'Can I have his bedroom?' Similarly, they may repeatedly ask the same questions. We all utilise inbuilt coping strategies, known as 'defence mechanisms', as protection against being overwhelmed by intense emotions. These natural ways of managing stress and difficult feelings operate at an unconscious level (Burgo, 2012). Hence the importance of the therapist being aware of the unconscious defences in the child's responses.

Play therapy is particularly helpful for these children due to the nurturing environment, the respectful, non-judgemental stance of the therapist and the absence of pressure to 'talk about it'. The fact that the child is 'in charge' can be healing in itself, given that he has been powerless to prevent or remedy the loss. 'The healing power of play cannot be underestimated' (Gil, 1991:52).

Theories of loss

Bereavement refers to the state of loss, especially through death. Loss is similar, not necessarily through death (e.g. the separation/divorce of parents, moving house, death of a beloved pet, changing schools, loss of a sense of safety ...). Grief is the normal emotional response to a loss (Stokes, 2004). Mourning – often interchangeable with 'grieving' – is the complex psychological process involved following that loss (i.e. of accepting the reality and implications of such, and adapting to those changes).

A number of influential theories of loss have shaped therapeutic practice in this area.

Kubler-Ross (1969) originated the Five Stages of Grief, in which the bereaved person moves through key emotional responses to their loss:

1. Denial
2. Anger
3. Bargaining
4. Depression
5. Acceptance

Worden (2003) proposed the Four Tasks of Mourning as:

1. To accept the reality of the loss
2. To work through to the pain of grief
3. To adjust to an environment in which the deceased is missing
4. To emotionally relocate the deceased and move on with life.

While not originally intended to be linear models, the implied order of these theories both tend to suggest a distinct beginning and end, with a specific sequence to follow, along with the inherent possibility of failure when the bereaved might become 'stuck' at one of those stages. Worden (2003:15) supports this idea when he states that 'It is essential that the grieving person accomplish these tasks before mourning can be completed'.

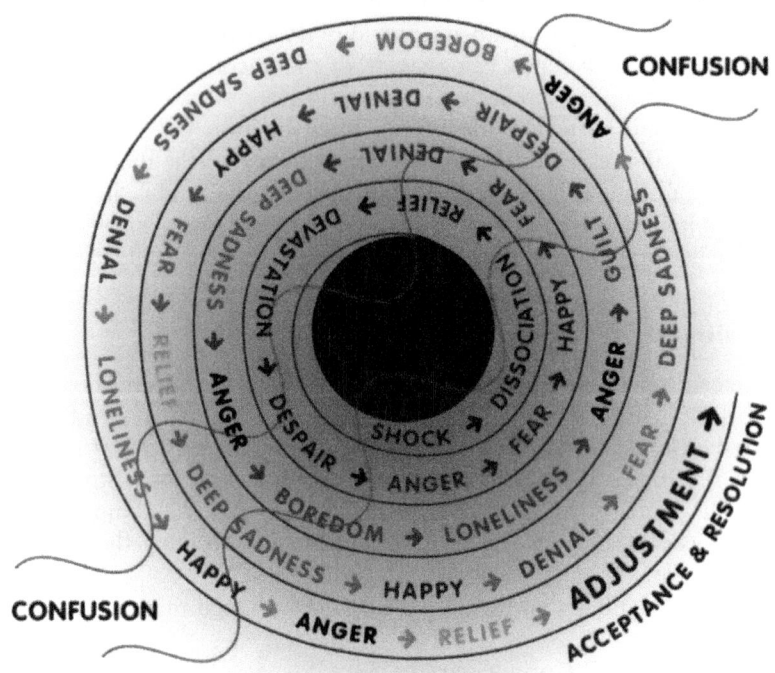

Figure 15.1 Upward Spiral of Grief © Gilbert 2004. Reproduced with kind permission.

The theories that most influence my own practice are the Bowlby/Parkes Attachment Model of Bereavement and the Upward Spiral of Grief (Figure 15.1).

Bowlby and Parkes (1970) described the Four Phases of Grief in children as: **Numbness** ⟷ **Yearning** ⟷ **Disorientation & Despair** ⟷ **Reorganisation.** They suggest overlapping phases of grief, rather than prescriptive, sequential stages. This notion allows for the fluidity of children's grief over time, as they move in and out of the overwhelming nature of their loss.

I find the Upward Spiral of Grief (Gilbert, 2018) particularly helpful as it is clear and direct, engenders a sense of hope, and children themselves 'get it'. 'Upward' denotes directional movement away from the dark 'starting point'; the 'scattered' range of emotions seems more realistic than a clear-cut pathway in neat, predictable steps. This concept normalises the repeated resurfacing of emotions as an ongoing part of the upward process, rather than a backward step. 'It does not mean that you have gone back to the black hole in the beginning. **Life will never be the same. It's different. And that's OK**' (Gilbert, 2018:3).

There is no 'right' or 'wrong' way to grieve; it is a personal journey that cannot be prescribed. Smith and Pennells (2000) emphasise that mourning remains an ongoing experience throughout our lives.

The concepts of 'acceptance' and 'moving on' can be misunderstood as meaning to 'leave behind' ... to 'forget'. Prince William was aged 15 when his mother died in a car accident. Many years later, whilst visiting a hospice, he said to a 14-year-old boy whose mother had died the previous year:

> Time makes it easier ... I still miss my mother every day and it's twenty years after she died ... It's okay to feel sad; it's okay for you to miss her.[1]

This process is not about forgetting the person. It is about acknowledging, albeit reluctantly, 'this has really happened' and gradually learning to live without them.

Working with the wider system

The systemic perspective considers the world in terms of social systems, relationships and integration, with the immediate system being the child's family (Hoffman, 1981). Whilst the child is often perceived as 'the problem', it is vital to consider the presenting issues in a relational context.

The involvement of parents/carers to support the therapeutic intervention is important in promoting the effectiveness of the eventual outcome for the child (Ryan & Wilson, 2000). Due to the presenting issues of the child invariably relating to perceived 'bad/unacceptable behaviour', many families have experienced criticism and, quite understandably, may approach the first meeting with trepidation and a defensive stance. I tend to adopt the systemic therapy concept of the 'one-down position' (Fisch & Schlanger, 1999) whereby I regard the parent as the expert on their child and I therefore need their help in understanding what has brought them to this point. It is vital that the parent feels accepted and respected, and an attitude of 'respectful curiosity' can facilitate such.

For assessment (BAPT Core Competence 18, see Appendix 1), I meet first with the parents, then with the parents and child together, then with the child individually. Inclusion of the parents with the child can be particularly useful in giving a glimpse of insight into the relational dynamics, as well as being more helpful for the child than meeting this 'new person' alone. It also provides the opportunity to model sensitive and supportive responses to the child.

Alongside regular parental reviews, occasional family meetings have proved beneficial in enabling a greater understanding of each other and a sense of working together. For example, parents are often unaware of the capacity of a young child to remember significant events; are convinced that 'he won't remember that – he was only little', and therefore will have been unaffected by it. Meeting together to focus on a 'time-line', beginning with the child's birth, I wonder at each point what both parents felt and how the child might have felt at the time. This invariably proves significant in developing closer relationships and a more open expression of emotions generally within the family.

Another helpful activity is 'Family Changes' whereby I read out a story and family members use puppet re-enactment (Lowenstein, 2006). For example, a family who experienced parental death by suicide were able to demonstrate reactions when told, including associated thoughts and feelings.

Therapist's use of self

Entering each session free of distractions allows the therapist to be fully attentive, and is central to the intervention being child-focussed (Axline, 1969). Hence the need to find a way of ensuring all associated facts, thoughts and feelings are left outside the therapy room door, thereby enabling the therapist to be completely available to the child (Kirschenbaum, 2007).

The area of bereavement and loss, including the temptation to 'rescue' the child, can pose a considerable challenge to the play therapist. We have all encountered some sort of loss in our lives, and our minds automatically revert to them. Accompanying a grieving child may reactivate feelings about our own past losses (Worden, 2003) and if the child's situation is beyond our personal experience, we may have strong views as to how it might (or, indeed, 'must') be for the child. This is where preconceived ideas can be rooted, and not necessarily part of our awareness; thus personal therapy and professional supervision are essential (BAPT Core Competences 13 & 14, see Appendix 1).

Occasions will arise when we need to 'speak the unspeakable' (McCarthy, 2008). For example, initial meetings when it is important to ensure that the child is clear about our understanding of why they have come – that we are open with the child about what we already know. This is essential to developing a trusting relationship, as well as demonstrating that nothing 'terrible' happens if the loss is mentioned, which is a worry that children often have. Awareness of both self and the child are vital to maintaining professional distance – to empathise with the child without becoming overwhelmed oneself by their feelings of distress (Kirschenbaum, 2007).

We have our personal opinions, but that is all they are: there is no room for such in the therapeutic arena. I attempt to redress the balance by holding uppermost what is in the child's best interests, focussing upon what the child is trying to communicate, and reminding myself that 'the therapeutic journey belongs to the child' (Cattanach, 1994:52).

Trusting the child's inner process

The play therapist chooses to trust that the child knows what she needs at any given time, and that she has the capacity to get those needs met in the most appropriate way. Confidence in 'the actualising tendency' (Kirschen-baum, 2007) is crucial. Indeed, the innate striving towards growth and maturation is a fundamental tenet of play therapy and facilitates the process of mourning and recovery.

Play symbolically reflects something of the child's internal world, thereby enabling safe expression of otherwise overwhelming feelings, and the possibility of increased mastery through the themes that emerge. 'It provides a medium for the growth of a sense of self, competence and confidence in the surrounding world' (Chazan, 2002:19). My work with Daisy illustrates this.

Daisy

Daisy (aged 6) and Beth (aged 8) were referred by their mother five months after a traffic accident that resulted in the death of their father (who was driving at the time). Daisy had changed considerably since the event: the contented, happy little girl had become a rampaging, raging bull. I worked with the family for nine months. Two years later, Daisy asked Mum if she could see me again. Play therapy was agreed.

From the outset, Daisy was particularly drawn to the doll-house and figures, and began to enact an elaborate family scenario which lasted over five sessions.

Shortly before the fourth session ended, a brief scene between the parents took place in which Dad was ready to leave for work and called out that he was taking the car. Mum responded that he couldn't, as she needed it 'to take the kids to school'. As the engine started, Mummy said (in an almost 'matter-of-fact' manner) 'I'm a good driver, because Daddy just crashes'.

The next week, Daisy took on the role of Mum when she commented about being a good driver, ending with an incredibly long, loud, high-pitched scream to her husband: 'You always crash the car!!!' She repeated this several times. Daisy sighed, then calmly concluded, 'I think we can leave it there now'.

Reflections: The following session, Daisy informed me that she no longer needed to see me. Without being able to say exactly what prompted this decision, it seemed that the previous session had given her a sense of completion. By entering fully into role play to express anger to her Dad about his driving, whilst maintaining psychological safety through remaining in the role of 'Mum', this little girl had done what was necessary, at least for now.

Based upon the Four Phases of Grief model, Daisy initially appeared to manage well ('Numbness' characteristically gives this impression). After several weeks, as the reality of her loss began to dawn, her sense of bewilderment and rage seemed all-pervasive ('Yearning' typically involves intense feelings being acted out towards others). Two years later, her play indicated a shift to more personalised anger, firstly portrayed symbolically, and then taken on by herself in the role of Mum, now in the present tense. This supported her in being able to own and express her thoughts and feelings regarding not only Dad's death, but also her perception of his responsibility in that. As the harsh reality continues to sink in, deep sorrow and anguish would likely surface (encompassed in 'Disorientation and Despair'). I am sure that Daisy will continue her 'journey' in the way that is best for her.

I firmly believe that, given an appropriate environment and the security of the therapeutic relationship, our clients will draw from each session what they need at that time. Play therapy provides optimum conditions for growth (Axline, 1969). The fact that Daisy took the initiative in asking for further professional help two years later, demonstrates how the child will instinctively discern, albeit on an unconscious level, her own therapeutic timescale. It confirms that 'the child knows best'.

Working flexibly within child-centred practice

It is easy to agree enthusiastically on the importance of flexibility and being child-led. We never know, however, where exactly the child will take us, and this example illustrates the challenge when 'following' entails adapting established boundaries.

Hayden

Hayden's mother had unexpectedly left the family 3 months ago. Aged 7, he was displaying signs of 'separation anxiety' in relation to his father (Mick).

Hayden's opening ritual each week was to kick off his shoes and dash to the other side of the room, landing on a pile of large, soft cushions. (He described this as 'getting rid of my angry energy'). He then picked up the mega-sized crocodile, using it in different ways each week (e.g. hungry, mean, friendly crocodile, hoover, oar, cricket bat). He called it 'The Croc of the Week': my task was to guess what it was each time.

Apart from the possible symbolism of different aspects of Mum, I sensed this was about far more than 'The Croc' itself, but also about testing how attentive and trustworthy I was to him. How much 'control' did he really have? Would I accept and follow where he led? Hayden clearly benefitted from releasing his 'angry energy' before proceeding further, confident that I could safely contain those emotions (Symington & Symington, 1996).

Session 6

Hayden was reluctant to come with me today, so Dad joined him … He used mainly symbolic play, with some representation through drawing;

themes revolved around destruction and devastation. The emotional content focussed on Hayden's feelings when told Mum was leaving. He communicated clearly and safely through the metaphor of play, with verbal clarification in response to my reflections and checking out meanings directly with him.

Hayden spontaneously drew pictures of the family before and after Mum left. He chose four 'Moody Bears' faces: sad, angry, confused and scared. ('Moody Bears' are wooden figures portraying different feelings by facial expression). Slowly taking the happy and laughing faces, Hayden laid a finger across each and pushed them to the far end of the table.

THERAPIST: Perhaps it's difficult to imagine being happy again?

CHILD: Yes … *(He held another face: surprised.)*

THERAPIST: I wonder whether you were surprised when you were told Mummy was leaving?

CHILD: Yes … very, very surprised … *(Hayden then drew a heart and tore the paper.)*

THERAPIST: That looks like a heart torn apart …
(He nodded, then pretended to remove his own heart and break it).

THERAPIST: Perhaps Hayden has a broken heart?

CHILD: Yes, that's right.
(Dad then went to the toilet…)
Immediately, Hayden said: Right then … I know what I must do now!
(Removing his shoes, he repeatedly hurled himself at the cushions.)

CHILD: And "The Croc of the Week" is …. *(He raised the large crocodile like a plane above his head … 'zooming' loudly around the room. I guessed correctly.)*

CHILD: Imagine two very high towers (they've been on the telly) at the end of the room … What are they called?

THERAPIST: The Twin Towers?

CHILD: Correct … Now watch closely what happens …

THERAPIST: So the plane gets faster and faster and louder and louder and flies straight into the tower … SMASH! Then it flies into the other tower … BOOM!

CHILD: Exactly! This one totally collapsed … the other only half-collapsed … And what happened next?
(He ran away from the towers …)

THERAPIST: The people ran away as fast as they could.

CHILD: Correct again!
(Hayden opened his mouth wide, pointing to it …)

THERAPIST: And lots of rubble and dust went into their mouths?

CHILD: Yes, but that's not really it …

THERAPIST: And they were screaming.

CHILD: Now you're getting the point!

THERAPIST: And that's what you did when you were told about Mummy leaving?

CHILD: No ... but I wanted to ...

THERAPIST: So ... when you were told about Mummy leaving you felt like screaming and running out of the room.

CHILD: Yes, yes!

> *(Giving him permission to scream now if he wanted to, Hayden let out two lengthy, piercing screams ...)*

THERAPIST: And it was like your heart was broken? There was a big explosion inside you and your heart was broken in pieces?

CHILD: That's it – **NOW** you understand – that's what I've been trying to tell you all this time – that's the **WHOLE** point! *(Hayden chose to re-enact the above when Dad returned.)*

Reflections: Hayden had been confident working individually, whilst his father waited in a nearby room. This made me take particular notice of his reluctance now.

Whilst there are a range of approaches involving parents with their child, such as Filial Therapy (Van Fleet & Guerney, 2003), this had not been the approach used with Hayden. A parent joining the child's session would ordinarily cross the clear boundary of ensuring consistency and confidentiality of the session, yet I had a strong sense that this would be beneficial, rather than an interruption or intrusion of the child's space. Permitting this was an exception for this particular child at this particular moment – exercising clinical judgement based upon the concepts of being child-led and of 'self-actualisation' (Kirschenbaum, 2007). 'Internal supervision' (Casement, 1985) was intrinsic to responding to what I considered to be in Hayden's best interests.

With my play therapy practice being primarily non-directive, I would normally stay within the metaphor of the play (Mills & Crowley, 1986). Hayden, however, had invited some sort of interpretation through 'The Croc of the Week'. He wanted me to say what 'The Croc' represented each time – to identify my sense of his perspective in that moment ... what it meant to him. He made a direct link to his broken heart, hence my decision to follow his lead beyond the metaphor (Dorfman, 1996).

It was interesting that Hayden did not slip into his familiar 'opening ritual'. On some level, perhaps, he felt unsafe at discharging such overwhelming anger with Dad there. He set the theme by drawing and utilising the 'Moody Bears' in the context of being told Mummy was going.

His description of the towers falling seemed particularly poignant, given that one parent 'disappeared' completely whilst the other partially 'collapsed'.

Equally significant was Hayden's response as soon as his Dad left the room. Hayden had not forgotten the ritual: his need to reveal his feelings of sorrow and distress to Dad, in the safety of my presence, was paramount from the outset. Mick was meeting with me weekly regarding the needs of the children and appropriate responses to them. Witnessing Hayden's sorrow was unbearable, prompting him to leave the room; returning took immense courage. We spoke later by phone and discussed fully the next day. He also commenced personal counselling, which enabled him to support the children without becoming overwhelmed by his own emotions (Stokes & Stubbs, 2008).

Linking with the Upward Spiral of Grief image, Hayden gradually emerges from the 'black hole' of initial shock and confusion, into a 'whirlwind' of powerful emotions. With fluctuating intensity, he began to distinguish between them and express them, graphically 'without words' until he 'found his voice'. With no pressure of fixed expectations, this concept releases Hayden to feel what he does, when he does, both now and in the future.

This session reflects not only Hayden's progress, but also Mick's in terms of what he could tolerate himself. Dad was more able to 'hear' his son. They 'survived the worst', emotionally, and did so together. The play was painfully difficult, yet immensely cathartic. As they left, I heard Hayden triumphantly exclaim, 'Gosh, I'm tired, but I think that went really well today!'

Hayden never asked for Dad to enter a session again. Nevertheless, it was a pivotal part of the developing sequence throughout the whole intervention, whereby Hayden was enabled to express feelings to me ... then to Dad in my presence ... and finally to Dad at home. This indicates healthy 'upward' progress in the family system; empowering them, rather than encouraging dependence upon me. Mick's parting words at the final review were, 'Thank you for giving me back my son ...'.

Evaluating outcomes in play therapy

Evaluating recovery from loss can be complex because of the long-term nature of grieving and the lack of clear, distinguishable points in that journey. Even more so with children, due to the frequent changeability in responses and their difficulty articulating feelings.

The 'Body of Feelings' (my terminology) is a simple, child-friendly evaluation tool that I use with clients at the start and towards completion of the intervention. Children colour in the 'ginger-bread' body, indicating the location and size of their feelings (Heegaard, 1998). We review them together on our penultimate week, and I give the child a copy at the final session.

The reality is that even if significant changes are noticed by family, friends, school or therapist, the impact is likely to be diminished if the child himself is unaware of them. Participating in this activity ensures that the child becomes conscious of such changes themselves.

The following is based upon comparison of 9 year old Josh's 'Before Therapy' and 'After Therapy', 20 months after his mother's suicide.

Before Therapy

- Your arms, chest and legs were 'blue' ... FULL OF SADNESS
- Your head and your stomach were 'red' ... SO MUCH ANGER
- Your hands and your feet were 'black' ... REALLY SCARED

After Therapy

- Your arms, chest and legs were 'yellow' ... full of HAPPY FEELINGS
- Your head and your stomach were 'blue', with SADNESS
- Your feet were 'red' ... showing ANGRY FEELINGS
- Your hands were 'green', although you didn't say what that was ...

Reflecting upon these, Josh noticed that his original anger was now replaced by the same amount of sadness; his feet now held that anger, but there wasn't as much as before. There was nothing black – those scared feelings had gone. He was now able to have happy feelings – there was no happiness at all before.

I believed it was important to follow through on Josh not saying what his 'green hands' indicated. Below are my verbatim notes that I shared with him.

> I wondered what the colour of your hands might mean. 'Jealous', you whispered. I commented that we're often told that it's not a good thing to be jealous – that it's 'wrong'. There are times though when it is so understandable to feel jealous that it would be very surprising if you didn't have those feelings ...
>
> I said that we both knew that I don't always get things right, but I wondered if you'd let me have a guess about it. You nodded.
>
> I wondered whether, when you came out of school you felt jealous when you saw other children running to their mums. You knew that your Mum would never be there to meet you again. 'Yes', you replied.
>
> I also wondered whether you might feel jealous when you were playing at friends' houses and heard their mums calling out to them. You knew that you would never hear your Mummy's voice calling your name again. You looked straight at me, saying, 'Yes – that's it! You've got it!' You breathed out a huge sigh of relief and smiled – it really was OK for you to feel jealous after all ...

Evaluation is crucial to ensuring the highest levels of professional standards (BAPT Core Competence 31, see Appendix 1) and effectiveness of interventions, including feedback from clients themselves. Josh said that before therapy he thought that he would always feel like that. It was good for him to see that things had changed, without his realising it was happening.

Conclusion

Children are often the 'forgotten mourners' (Smith & Pennells, 1995) and they need to be able to work through their grief and to know that supportive adults understand and respect their need to do so (Dreikurs & Stolz, 1987). There can be serious repercussions if issues relating to bereavement and loss are not adequately managed – if children are not able to 'make sense' of their experience ... Significant losses, and the manner they are dealt with, will affect not only the child but also the adult they will become (Mallon, 1998).

Tempted as we might be to 'protect' our children from distress, it is only through the actual experiencing of the natural emotional pain intrinsic to each 'journey of grief' that adequate healing can be attained (Worden, 1996). With encouragement and sensitive support, grieving children can develop strategies for managing loss not only now, but in the future.

> Loss and pain are inescapable, but permanent damage should not be.
>
> (Weiss, 1988:50–51)

Summary

- Children are never too young to grieve.
- There is no right or wrong way to grieve.
- Play therapy supports the grief process towards recovery particularly well.
- Children need to feel included, heard and reassured.
- Children need to be encouraged to express their feelings fully, to ask any questions they may have.
- Children need truthful, clear and age-appropriate responses from adults.
- It is the child's journey; the child knows best!

Further reading

Cusick, T. & Hepworth, S. (2004) *When Someone Dies: Questions Children Ask about Bereavement and Grief.* Dewsbury, UK: Eric. F. Box Ltd.

Grollman, E. (1993) *Straight Talk about Death for Teenagers: How to Cope with Losing Someone You Love.* Boston, MA: Beacon Press.

Mellonie, B. (1983) *Lifetimes: The Beautiful Way to Explain Death to Children.* Melbourne, FL: Bantam Books.

Romain, T. & Verdick, E. (2003) *What on Earth Do You Do When Someone Dies?* Minneapolis, MN: Free Spirit Publishing Inc.

Winchester, K. & Beyer, R. (2001) *What in the World Do You Do When Your Parents Divorce?* Minneapolis, MN: Free Spirit Publishing Inc.

Supporting a child when ... A range of publications by Winston's Wish, offering support for a child or young person who has been bereaved or who is facing the possible death of a family member: guidance for families and professionals – www. winstonswish.org.uk

Note

1 Reproduced with kind permission from HRH Prince William, The Duke of Cambridge.

References

Axline, V. (1969) *Play Therapy.* New York: Ballantine Books.

Bowlby, J. & Parkes, C. M. (1970) Separation and loss within the family. In: Anthony, E. J. (ed.) *The Child in His Family.* New York: John Wiley. pp. 197–216.

Burgo, J. (2012) *Why Do I Do That? Psychological Defense Mechanisms and the Hidden Ways They Shape Our Lives.* Chapel Hill, NC: New Rise Press.

Casement, P. (1985) *On Learning from the Patient.* London: Routledge.

Cattanach, A. (1994) *Play Therapy: Where the Sky Meets the Underworld.* London: Jessica Kingsley Publishers.

Chazan, S. (2002) *Profiles of Play: Assessing and Observing Structure and Process in Play Therapy.* London: Jessica Kingsley Publishers.

Di Ciacco, J. (2008) *The Colors of Grief: Understanding a Child's Journey through Loss from Birth to Adulthood.* London: Jessica Kingsley Publishers.

Dorfman, E. (1996) Play therapy. In: Rogers, C. (ed.) *Client-Centred Therapy: Its Current Practice, Implications and Theory.* London: Constable. pp. 235–277.

Dreikurs, R. & Stolz, V. (1987) *Children: The Challenge.* New York: Plume Books.

Dyregrov, A. (2008) *Grief in Children: A Handbook for Adults.* (2nd ed.) London: Jessica Kingsley Publishers.

Fisch, R. & Schlanger, K. (1999) *Brief Therapy with Intimidating Cases: Changing the Unchangeable.* San Francisco, CA: Josey-Bass.

Gil, E. (1991) *The Healing Power of Play: Working with Abused Children.* New York: The Guilford Press.

Gilbert, S. (2015) *Diagram of 'Spiral of Grief'.* London: Grief Encounter Publications.

Gilbert, S. (2018) *Grief Encounter: A Workbook to Encourage Conversations about Death between Children and Adults.* (5th ed.) London: Grief Encounter Publications.

Heegaard, M. (1998) *When Someone Very Special Dies: Children Can Learn to Cope with Grief.* Minneapolis, MN: Woodland Press.

Hoffman, L. (1981) *Foundations of Family Therapy: A Conceptual Framework for Systems Change.* New York: Basic Books.

Kirschenbaum, H. (2007) *The Life and Work of Carl Rogers.* (2nd ed.) Ross-on-Wye, UK: PCCS Books.

Kubler-Ross, E. (1969) *On Death and Dying.* New York: The Macmillan Company.

Lowenstein, L. (2006) *Creative Interventions for Bereaved Children.* Toronto, ON: Champion Press.

Mallon, B. (1998) *Helping Children to Manage Loss: Positive Strategies for Renewal and Growth*. London: Jessica Kingsley Publishers.

McCarthy, D. (ed.) (2008) *Speaking about the Unspeakable: Non-Verbal Methods and Experiences in Therapy with Children*. London: Jessica Kingsley Publishers.

Mills, C. & Crowley, R. (1986) *Therapeutic Metaphors for Children and the Child within*. London: Brunner-Routledge.

Ryan, V. & Wilson, K. (2000) *Case Studies in Non-directive Play Therapy*. London: Jessica Kingsley Publishers.

Smith, S. C. (1999) *The Forgotten Mourners: Guidelines for Working with Bereaved Children*. (2nd ed.) London: Jessica Kingsley Publishers.

Smith, S. C. & Pennells, S. M. (1995) *The Forgotten Mourners: Guidelines for Working with Bereaved Children*. London: Jessica Kingsley Publishers.

Smith, S. C. & Pennells, S. M. (eds.) (2000) *Interventions with Bereaved Children*. (3rd impression.) London: Jessica Kingsley Publishers.

Sories, F., Maier, C., Beer, A. & Thomas, V. (2015) Addressing the Needs of Military Children through Family-Based Play Therapy. *Contemporary Family Therapy*, 37 (3), pp. 209–220. doi:10.1007/s10591-015-9342-x

Stokes, J. (2004) *Then, Now and Always: Supporting Children as They Journey through Grief*. Cheltenham, UK: Winston's Wish.

Stokes, J. & Stubbs, D. (2008) *A Child's Grief: Supporting a Child When Someone in Their Family Has Died*. (3rd ed.) Cheltenham, UK: Winston's Wish.

Symington, J. & Symington, N. (1996) *The Clinical Thinking of Wilfred Bion*. London: Routledge.

Van Fleet, R. & Guerney, L. (eds.) (2003) *Casebook of Filial Therapy*. Boiling Springs, PA: Play Therapy Press.

Walsh, F. & McGoldrick, M. (eds.) (2004) *Living Beyond Loss: Death in the Family*. (2nd ed.) New York: Norton.

Weiss, R. S. (1988) Loss and recovery. *Journal of Social Issues*. 44 (3), pp. 37–52. doi:10.1111/j.1540-4560.1988.tb02075.x

Wells, R. (2007) *Helping Children Cope with Grief: Facing a Death in the Family*. (2nd ed.) London: Sheldon Press.

Worden, J. W. (1996) *Children and Grief: When a Parent Dies*. New York: The Guilford Press.

Worden, J. W. (2003) *Grief Counselling and Grief Therapy: A Handbook for the Mental Health Practitioner*. (3rd ed.) London: Routledge.

Chapter 16

Integrative approaches to working with trauma

Lisa Waycott and Clare Carbis

Chapter overview

In this chapter, we reflect on our therapeutic practice when working with a child who has experienced developmental trauma as a result of neglect and abuse. A definition of developmental trauma will be provided and we will present our integrative model of working, based on a case study of a 7-year-old boy's journey through the therapeutic process, utilising child-centred play therapy, attachment-focused therapy and therapeutic life story work. Techniques and approaches used in our work with children will be integrated throughout the chapter. The importance of the role of the child's caregiver will also be explored and the value of psycho-educational work with children and their caregivers will be described. The anonymised case study is presented here with consent from the child's Foster Carer and Social Worker.

Developmental trauma

A child's brain begins developing whilst in utero. Research indicates that the mother's exposure to high levels of stress during the pregnancy can result in long-term effects on a child's neurodevelopment (Talge, Neal & Glover, 2007). Children who have experienced developmental trauma have undertaken much of their early development in an environment with ongoing perceived danger and inadequate care, leading the child to believe that the world is an unsafe and unpredictable place. Children therefore often develop strategies in order to help them feel safe, which can present and be described as 'challenging behaviour'. For example, the child who has experienced neglect may 'tend to hoard or hide food "just in case" where supplies have been unpredictable or absent in the past' (Archer & Gordon, 2006:115).

Developmental trauma has been linked to children having low self-esteem, low impulse control, poor concentration, hypervigilance and difficulties with emotional regulation (Schwarz & Perry, 1994), negatively affecting a child's social, cognitive, emotional and behavioural development (Van der Kolk, 2005). Schwarz and Perry (1994) state that in addition to

PTSD, those who have experienced developmental trauma are at greater risk of developing Attention Deficit Hyperactivity Disorder, major depression and Borderline Personality Disorder. Furthermore, this impacts on a child's ability to form secure attachments and trust caregivers to meet their unmet developmental needs (Archer & Gordon, 2013). It is important that understanding of the impact of developmental trauma informs therapeutic intervention and process.

Child centred play therapy

We often consider non-directive play therapy (Axline, 1947) to be a starting point when working with children who have experienced developmental trauma (Yasenik & Gardner, 2012) as this approach allows the child to develop a therapeutic relationship within a safe therapeutic space (Barnes, 2007). Within this environment the child can express their internal world, often through the use of projective and symbolic play (Wilson, Kendrick & Ryan, 1992). A non-directive approach allows the child to have an appropriate level of control over the content of their sessions, so they are able to control the pace and content of their own therapeutic process. Our approach to working with children is underpinned by humanistic theory based on the work of Rogers (1951) and Axline (1947). However, we consider our application of play therapy to practice to be integrative and tailored to the individual therapeutic needs of the child and their caregivers.

An integrative approach

It is evident from current research literature that a single model of intervention is not effective in addressing the complex needs of children who have experienced developmental trauma (Gil, 2006; Goodyear-Brown, 2010; Schaefer, 2001; West, 1992). Therapeutic work with children and young people needs to be adapted to meet the individual's needs. Therefore, children and young people need to be assessed prior to the therapeutic intervention commencing, in order to establish the most appropriate intervention (BAPT Core Competence 18, see Appendix 1). We do this by undertaking a Family Assessment, which is the initial stage of The Stepping Stones (Child Therapy Consultants) Integrated Model (Waycott, Carbis & McInnes, 2015).

When using a non-directive approach, children who have experienced developmental trauma can become stuck in post-traumatic play (Dripchak, 2007; Gil, 1991; Levine, 1997). Such re-traumatising play, in which children are not in control of their play re-enactments and seem compelled to repeat their highly distressing experiences, may induce further suffering and psychological damage in children. Schaefer (1994:305) states that 'the cycle of retraumatising play must be broken by active intervention from a therapist who directs the trauma play so as to create a sense of mastery'.

Prominent child therapists support the need for more integrative training programmes within the field of child therapy (Schaefer, 2001; West, 1992). Play therapists using integrative approaches require training and knowledge in the use of different therapeutic models and how to apply them to practice, for example trauma and neurobiology (e.g. Perry, 2009), attachment-based interventions such as Theraplay[1] (Jernberg & Booth, 2010) and Filial Therapy (Van Fleet, 2005), Therapeutic Life Story work and Psycho-education.

When working with children who have experienced developmental trauma and have attachment difficulties, the research indicates that the most significant adults for a traumatised child to form an attachment to are their caregivers (Barnes, 2007; Hughes, 2009; Jernberg & Booth, 2010) and not an individual therapist. Play therapists using an integrative approach need to be able to adapt to unpredictable situations which arise in the therapeutic process, including managing and responding to distress and on occasions, aggressive or sexualised behaviours. The use of effective clinical supervision is essential when working with traumatised clients and often requires the therapist to undertake further personal therapy if triggered by clients' presentation and experiences (Dripchak, 2007).

Our Integrated Model (Waycott, Carbis & McInnes, 2015) has been informed by knowledge of child development, trauma, attachment and systemic theory and research, and our clinical experiences of delivering a variety of therapeutic interventions. The approach will be explored through a discussion of the case of Ollie.

Introducing Ollie

Ollie was 7 years old and living in foster care when he was referred for therapeutic intervention by his social worker due to concerns school had reported, such as 'him tying a scarf around his neck', 'asking if anyone would miss him if he died', 'asking himself how long it would take to die if he were shot' and 'harming himself by scratching'. Ollie was diagnosed with developmental delay. His foster carer, Kate, reported that he rarely presented with challenging behaviours within placement, however she was concerned that he blamed himself for the separation from his birth parents and she had observed that at times he could be overfamiliar with people he did not know. The local authority accommodated Ollie when he was six years old, due to a history of neglect and emotional abuse. He was placed with Kate and has remained with her throughout his therapeutic journey.

During an initial consultation session between the play therapist, social worker and foster carer, Ollie's history and reported presenting difficulties were discussed in order to assess the most appropriate therapeutic intervention. It was agreed that Ollie would attend 20 individual weekly play therapy sessions, followed by 14 sessions with his foster carer, which would focus on trauma and attachment. In addition, the therapist would provide carer consultation sessions and regular therapy review meetings throughout the process. Starting with a child-centred approach allowed Ollie a safe space to process his experiences and feelings, prior to the therapist enabling him to cognitively process his experiences within a more focused framework whilst enhancing his attachment to his primary caregiver.

From the start, Ollie presented as over-familiar and over-confident in his interactions with the therapist; he showed little anxiety leaving his foster carer and going to the playroom with the therapist on his first or subsequent sessions. Ollie presented as hyper-vigilant (Perry et al., 1995) during sessions, for example if he heard a noise within the building he would immediately ask what was happening (Prichard, 2016). Children who have experienced trauma can develop a heightened state of sensory sensitivity and enhanced behaviours in detecting information that is reminiscent of the trauma they have experienced.

Ollie approached play therapy sessions in an enthusiastic manner, engaging the therapist in play and responding appropriately to the therapist's boundaries. He enjoyed exploring the toys in the playroom and was able to focus on one play activity for some length of time. Ollie often appeared to approach his play therapy sessions with an agenda and primarily engaged the therapist in high-energy dramatic role-play, making use of dressing up costumes and props, soft toy animals, monsters and puppets in his play. Ollie would use different voice tones when speaking as different characters and would direct the therapist as to how he wanted her to engage in the play. Ollie's play could be frantic and chaotic at times quickly switching between roles. He also engaged in sensory and embodiment play and appeared to value the opportunity to engage in messy play, which perhaps suggested gaps in his early play experiences (Jennings, 2011).

Play therapists look for themes in a child's play, as an indication of what the child may be trying to communicate (Ryan & Edge, 2011). Themes in Ollie's play centred on parent-child relationships, power imbalances between 'scary'/'nasty' characters (including a monster) and the 'victim', and death. There was a sense of power imbalance within Ollie's play, with stronger characters dominating weaker characters. Ollie often played the role of a father figure making comments such as 'go away, you're not my son any more' and 'I'm not your dad any more – I'm on their team'. The child or baby doll in the play was often being told off for 'not listening' and whilst in role as 'parent' Ollie made comments such as 'you're a nasty person' and 'no one ever loves you'. Goodyear-Brown (2010) suggests that when children feel inadequate to defeat their perpetrator themselves they often enlist a helping symbol, such as a puppet to fight on their behalf in order to gain mastery.

It became apparent whilst undertaking therapeutic life story work, that the themes within Ollie's play therapy sessions were rooted in his early experiences. Due to the nature of Ollie's dramatic play, the therapist ensured the play was stopped five minutes before the end of the session and time was spent de-roling, in which both the child and therapist consciously come out of the roles they have been playing and back into the present (Lassken, 2017).

Over the course of the play therapy sessions the therapist felt it was helpful to integrate focused therapeutic techniques specifically to help Ollie process, understand and manage his trauma and family relationships. For example, the use of a dream-catcher and creating an ecomap using toys.

Dream-catcher

During an early session Ollie shared with the therapist that he had been having nightmares. It is not uncommon for children who have experienced trauma to experience a range of sleep disturbances, including nightmares or night terrors (Goodyear-Brown, 2010). There is a dream-catcher in the window of the playroom and Ollie requested to make one; this was a familiar object to him. Dream-catchers originate from Native Americans and involve a 'web' being created with thread within a hoop or ring which is decorated with feathers and beads. Dream-catchers are often hung in bedroom windows and are said to catch bad dreams and prevent them getting through (Mallon, 2002). During the following session the therapist had appropriate craft materials available for Ollie to create a dream-catcher. Ollie was allowed to take this home and both he and Kate reported that there had been a reduction in nightmares. Typically, purely non-directive play therapists do not allow children to take items or things they have made from the play room until the end of the therapeutic process (West, 1992). In this case, the therapist allowed Ollie to take his dream-catcher home as it had a clear therapeutic purpose at this stage in the therapeutic process and Ollie was still at a developmental stage where he believed in magical thinking. The therapist believed that this gave Ollie a sense of empowerment in defeating his nightmares.

Family play genogram

Ollie had talked briefly about his birth family during play therapy sessions and expressed some confusion regarding his long-term care plans. During session 15 Ollie expressed some uncertainty regarding how to use his session. The therapist suggested the concept of choosing animals to represent 'people who are important' and creating a 'picture' by arranging them in the sand-tray (adapted from Buurma, 1999). Ollie began with his birth family, and then foster family and friends. Ollie talked openly about family members and appeared to have a good understanding of his family structure. It was also clear that his foster family and friends were very significant to him.

At this point, the therapist began reflecting on whether Ollie had processed as much of his trauma as he was able to within a child-centred play therapy approach. Ollie began asking the therapist more questions about his past and family and therefore it felt like an appropriate stage to prepare Ollie for the next phase of the therapeutic process.

Throughout the play therapy sessions the therapist needed to maintain clear boundaries and limits to ensure both Ollie and her own safety. Working therapeutically with a child who has experienced developmental trauma and is using their sessions to explore this through role-play is physically and emotionally demanding. Regular clinical supervision (Ray, 2011) was essential for the therapist to explore themes and best responses to Ollie's play. It was also important to identify any issues of transference or countertransference, and ultimately ensure safe and ethical practice (BAPT Core Competence 13, see Appendix 1).

Stepping Stones (child therapy consultants) integrated model

On completion of the individual play therapy sessions, Ollie and his long-term foster carer, Kate, undertook further therapeutic work which focused on helping Ollie form a positive attachment to Kate and providing him a safe therapeutic space to process his traumatic experiences. Establishing clear therapeutic boundaries and contracting with the child and their caregiver is essential, in order for the child to feel safe and contained, therefore creating a therapeutic space which enables the child to process their developmental trauma and begin to heal (Axline, 1947; Landreth, 2001; West, 1992).

At this stage of the process, a new therapist was allocated as the therapist who had undertaken the play therapy sessions was no longer able to continue with the work due to personal circumstances. The therapeutic space remained familiar to Ollie as a place where he felt contained and safe (Cattanach, 2003) in the presence of his foster carer. In Ollie's case, he appeared to be able to establish a therapeutic relationship with the new therapist, over the initial sessions together.

Ollie and Kate attended 14 sessions over a period of nine months. During these sessions the therapist introduced Theraplay (Jernberg & Booth, 2010) activities focusing on Ollie's need for nurture and structure, to encourage a positive attachment between him and Kate. In this model the therapist has an adaptable therapeutic plan with a number of therapeutic activities for each session, selected in order to meet the therapeutic needs of the child and measure clinical outcomes. This would include: the child's ability to process their trauma, the child's ability to express and connect to their internal thoughts and feelings, the caregiver's ability to respond to the child's behaviours and emotional needs and to enhance the child's attachment to a significant caregiver. Ollie responded positively to the playful nature of the Theraplay-based activities, especially those on the nurture dimension, however he initially struggled whilst engaging in the structured activities possibly due to his 'need' to be in control. Ollie became more able to engage in the structured activities as the process progressed and he experienced that Kate providing structure was a safe experience.

Therapeutic techniques were used to help Ollie feel safe in the therapeutic space and to help him express himself. The techniques used with Ollie included: My Safe Hand; Feelings Balloons; Fight, Flight, Freeze technique; and, creating a Self-care box. In addition, the therapist used ending techniques to evaluate clinical outcomes for Ollie and Kate.

My Safe Hand

My Safe Hand technique (an adaptation of the Safety Hand Technique by Hobday & Ollier, 1998) is used to assess the child's understanding of the concept of 'feeling safe' and to identify the people they consider capable of keeping them safe. For this technique, Kate was asked to draw around Ollie's hand. The therapist then explored with Ollie the concept of feeling safe. If the therapist is satisfied that the child understands this concept, the child is invited to write the names of adults they believe keep them safe on each finger and thumb on the child's hand image. If the child wants to include peers or siblings, the therapist might discuss whether or not they are an appropriate person to go to if they feel unsafe. Ideally, the therapist would like to see the child identify five appropriate safe adults.

Ollie was asked to identify the person on the hand that he would call first if he felt unsafe; Ollie identified Kate. Should a child want to include the therapist as a safe person early in the therapeutic process, the therapist may consider the child's intention. This could potentially reflect a child's possible attachment style and patterns of behaviour, for example, a child who feels they need to please or are overfamiliar towards adults.

Feelings Balloons

In order to help Ollie and Kate develop strategies to best manage Ollie's feelings of anger and frustration in the placement, the therapist used Feelings Balloons (adapted from Balloons of Anger, by Horn, cited in Kaduson & Schaefer, 1997:250–253). Ollie was given a balloon and asked to blow 'all his wobbly feelings of anger, sadness and fear into the balloon', when all the feelings are in the balloon, he was asked to 'let the balloon go'. Ollie practised this strategy at home and often requested balloons in the sessions when he started to feel overwhelmed.

Fight, Flight and Freeze

The therapist introduced Ollie to four animals to explain the concept of the fight, flight and freeze (Archer & Gordon, 2006; Perry, 2009) responses to potential perceived danger. A large dinosaur was used to represent the potential danger. Fight was represented by a lion, flight by a horse and freeze by a lamb (Waycott, 2016). The therapist used a simple narrative to explain that each of the animals, like people, would react in a different way to feeling fearful or under attack. The therapist explained

> if the large dinosaur, approached the lion the lion would react by trying to fight the dinosaur, if the dinosaur approached the horse, the horse would run and hide and if the dinosaur approached the lamb, the lamb would be stuck and freeze.

The therapist then asked how Ollie would react if the dinosaur approached him, Ollie stated 'I would be like the lion and fight him off'. Ollie's response fitted with his reactions to his perception of potential threats at school and home. This also fitted with play themes within his individual play therapy. At this stage Ollie became consciously aware of his behaviours and how they related to his past traumatic experiences (Rees, 2009).

Therapeutic life story work

Once the therapist had established a relationship with Ollie the next stage of the intervention focused on helping him to process his life story. In the case of Ollie, the therapist used a toy train and track to explore Ollie's life story through play. Our approach to therapeutic life story work has been influenced by the work of Ryan and Walker (2007), Rose (2012), Rose and Philpot (2005) and Rees (2009). During the sessions the therapist shared significant information about his life experiences and Ollie was invited to use images which he had created to represent his feelings and play to process the information (see Figure 16.1).

The narrative starts with sharing information about the child's birth, including their birth certificate. As part of this process with younger children a baby doll is introduced (Platteuw & Waycott, 2012). Ollie was asked to choose a baby doll to represent him (from a selection of culturally appropriate dolls). The therapist explained to Ollie that the baby doll represented him and asked Ollie to think about what a baby needs to be cared for. From this point the doll is then only referred to by the child's name. A range of real baby items for example a bottle and dummy are provided

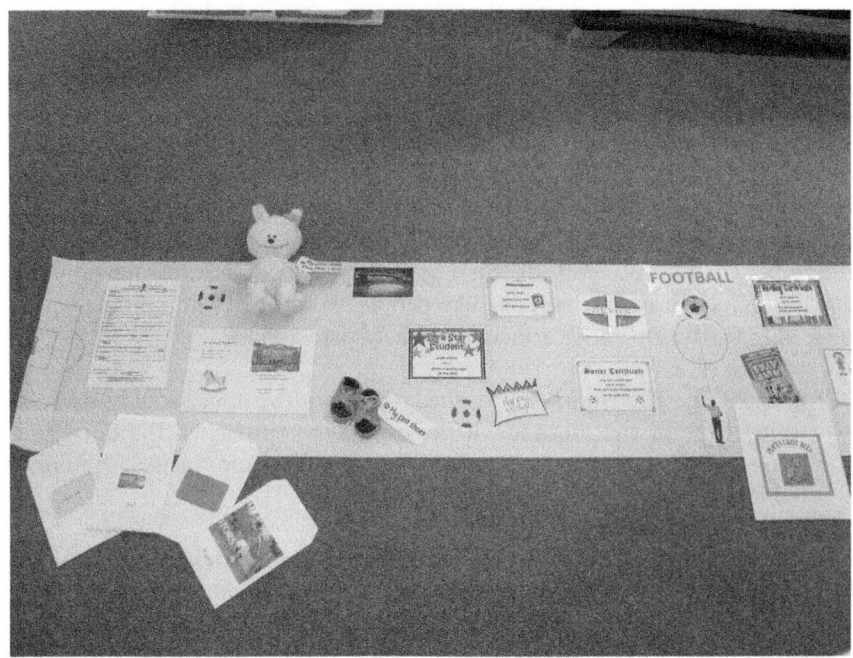

Figure 16.1 Example of a play-based exploration of life story

so that the baby's needs can be explored through the use of projective and role play (Murray, as cited in Kaduson & Schaefer, 1997:236). Ollie was able to assist in nurturing the baby doll; he decided that the baby needed to be changed, fed and bathed. The therapist responds using a child-centred approach, however, if the child's play became aggressive or harmful towards the baby doll the therapist would challenge this play because the doll represents the child. Through the use of reflections, the therapist would explore how the baby may feel based on the child's play of the care provided.

The purpose of this technique is to help children to develop self-nurture through the use of projective play and to focus on enhancing a healthy and secure attachment between the child and their caregivers. This is a helpful technique for children who have unmet developmental needs due to early developmental trauma and neglect and who are often initially unable to tolerate or accept direct nurture from their caregivers (Platteuw & Waycott, 2012). We have observed that through using the baby dolls, the child is often curious to explore for themselves those nurturing experiences which have been played out with the dolls, for example the child may use the bottle or dummy. It is not uncommon for children to display regressed behaviours within the sessions and at home. It is essential that prior to introducing the baby dolls to the child that the therapist provides psycho-educational advice and support to the child's caregivers in relation to the concept of therapeutic regression (Landreth, 2001; West, 1992) in order that they are adequately prepared to assist the child in caring for the doll in the therapy sessions and within the home.

Ending techniques

The final sessions are used to prepare the child and their caregiver for the ending of the therapeutic intervention and to evaluate therapeutic outcomes with the child, their caregivers and other professionals involved with the child and family (BAPT Competence 21, see Appendix 1). It is crucial that therapists plan in advance to prepare the child for the final stages of therapy and how the ending of the therapy will be managed (McMahon, 1992; West, 1992). Deciding to end the therapy can often present difficulties and dilemmas for the therapist. It is essential that the therapist is aware of their own feelings about ending therapy and the feelings of the child. It is important that the decision to end the therapy is done in the best interests of the child and their caregivers and not based on the needs or feelings of the therapist.

Terminating therapy can be especially challenging for children who have experienced developmental trauma and have attachment difficulties, as they have often experienced a number of abrupt and traumatic endings throughout their life, including removal from their birth family, multiple placement moves, and changes of schools and loss of peer relationships (Platteuw, 2011, cited in Taylor De Faoite, 2011). Further attention should be focused on evaluating the therapeutic process and acknowledging the child's achievements during therapy (Jones, Casado & Robinson, 2003). Useful techniques to acknowledge the child's achievements include the Tower of Achievement and Farewell Pass the Parcel.

To prepare a child for the ending of the therapeutic process, West (1992) suggests it is helpful to create a countdown chart which the child is invited to colour in at the start of each session. A count-down chart can be made by the therapist with the child during a session and designed to reflect a character or object pertinent to the child that the child can identify with. In the case of Ollie the therapist introduced a countdown chart for the remaining five individual sessions and at the start of the second phase of intervention. Ollie was invited to add an image to his countdown chart at the start of each of the therapeutic sessions.

During the penultimate session Ollie and his foster carer were invited to create their Tower of Achievement (Waycott & Carbis, 2014, adapted from Termination Party Techique, Leben, 2009). Using large plastic blocks Ollie, Kate and the therapist each wrote positive messages on post-it notes to highlight areas of achievement in Ollie's therapy and home/school life. The following are examples from Ollie and his carer:

'You are able to listen to me (Kate)'
'I can talk about my feelings'
'I am better at showing my angry feeling safely'.

It is also helpful to ask the child and their caregiver to think of any changes the parental figure has made that has impacted on the family unit. For example:

'Kate is really good at taking care of me'
'I feel safe with Kate'
'You have learnt how to trust each other and work together as a team'.

The final session was used to celebrate Ollie's achievements and journey through his therapy. A tea party was held (West, 1992), which had been planned with Ollie in the previous session. A tea party has proven to be successful when working with children who are looked after or adopted who often have experienced unplanned or negative endings.

The therapist introduced Ollie and Kate to Farewell Pass the Parcel (adapted from Farewell Fortune Cookies Technique, Kenny-Noziska, 2008). This technique is based on the popular British children's party game, 'Pass-the-parcel'. In preparation for the game, an ending gift is wrapped within several layers of wrapping paper. Smaller gifts can be placed between all other layers of wrapping and each gift has a question attached which reflects an aspect of the therapeutic process or the child's newly learnt skills. Examples of questions to use in this game may include:

i.   what will you miss about therapy?
ii. who is someone who keeps you safe?
iii. what have you learnt about yourself?
iv. what do you do when you are feeling sad?

Self-care boxes

As part of the therapeutic process the therapist, child and their caregiver work together to create a self-care box which contains items to help the child find safe ways to express and take care of themselves. The self-care box is tailor-made to meet the individual needs of the child based on their presentation, behaviours and developmental ability to use the strategies as observed in the sessions by the therapist (see Figure 16.2). Ollie's self-care box contained the following items: balloons (Feeling Balloons strategy), hand lotion and paper to create hand prints, sachets of hot chocolate (which Ollie would request in the sessions to keep him 'warm inside'), a packet of tissues to remind Ollie that it is okay to show our sad and hurt feelings, and a fidget toy to help Ollie focus. There is some debate amongst therapists about the appropriateness of giving and receiving ending gifts (Ray, 2011; West, 1992). We consider ending gifts to be appropriate if there is a clear therapeutic link between the gift chosen for the child and the child's therapeutic process. Ollie's ending gift was his self-care box and his life story book.

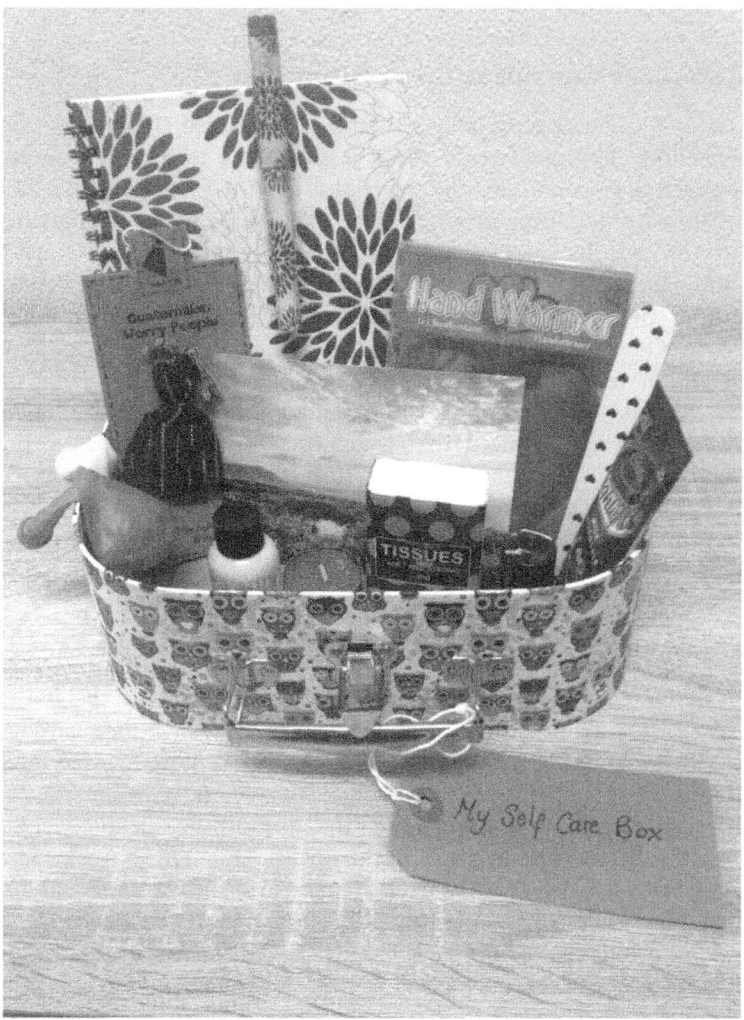

Figure 16.2 Example of teenage girl self-care box

1. A note book and pen to write down my thoughts and feelings
2. Tissues to remember it is okay to cry and feel upset
3. A punch balloon to let go of my angry feelings
4. Balloons to release my sad, angry and anxious feelings
5. A heart stone to remember I am loved and valued by the people who care about me
6. Information to read about growing up and keeping myself safe from further harm
7. Lots of lovely things to pamper myself when I need cheering up
8. Hot chocolate to keep me warm

Parent/carer consultation sessions

As part of the therapeutic intervention Kate attended three carer consultation sessions. The purpose of these sessions was to explore concepts of developmental re-parenting, the principles of PACE: Playfulness, Acceptance, Curiosity and Empathy (Hughes, 2009) and how to apply them in practice through the use of role-play between the therapist and Kate. Practical strategies were implemented in order to manage Ollie's behaviours within the placement. Additional consultation and guidance was also offered to Ollie's school to ensure consistency of strategies used within school and home. Empirical research and literature supports the notion that to provide effective therapeutic outcomes for children and young people, their caregivers need to be connected to the therapeutic process (Baggerly, Ray & Bratton, 2010; Bratton et al., 2005; Landreth, 2001; West, 1992). In order to provide effective outcomes for children it is essential that the child's caregivers have an understanding of what the therapy is and how it works in practice.

Summary

- Play therapy interventions should be tailored to meet the individual needs of the child and their family, particularly where they have experienced developmental trauma and may require a more focused intervention in order to make sense of their past experiences.
- Integrative approaches, including the use of therapeutic techniques, attachment-based therapy and therapeutic life story work, may be necessary in order to help a child gain a cognitive understanding of their experiences.
- Using an integrative approach requires knowledge of a broad range of theories and how to apply them in a flexible manner. Choice of specific techniques is in response to the child's and family's engagement and individual needs and should be developmentally and culturally appropriate, within the context of the child's overall therapeutic journey.

- Clinical supervision and personal therapy are of great importance whilst working with children who have experienced developmental trauma. The therapist should be especially aware of transference and counter-transference issues whilst working with this client group.
- The child is not viewed in isolation, but rather within their family and social system. It is important that parents/carers and professionals are involved in regular therapy review meetings. Parents/carers are provided with psycho-educational support and are involved in the child's therapy sessions, to explore their life narrative and undertake attachment-based interventions.

Note

1 Theraplay is a registered service mark of The Theraplay Institute, Evanston, IL, USA

Further reading

Archer, C., Drury, C. & Hills, J. (2015) *Healing the Hidden Hurts: Transforming Attachment and Trauma Theory into Effective Practice with Families, Children and Adults.* London: Jessica Kingsley Publishers.

Goodyear-Brown, P. (2010) *Play Therapy with Traumatized Children: A Perspective Approach.* Hoboken, NJ: John Wiley & Sons.

Jernberg, A.M. & Booth, P.B. (2010) *Theraplay: Helping Parents and Children Build Better Relationships through Attachment-Based Play.* (3rd ed.) San Francisco, CA: Jossey-Bass Publishers.

References

Archer, C. & Gordon, C. (2006) *New Families Old Scripts: A Guide to the Language of Trauma and Attachment in Adoptive Families.* London: Jessica Kingsley Publishers.

Archer, C. & Gordon, C. (2013) *Re-Parenting the Child Who Hurts: A Guide to Healing Developmental Trauma and Attachments.* London: Jessica Kingsley Publishers.

Axline, V. (1947) *Play Therapy.* New York: Ballantine Books.

Baggerly, J.N., Ray, D.C. & Bratton, S.C. (Eds.) (2010) *Child-Centred Play Therapy Research: The Evidence Base for Effective Practice.* Hoboken, NJ: John Wiley & Sons.

Barnes, A. (2007) Integrative work with children in long-term placements. *British Journal of Play Therapy.* 3, pp. 40–51.

Bratton, S., Ray, D., Rhine, T. & Jones, L. (2005) The efficacy of play therapy with children: A meta-analytic review of outcome research. *Professional Psychology: Research and Practice.* 36 (4), pp. 376–390.

Buurma, D. (1999) *The Family Play Genogram: A Guidebook.* Summit, NJ: Family Play Therapy Press.

Cattanach, A. (2003) *Introduction to Play Therapy*. London: Routledge.

Dripchak, V. (2007) Posttraumatic play: Towards acceptance and resolution. *Clinical Social Work Journal*. 35, pp. 125–134.

Gil, E. (1991) *The Healing Power of Play: Working with Abused Children*. London: Jessica Kingsley Publishers.

Gil, E. (2006) *Helping Abused and Traumatized Children: Integrating Directive and Non – Directive Approaches*. New York: Guilford Press.

Goodyear-Brown, P. (2010) *Play Therapy with Traumatized Children: A Perspective Approach*. NJ: Wiley & Sons.

Hobday, A. & Ollier, K. (1998) *Creative Therapy: Activities with Children and Adolescents*. Leicester: British Psychological Society.

Hughes, D. (2009) *Attachment Focused Parenting: Effective Strategies to Care for Children*. New York: W.W. Norton & Co.

Jennings, S. (2011) *Healthy Attachments and Neuro-dramatic Play*. London: Jessica Kingsley Publishers.

Jernberg, A.M. & Booth, P.B. (2010) *Theraplay: Helping Parents and Children Build Better Relationships through Attachment-Based Play*. (3rd ed.) San Francisco, CA: Jossey-Bass Publishers.

Jones, K.D., Casado, M. & Robinson, E.H. (2003) Structured play therapy: A model for choosing topics and activities. *International Journal of Play Therapy*. 12 (1), pp. 31–47.

Kaduson, H. & Schaefer, C.E. (Eds.) (1997) *101 Favourite Play Therapy Techniques*. New York: Jason Aronson.

Kenny-Noziska, S. (2008) *Techniques, Techniques, Techniques: Play-Based Activities for Children, Adolescents and Families*. West Conshohocken, PA: Infinity Publishing.

Landreth, G. (2001) *Innovations in Play Therapy: Issues, Process and Special Populations*. New York: Brunner-Routledge.

Lassken, S. (2017) Persona non grata: A systematic review of de-roling in drama therapy. *Drama Therapy Review*. 3 (2), pp. 165–179.

Leben, N.Y. (2009) Termination party. In: Lowenstein, L. (Ed.). *Assessment and Treatment Activities for Children, Adolescents, and Families: Practitioners Share Their Most Effective Techniques*. Toronto: Champion Press, p. 179

Levine, P. (1997) *Waking the Tiger: Healing Trauma*. Berkeley, CA: North Atlantic Books.

Mallon, B. (2002) *Dream Time with Children: Learning to Dream, Dreaming to Learn*. London: Jessica Kingsley Publishers.

McMahon, L. (1992) *The Handbook of Play Therapy*. London: Routledge.

Perry, B. (2009) Examining child maltreatment through a neurodevelopmental lens: Clinical applications of the neuro-sequential model of therapeutics. *Journal of Loss and Trauma*. 14, pp. 240–255.

Perry, B., Pollard, R.A., Blakley, T.L., Baker, W.L. & Vigilante, D. (1995) Childhood trauma, the neurobiology of adaptation, and 'use-dependent' development of the brain: How 'states' become 'traits'. *Infant Mental Health Journal*. 16 (4), pp. 271–291.

Platteuw, C. & Waycott, L. (2012) *Therapeutic Life Story Work: Using Play to Help Children and Young People Explore their Life Narratives*. 2nd International Play Therapy Conference, 28th June 2012, Dunboyne Castle, Dublin, Ireland.

Prichard, N. (2016) Stuck in the dollhouse: A brain-based perspective of post-traumatic play. In: Le Vay, D. & Cuschieri, E. (Eds.). *Challenges in the Theory and Practice of Play Therapy.* London and New York: Routledge. pp. 71–85.

Ray, D. (2011) *Advanced Play Therapy.* New York: Routledge.

Rees, J. (2009) *Life Story Work for Adopted Children: A Family Friendly Approach.* London: Jessica Kingsley Publishers.

Rogers, C. (1951) *Client Centred Therapy.* London: Constable.

Rose, R. (2012) *Life Story Work Therapy with Traumatized Children: A Model of Practice.* London: Jessica Kingsley Publishers.

Rose, R. & Philpot, T. (2005) *The Child's Own Story: Life Story Work with Traumatized Children.* London: Jessica Kingsley Publishers.

Ryan, T. & Walker, R. (2007) *Life Story Work: A Practical Guide to Helping Children Understand Their Past.* London: BAAF.

Ryan, V. & Edge, A. (2011) The role of play themes in non-directive play therapy. *Clinical Child Psychology and Psychiatry.* 17 (3), pp. 354–369.

Schaefer, C.E. (1994) Play therapy for psychic trauma in children. In: O'Connor, K.J. & Schaefer, C.E. (Eds.). *Handbook of Play Therapy, Vol II.* Chichester: Wiley. pp. 297–318.

Schaefer, C.E. (2001) Prescriptive play therapy. *International Journal of Play Therapy.* 19(1), pp. 57–73.

Schwarz, E. & Perry, B.D. (1994) The post-traumatic response in children and adolescents. *Psychiatric Clinics of North America.* 17 (2), pp. 311–326.

Talge, N., Neal, C. & Glover, V. (2007) Antenatal maternal stress and long-term effects on child neurodevelopment: How and why? *Journal of Child Psychology and Psychiatry.* 48 (3–4), pp. 245–261.

Taylor De Faoite, A. (2011) *Narrative Play Therapy: Theory and Practice.* London: Jessica Kingsley Publishers.

Van der Kolk, B. (2005) Developmental trauma disorder: Towards a rational diagnosis for children with complex trauma histories. *Psychiatric Annals.* 35 (5), pp. 401–408.

Van Fleet, R. (2005) *Filial Therapy: Strengthening Parent-Child Relationships through Play.* Sarasota, FL: Professional Resource Press.

Waycott, L. (2016) *Therapeutic Play in School.* Mental Health and Wellbeing in School Conference, 23rd May 2016, Cardiff, UK.

Waycott, L. & Carbis, C. (2014) *The Integration of Therapeutic Techniques within Play Therapy.* BAPT Annual Conference, 20th June 2014, Birmingham, UK.

Waycott, L., Carbis, C. & McInnes, K. (2015) Developmental trauma and attachment: An integrative therapeutic approach. In: Archer, C., Drury, C. & Hills, J. (Eds.). *Healing the Hidden Hurts: Transforming Attachment and Trauma Theory into Effective Practice with Families, Children and Adults.* London: Jessica Kingsley Publishers. p. 102

West, J. (1992) *Child Centred Play Therapy.* London: Arnold.

Wilson, K., Kendrick, P. & Ryan, V. (1992) *Play Therapy. A Non-directive Approach for Children and Adolescents.* London: Balliere Tindall.

Yasenik, L. & Gardner, K. (2012) *Play Therapy Dimensions Model.* London: Jessica Kingsley Publishers.

Chapter 17

Play therapy and Polyvagal Theory

Towards self-regulation for children with paediatric medical trauma

Stuart Daniel

Chapter overview

The Polyvagal Theory offers us a re-visioning of the human autonomic nervous system – a three-tiered model of adaptive strategies, with each of the three systems coming on-line in succession depending on an immediate evaluation of threat. Understanding the relationship between these systems helps us understand the roots of trauma – the co-occurrence of fear and inescapability – and the mechanisms of chronic Posttraumatic Stress. Understanding the nature of our two defence systems – the Mobilisation System (fight/flight) and the Immobilisation System (dissociation and behavioural 'shut-down') – helps us get a sense of how a traumatised child experiences the world. Exploring the relationship between our prosocial system (the Social Engagement System) and our two defence systems – primarily that our defence systems are enabled at the expense of health, homoeostasis, and flowing social ability – helps us get a feel for the social impact of trauma. Understanding that this relationship has a therapeutic inverse – i.e. that consciously supporting a child's Social Engagement System in therapy will down-regulate his defence systems – gives us a valuable perspective on co-regulation in Play Therapy. From the Polyvagal perspective, supporting children through difficult experiences back to a shared calm state is a natural goal of Play Therapy – an extension of the natural goal of healthy play. Through many such shared experiences over time, the dys-regulated child is effectively exercising, and so strengthening, his *vagal brake*, moving towards self-regulation. As I explore the vagal brake at various stages within the dynamics of the Play Therapy relationship, I will be discussing the following principle concepts: the face–heart connection; sensitive musicality in communication; vitality matching; and a somatic trajectory in Play Therapy. At key points in the chapter, I bring in examples from Josh's experience in Play Therapy[1] to illustrate these concepts.

Paediatric medical trauma and the Polyvagal Theory

Almost all medical procedures are experienced as aversive by children and, sadly, many procedures are still undertaken in ways that can have traumatic effects (Azeem et al. 2015). The dynamics of childhood medical trauma can be described by the co-occurrence of two qualities: overwhelming fear and inescapability (either physical or perceived) (Kazak et al. 2006, Levine 2017, Levine & Kline 2006, Van der Kolk 2015). Several treatment experiences have the potential to meet these co-occurring criteria: primarily, any frightening procedure which involves being physically restrained, and/or intense and immobilising toxic/physical shock, but also potentially MRI scans with limited (not general) anaesthetic (Porges & Daniel 2017). Despite many intelligent, child-friendly hospital protocols, physical restraint continues to be used on a daily basis in many paediatric wards. Studies by Diseth (2005) illustrate that children forced to undergo medical procedures, particularly in the context of their families holding them down, present with significantly more dissociation than children treated less invasively. As many as 30% of medically ill children go on to develop symptoms of chronic post-traumatic stress (Forgey & Bursch 2013).

A central framework for us here, in our understanding of medical trauma and of Play Therapy as an intervention, will be the Polyvagal Theory – a powerful re-visioning of the human autonomic nervous system (Porges 2009, 2011, 2018). The Polyvagal Theory explains how we have evolved to live in a quickly changing social environment – an environment in which some people represent safety, some threat, and some the uncertainty of both. We live best and are most healthy when we are at ease, safely connected to other people. The Polyvagal Theory emphasises our life-long human drive to calm our neural defence systems by detecting features of safety in others. This drive is the central impulse within social behaviour and is present from birth, when an infant communicates the need to be soothed and regulated in partnership with her care-giver. However, we also need to be ready to respond to danger in an instant. To shift quickly between adaptive states, humans have evolved a three-tiered hierarchy of survival-oriented systems, each system an organism-wide response to the immediate environment (see Figure 17.1).

When we detect features of safety, our defence systems are dampened and the first of the three tiers comes on-line – the Social Engagement System. When this happens, two important dynamic responses are expressed. Firstly, bodily state is regulated in an efficient manner to promote health, growth, and restoration (visceral homoeostasis). This occurs when the influence of mammalian myelinated vagal motor pathways on the cardiac pacemaker increases. Increasing the influence of these vagal pathways slows heart rate, inhibits the fight–flight mechanisms of the sympathetic nervous system, dampens the stress response system of the hypothalamic–pituitary–adrenal (HPA) axis, and reduces inflammatory reaction (Porges 2009, 2011, 2018). Secondly, system-

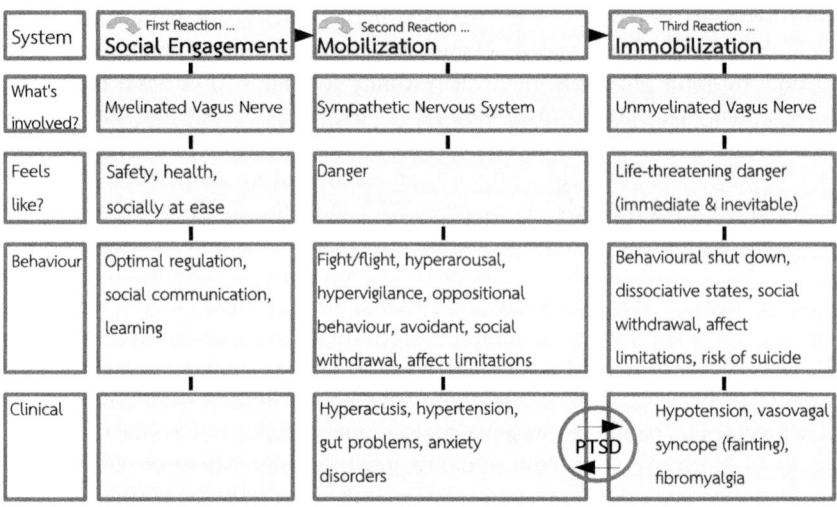

Polyvagal Theory

How humans adapt and regulate in the face of safety or danger

We react to our environment, continually trying to keep safe...

As we detect changes, possible danger, a hierarchy of adaptive systems comes into play...

System	First Reaction ... **Social Engagement**	Second Reaction ... **Mobilization**	Third Reaction ... **Immobilization**
What's involved?	Myelinated Vagus Nerve	Sympathetic Nervous System	Unmyelinated Vagus Nerve
Feels like?	Safety, health, socially at ease	Danger	Life-threatening danger (immediate & inevitable)
Behaviour	Optimal regulation, social communication, learning	Fight/flight, hyperarousal, hypervigilance, oppositional behaviour, avoidant, social withdrawal, affect limitations	Behavioural shut down, dissociative states, social withdrawal, affect limitations, risk of suicide
Clinical		Hyperacusis, hypertension, gut problems, anxiety disorders	Hypotension, vasovagal syncope (fainting), fibromyalgia

Figure 17.1 The Polyvagal Theory – a 3-tiered model of the human autonomic nervous system

wide influences promote effective prosocial behaviour, co-regulation, and relationship. How? Through evolutionary bootstrapping processes, the brain-stem nuclei which orchestrate calm states and a happy heart (via regulation of the myelinated vagus), were integrated with the nuclei which orchestrate expressive and receptive social gestures (via regulation of the striated muscles of the face and head – specifically the muscles controlling facial expression, listening, and prosodic vocalisations). This integrated connection enables a bidirectional coupling (a communication and mutual-regulation) between spontaneous social engagement behaviours and bodily states – the *face-heart connection* (Porges 2007).

On initial orienting, in response to threat, or as result of chronic trauma, the second of our two systems activates – the defensive Mobilisation System. The actions of the Mobilisation System correlate closely with the classically conceived sympathetic nervous system and orchestrate fight/flight responses.

When a child experiences intense fear, coupled with inescapability, this initial Mobilisation response is redundant to her – a physically restrained child or a baby, for instance, cannot fight or flee. Here the child's Immobilisation System is activated. This is the human body's phylogenetically ancient response to the detection of an inevitable and significant threat to physical integrity and/or imminent death. The Immobilisation System recruits the unmyelinated vagal motor pathways to the heart to produce an immediate and massive slowing of heart rate (bradycardia), often the cessation of breathing (apnoea), and is often associated with fainting (vasovagal syncope). This reaction is metabolically conservative, rapidly withdrawing resources from the highly-oxygen-dependent central nervous system. The result – which may involve feigning death, behavioural shut-down, and dissociation – is an organism that appears to be inanimate.

The neuro-behavioural patterns of children suffering Posttraumatic Stress Disorder (PTSD) after medical illness, trend towards immobilisation and/or mobilisation responses (Levine & Kline 2006, Porges 2018). Traumatised children can be hyper-vigilant, hyper-aroused, quick to anger and slow to calm (highly mobilised), or dissociated (immobilised), or a mixture of both (Levine 2017, Porges 2018, Van der Kolk 2015). It is also important to note here that humans recruit their defence systems *at the expense* of calm states, social ability, health, growth, and restoration (Porges 2011, 2018). Once either of the two defence systems is reflexively employed, the Social Engagement System is temporarily disabled, which shuts down all co-ordinated regulation of prosocial behaviour. Simply put, a human who feels safe is an effective social being, while a human who feels threatened is severely compromised socially. A child with PTSD has *chronic* difficulties relating to others and in discerning the environment as safe (Levine & Kline 2006, Porges 2018, Porges & Daniel 2017). Fortunately, the relationship between defence and social engagement can be playfully inversed. We can consciously support the Social Engagement System to down-regulate chronic defence patterns as part of the Play Therapy process (Porges & Daniel 2017). More on this later.

Let's now turn to Josh's first session in Play Therapy to illustrate our use of the Polyvagal Theory in understanding trauma.

Josh, who was nine years old at the time, was referred for Play Therapy with the following profile: social withdrawal punctuated by episodes of extreme anger and violence; hyper-vigilance; difficulty sleeping; difficulty making friends; problems at school and home. When Josh was four, he had been through an eighteen-month treatment for leukaemia. He had been regularly physically restrained for certain medical procedures.

In our first session together, Josh drifted into the room like a shadow. He pushed the toy ambulance around with his left foot, then sat in the corner near the tent. He glanced at me then scuffled the wall with his trainers. I sat down nearby. The Polyvagal Theory gives us some clues about what Josh might have been feeling. At this point Josh is likely to be experiencing one of two defensive patterns – immobilisation or mobilisation – or fluctuating between periods of both. Josh could have a sense of generalised anxiety whilst also feeling vaguely disconnected from his emotional surrounding – experiencing dissociation. In this immobilised state his senses will be numbed, his thoughts ambiguous, his ability to detect and engage in flowing interaction highly limited – his impulse to do so, zero. Alternatively, Josh could be feeling highly mobilised, like a box of fireworks ready to explode. Although seemingly turned inwards, Josh might be scanning every aspect and moment of his environment for cues of risk and danger. Internally, his heart rate might be elevated, his breathing shallow and rapid, his viscera, blood vessels, and muscle tone constricted ready for action. In this mobilised state Josh is likely to perceive almost everything as a threat. The Polyvagal Theory explores why this might be the case. In the process of risk detection, external cues are by no means our only source of information. Information from inside the body (specifically, afferent feedback from the viscera) provides a major mediator of the accessibility of prosocial circuits associated with social engagement behaviours. Functionally, visceral states distort or colour our perception of other people.

Engaging traumatised children in play therapy

The face-heart connection and communicative musicality

The human *face-heart* connection (Porges 2007) concurrently enables an individual to signal *safety* through patterns of facial expression and vocal intonation, to detect signs of safety, and potentially calm an agitated other to form a social relationship. Let's take the example of voice. In the same way a mother uses her voice to sooth her infant, we as Play Therapists can communicate safety through ours. Dan Hughes (2004, 2011) talks of using his 'story teller's voice' in therapy – a melodic vibrant pattern which avoids monotone or flatness. When we use a voice like this in therapy, the child's brain dampens her Mobilisation System response and facilitates a calming effect on her heart via ventral vagal influences. In parallel to this calming effect, the regulation of the muscles of the face, head, and vocal apparatus is enhanced to enable reciprocal interactions to deepen between the child and therapist. Here we have consciously leveraged an aspect of the face–heart connection – specifically a sensitive musicality in voice – to support a traumatised child through difficult emotions, down-regulating stress responses back to a shared calm state.

Back to Josh's first session:

> I sat on the floor near Josh, trying to get some sense of his internal experience. I work with the basic principles of Child-Centred Play Therapy as a foundation: acceptance, non-judgement, empathy, and emotional honesty (Landreth 2012). As I sat with Josh, I sometimes used whole–body gestures and empathic 'sighs' to accompany reflections like, 'just not sure what it's all about in here' and, 'feeling kind of weird, what am I doing in here …' I knew that the musicality in my voice – the rhythmic pulse, the contours of volume, and in particular the quality of intonation – would be a crucial factor in helping Josh feel safe. In a state of immobilisation Josh would probably respond to very little, but he would need the background tone to be playful, peaceful, and musical (never monotone) to give him the best chance in engagement. I used to think that my deep voice would be a calming, perhaps fatherly presence in the playroom. The Polyvagal Theory told me otherwise. If Josh was in a mobilised state, hyper-vigilant and prone to interpreting any stimulus as a threat, then a deep voice was a no-go. A deep male voice, like the bass hum of an MRI scanner, could easily be felt as a tiger's growl. So I kept my voice light and musical.

The vagal brake

From the Polyvagal perspective, supporting a child through difficult experiences and back down to a shared calm state is a natural goal of Play Therapy – a natural extension of the goal of healthy play (Porges 2015, Porges & Daniel 2017). In doing so, we provide the dysregulated child with opportunities to exercise, and so strengthen, his *vagal brake* (Porges 2015, Porges et al. 1996). The strength of a child's *vagal brake* refers to the degree to which a child's nervous system is tuned to support his Social Engagement System and down-regulate his defense systems – basically his ability to self-regulate in the face of stress. By exercising the vagal brake over time, a child's autonomic system is slowly entrained towards a dampening of defensive responses and an awakening of the Social Engagement System (ibid.).

As Play Therapists we bring a conscious playfulness to opportunities for this neural exercise of the vagal brake. It is not as if we create difficult experiences for the children we work with – but we do see the power in these experiences when they arise and work with them respectfully. In what follows, I discuss some ideas to support this practice, talk about the vagal brake at various stages in the dynamics of the Play Therapy relationship, and continue with illustrations from Josh's Play Therapy.

> From our tentative connections in that first session, Josh had grown to trust me a little. In his third session, he felt safe enough to show some of his anger: safe enough to start to test this new adult in his life. Traumatised

children are always energised under the surface. Although sometimes seeming calm or even withdrawn, most traumatised children can snap into angry action in the blink of an eye. Josh was exploring the Lego basket, when seemingly out of nowhere (to my perspective), he stood up, kicked the chair and shouted, 'You don't know nothing about me'.

I felt a wave of nervousness, but I needed to respond. I knew how easy it would be to press Josh's reactive buttons and start a conflict. I did not want to be another reactive adult in Josh's life. Josh was often locked in a behavioural cycle with his parents. Naturally his parents found Josh's violent behaviour and anger hard to handle. Sometimes they reacted reflexively. And sometimes, out of necessity, they had to restrain their son physically. If you remember the root conditions of trauma – fear and inescapability – it is easy to see how physical restraint can often be a re-traumatising experience for a child. I also knew how easily a shallow attempt at empathy or being nice might be interpreted as an insult. But I did need to empathise with Josh. I knew that if Josh felt in-sync with me, felt togetherness even in his anger, then this shared experience would help bring Josh's Social Engagement System online. In turn, this would dampen Josh's mobilisation response a little. With his Social Engagement System primed, this would naturally open up more possibilities for interaction. And so on …

Vitality matching

An engaging, yet calming, 'story-teller's' voice is a useful baseline – a ground to return to in our quest to help a child towards self-regulation. But communicating empathy, togetherness, and acceptance as we travel with a child throughout flows of difficult emotion involves far more. As Play Therapists, the sensitive musicality of our voice (changing patterns of timbre, pitch, and volume) and of our bodies (changing patterns of position, intention, and intensity) give us a rich palate of ways in which we can stay in-sync with a child throughout her emotional world. A great way in which we can do this is through *vitality matching* (Stern 2010). *Vitality* is Dan Stern's concept for the energetic impetus of human action and interaction. In play, vitality flows in patterns of different shapes. Spontaneous games between an infant and her mother, for instance, often resemble a *vitality contour* – involving a shared heightening of excitement with a clear ending in resolution (Stern 1985, 2010). It is as if vitality provides the movement underlying the more obvious manifestations we call 'emotions'. Through vitality matching we can be with a child through a landscape of vitality without ever adding reactive fuel to specific emotional narratives. We can play with this idea in two ways. Firstly, when Stern talks of 'attunement' he is describing, 'matching and sharing dynamic forms of vitality, but *across* different modalities' (Stern 2010, p.42). For example if a traumatised child gives a loud staccato shout, I could make a quick, double-footed stomping jump on the ground. If he punches out at the air with a closed fist, I could make a loud but blunt 'huuugh' sound full of energy. Secondly, we can explore vitality-matching *within* the same modality – usually here within the modality of vocal sound. For instance, if a child is shouting and swearing angrily, I might try to make loud sounds alongside him which match the increasing energy contours of his vocalisation but which communicate none of the verbal content or angry vibe. Once we have shared the journey through a contour together, if needed, I can then use my face–heart connection to help the child return to calm state and so exercise his vagal brake.

Back to that moment in Josh's third session:

> ... So I replied to Josh with a sentence that started relatively high in pitch and loud in volume, and increased in both towards the end. It was full of energy, to some degree a desperate energy. It followed the vitality contour of anger, but was not angry in tone or content. Most of the communication was in the musicality. The words, much less significant, were:

> I don't even know anything about you.

> It was a useful moment in our relationship. Josh relaxed a little and let in a tiny bit of sadness. I sighed with him and let my body tone relax and drop. Together we had travelled our first difficult emotion, survived, and come out the other side in-sync and calm. I followed Josh's contour down with him, and matched the melancholic vitality underlying his sadness with the musicality in my voice, as I continued:

> But I'd love to know loads about you. You know in here you can talk to me about anything you want to, you can show me stuff with the toys, you can play in all kinds of ways.

> Josh calmed down. He stayed in the room and introduced the turtle – a significant character we'll meet a little later on. A difficult moment had become a chance for our relationship to develop and an opportunity for me to help Josh regulate back to a calm state, exercising his vagal brake.

A somatic trajectory

Next we take a look at the overall 'somatic trajectory' of Josh's progress in Play Therapy and explore a few more examples of vitality matching, each ending in a conscious exercise of Josh's vagal brake.

At a very young age, Josh had been traumatised by being repeatedly pinned down by his mother for the administration of frightening injections and inhalant anaesthesia (involving a mask over the nose and mouth). His tiny body had primed for fight/flight but then, on perceiving the futility of this, went into full dissociative shut-down. Peter Levine explains how, with no release and nowhere to go, Josh's energetic fight/flight impulse became locked into certain neuro-behavioural patterns – *unfulfilled* patterns that needed completion (Levine 2017, Levine & Kline 2006). Since his early trauma – and up until his resolution experiences in Play Therapy – Josh's brain and body had been continually, and unsuccessfully, seeking that completion (Levine 2017, Van der Kolk 2015). Unconsciously, in his dreams and in his play, Josh had revisited the experiences that frightened him so much. Equally unconsciously, Josh's body had sought the experience of breaking free, escaping, fighting back, running wild. The trauma-resolution sought is of the body and, in my experience in Play Therapy, often follows a 'somatic trajectory' – defined here as, increasingly embodied experiences towards a resolution of unfulfilled fight/flight patterns.

> In Josh's third session he introduced the turtle. Swimming in the sand tray, the turtle quickly found himself having difficulty breathing. Josh's body reflected the turtle's anguish: his face flushed; his speech quickened; his muscle tone tightened; his breathing became shallow and short. I matched the vitality of Josh's unspoken communication with an obvious shrinking and tensing of my posture, and a facial expression involving apprehension, expectation, and excitement. Above, when I talked about vitality-matching anger, I explored the possibility of replacing the child's words with empathic whole-body gestures as a way to connect without fuelling a particular narrative. Here, for Josh, my vitality-matching centred on the opposite function. Josh needed support in becoming conscious of his body's communication. So, along with my whole-body empathy, my vitality-matching brought words into the picture: [me: shallow breathing] 'Turtle can't breath down there, feeling scared, not sure what to do …' and, 'turtle's kind of stuck, can't breath, can't get out …'. Quite quickly turtle did break out of the suffocating water. Josh and I breathed deeply together as I added words and large, celebratory body movements to his sense of release. Wanting to support Josh completely through this contour of tension, release, celebration and then down to calm again (a great example of exercising the vagal brake) I modelled a physical shaking-out of tension and a subsequent slowing of breath to relax. Peter Levine (2010) describes the natural shaking-free that most animals spontaneously display after an experience of immobilisation. A traumatised child's body needs access to this release and, where appropriate, we can model and support this in Play Therapy. Josh tentatively picked up the threads of my modelled behaviour and we shook a little

together. He calmed slightly. Josh went on to incorporate the escape-shake-release-calm pattern more confidently into his play as our relationship deepened. As we went through similar play configurations repeatedly, Josh added various 'bad people' and hoards of enemies to the surface of the water. Each time he was giving turtle more to push against. The somatic experience of breaking free needs a physically energetic barrier to crash through. Josh was at the start of his somatic trajectory, but already he had brought that barrier into his play.

Josh had found his way into a progressive somatic trajectory with minimal support from me. But imagine if the turtle had remained trapped, suffocating under the water, with no escape. Imagine if this happened again and again in an energised but stuck loop, one in which the child becomes increasingly dysregulated. In such a situation I would be wondering about re-traumatisation. Re-traumatisation is something to be aware of, but not frightened by, when working with traumatised children. If a child is engaging in a repetitive loop of behaviour or play – one in which there is no evolution at all, and in which the child is increasingly disturbed or overwhelmed – then stepping out of a child-centred approach and into a focussed, supportive role to help the child shift gear is crucial (Levine & Kline 2006). Of course, this needs to be done carefully. I find Dan Hughe's rule-of thumb, 'Follow-Lead-Follow' useful here. Essentially child-centred, I *follow* the child's communication. But if I have a strong sense that the seed of something new is needed, I model or make that suggestion (*lead*) sensitively, always matching the child's vitality. It's then instantly back to *follow*, as I respond to the child's communication. The *lead* I would try initially, in the case of the trapped turtle, would be a simple suggestion, [me: shallow breathing, tense body posture, tentative expression] 'It's like the turtle can't breathe, feels frightened down there, maybe turtle wants to jump up and escape …'. Or, if suggestions are not helping, I might, very rarely (and in considered discussion with my supervisor), channel the child's play in a simplifying direction for a short while. In such instances I will be leveraging the power of the vagal brake through a calming embodied experience: breathing together; humming; tapping; clapping; rocking; rolling a ball together; changing postures (hopefully silly ones), can all help. To do this, I will match the vitality of the child's initial anguish but, instead of matching her contour, I will *lead* with my own contour into the supported experience and calming face-heart communication. On the very few occasions that I have needed to do this, the child has returned productively to her trauma theme with a little more self-regulatory capacity.

I find there is a general trend in the therapeutic somatic trajectory of most children suffering medical PTSD. As the child develops trust in our relationship, there is a movement: from play with toys, to play where events happen to me, and lastly to play where events happen to the child. In the latter two categories medically traumatised children often introduce doctor-patient play – a kind of emotional/embodied/symbolic surgery. Josh's play followed this trend.

> Eight sessions into his Play Therapy, Josh told me to lie down on 'the operating table'. As the doctor he gave me injections, anaesthetised me, and removed stones and black mud from my bones (remember his leukaemia diagnosis). I had many opportunities to empathise from the patient's perspective. I was vitality-matching Josh's immediate unconscious communication (his body tension, his fearful anticipation, his moments of clear dissociation). Again I brought words along with my body gestures, words to bring Josh's experience into his consciousness: 'Feels frightening, I just don't know what's going to happen', or, 'There's nothing I can do here, feel frightened and stuck', or, 'You know I just want to run away right now, but I can't'. After many 'operations', over many sessions, I felt a strong intuition to verbalise something I felt was intensely present in our shared emotional experience – it was a bit of a risk, but it felt right. In a stage whisper I mentioned to 'Child-Josh' (not 'Doctor Josh'), 'you know, I just want to jump off this damn operating table and run away'. And he let me! We escaped together and ran around the room in celebration! Exercising the vagal brake does not always trend to calm states, sometimes it culminates in playful joy!

> Eventually Josh found enough trust to become the patient himself. He instructed me, the Doctor, in his surgery. He had the resilience now to feel his pain in its most direct sense. My role was simply to stay strong, calm, and to do exactly what he told me. Josh underwent his 'operations' over the course of many sessions. Only once did he instigate the energetic and physical escape I had modelled when I was the patient. But this one escape, as the culmination of Josh's whole somatic trajectory, was enough. Again we celebrated in joy. Josh stayed in Play Therapy for a few more sessions. However, the impetus had gone from his trauma patterns and he was doing great at home. In our final session, number thirty-eight, Josh parked up the toy ambulance safely in the tent and said, 'Can I go now?'

Chapter summary

- The Polyvagal Theory supports our understanding of medical stress and PTSD through an understanding of the Mobilisation and Immobilisation systems and their oppositional relationship with the Social Engagement System.
- The face–heart connection enables us to down-regulate a child's stress response back to calm state.

- Repeated exercise of a child's Vagal Brake – where child and therapist travel together through difficult emotions back to calm state – is a natural goal of Play Therapy.
- Exercise of the vagal brake, over time, entrains a dysregulated child's neurophysiology towards self-regulation.
- Through sensitive musicality, the face-heart connection, and vitality-matching in Play Therapy we can support exercise of the vagal brake.
- The above concepts were explored within a proposed 'Somatic-Trajectory' in Play Therapy – defined as, increasingly embodied experiences towards a resolution of unfulfilled fight/flight patterns.

Note

1 'Josh' is a composite case study and the details given, although representative of real experiences with many children in Play Therapy, do not pertain to any one child.

Further reading

Dana, D. (2018). *The Polyvagal Theory in Therapy: Engaging the Rhythm of Regulation.* New York: W.W. Norton & Co. A powerful translation of the insights of Polyvagal Theory into practicable therapeutic exercises and principles for work with traumatized individuals.

Daniel, S. and Trevarthen, C. (eds.) (2017) *Rhythms of Relating in Children's Therapies: Connecting Creatively with Vulnerable Children.* London: Jessica Kingsley Publishers. A multi-author compilation exploring the concept of musicality and 'rhythms of relating' in therapeutic work with children in many settings and across many creative modalities.

Levine, P. and Kline, M. (2006).*Trauma through a Child's Eyes: Awakening the Ordinary Miracle of Healing.* Berkeley, CA: North Atlantic Books, U.S. Peter Levine's insights on trauma and trauma-treatment explored and expanded upon for application in work with traumatized children.

Porges, S.W. (2011). *The Polyvagal Theory: Neurophysiological Foundations of Emotions, Attachment, Communication, and Self-Regulation.* New York: W.W. Norton & Co. The original compilation of Stephen Porges's papers detailing his groundbreaking Polyvagal Theory.

References

Azeem, M.W., Reddy, B., Wudarsky, M., Carabetta, L., Gregory, F., and Sarofin, M. (2015). Restraint reduction at a pediatric psychiatric hospital: A ten-year journey. *Journal of Child and Adolescent Psychiatric Nursing*, 28 (4), pp. 180–184.

Diseth, T.H. (2005). Dissociation in children and adolescents as reaction to trauma – An overview of conceptual issues and neurobiological factors. *Nordic Journal of Psychiatry*, 59 (2), pp. 79–91.

Forgey, M. and Bursch, B. (2013). Assessment and management of pediatric iatrogenic medical trauma. *Current Psychiatry Reports*, 15 (2), pp. 1–9.

Hughes, D. (2004). An attachment-based treatment of maltreated children and young people. *Attachment and Human Development*, 3 (6), pp. 263–278.

Hughes, D. (2011). *Attachment-Focussed Family Therapy Workbook*. (Pap/DVD Wk edition). New York: W.W. Norton & Co.

Kazak, A.E., Kassam-Adams, N., Schneider, S., Zelikovsky, N., Alderfer, M.A., and Rourke, M. (2006). An integrative model of pediatric medical traumatic stress. *Journal of Pediatric Psychology*, 31 (4), pp. 343–355.

Landreth, G.L. (2012). *Play Therapy: The Art of the Relationship*. New York: Routledge.

Levine, P. (2010). *In an Unspoken Voice: How the Body Releases Trauma and Restores Goodness*. Berkeley, CA: North Atlantic Books, U.S.

Levine, P. (2017). Somatic experiencing®: A body oriented approach to the treatment of traumatized infants and children. In: S. Daniel and C. Trevarthen (eds.). *Rhythms of Relating in Children's Therapies: Connecting Creatively with Vulnerable Children*. London: Jessica Kingsley Publishers.

Levine, P. and Kline, M. (2006). *Trauma through a Child's Eyes: Awakening the Ordinary Miracle of Healing*. Berkeley, CA: North Atlantic Books, U.S.

Porges, S.W. (2007). The polyvagal perspective. *Biological Psychology*, 74 (2), pp. 116–143.

Porges, S.W. (2009). The Polyvagal Theory: New insights into adaptive reactions of the autonomic nervous system. *Cleveland Clinic Journal of Medicine*, 76 (Suppl 2), pp. 86–90.

Porges, S.W. (2011). *The Polyvagal Theory: Neurophysiological Foundations of Emotions, Attachment, Communication, and Self-Regulation*. New York: W.W. Norton & Co.

Porges, S.W. (2015). Play as a neural exercise: Insights from the Polyvagal Theory. In: D. Pearce-McCall (ed.). *The Power of Play for Mind Brain Health*. Available from: http://mindgains.org/ [Accessed on 02.09.2017]

Porges, S.W. (2018). Polyvagal Theory: A primer. In: S.W. Porges and D. Dana (eds.). *Clinical Applications of the Polyvagal Theory: The Emergence of Polyvagal-Informed Therapies*, p. 50. New York: W.W. Norton & Co.

Porges, S.W. and Daniel, S. (2017). Play and the dynamics of treating pediatric medical trauma: Insights from Polyvagal Theory. In: S. Daniel and C. Trevarthen (eds.). *Rhythms of Relating in Children's Therapies: Connecting Creatively with Vulnerable Children*, p. 113. London: Jessica Kingsley Publishers.

Porges, S.W., Doussard-Roosevelt, J.A., Portales, A.L., and Greenspan, S.I. (1996). Infant regulation of the vagal 'brake' predicts child behavior problems: A psychobiological model of social behavior. *Developmental Psychobiology*, 29(8), pp. 697–712.

Stern, D.N. (1985). *The Interpersonal World of the Infant*. New York: Basic Books.

Stern, D.N. (2010). *Forms of Vitality: Exploring Dynamic Experience in Psychology, the Arts, Psychotherapy, and Development*. Oxford: Oxford University Press.

Van der Kolk, B.A. (2015). *The Body Keeps the Score: Mind, Brain and Body in the Transformation of Trauma*. New York: Penguin.

Chapter 18

Working with child trauma through EMDR and play therapy

Debra May

Chapter overview

In this chapter I will describe how Simon, a five-year-old boy suffering with Post Traumatic Stress Disorder (PTSD) was able to make sense of a serious car accident with the use of Eye Movement Desensitisation Reprocessing (EMDR) and play therapy. I will explain how trauma can impact on a child. I will describe what EMDR is and how it helped Simon to process trauma-related dissociative thoughts and feelings, often in the form of nightmares and flashbacks of frightening images. I will discuss how the child then benefitted from play therapy to explore his internal struggles following the accident. I conclude that EMDR and play therapy work well together, although each had a different focus and role in this intervention. Signed parental consent was gained to include the clinical material in relation to this case for education and training purposes, with the understanding that the names of the child and his family are anonymised. I have also been mindful that the child may read this chapter in the future and recognise his personal story.

EMDR

EMDR is a therapeutic approach developed by Francine Shapiro (2001) from her work with Vietnam War veterans to treat trauma symptoms in an individual. It is one of the trauma therapies recommended for Post-Traumatic Stress Disorder (PSTD) by the National Institute for Health and Care Excellence (NICE) (www.nice.org.uk, 2018). In addition, from a worldwide perspective, EMDR is gaining recognition for providing trauma therapy both at the front end of mass disasters worldwide and for adults and children who have been involved in personal traumatic experiences (Bucan-Varatanovic & Sabanovic, 2017; Carriere, 2014; Colelli, 2003). The World Health Organisation (WHO), a specialist agency of the United Nations, recommends EMDR as a treatment of choice for trauma to support the work of trauma aid organisations (Crowley, 2016). To become an accredited EMDR practitioner, a professional must

be registered with an EMDR approved professional body to undertake certified training and supervision to ensure competency in using EMDR (EMDR
UK & Ireland, 2018).

EMDR follows a protocol to help an individual reprocess a traumatic
memory, with its associated dissociative symptoms, into an ordinary, coherent memory that does not cause dissociation (Ghnassia Damon, 2008; Shapiro, 2001). If required, a 'Developmental Protocol' (Morris-Smith &
Silvestre, 2007) provides age-related protocols that are adapted to the
child's developmental stage. A child can draw, use toys and sand trays, or
use key words to express what is 'troubling them' or making them feel
afraid. The child's parent or trusted adult is usually in the therapy room
with the child for their support (Lovett, 1999; Morris-Smith, 2011).

The adaptive information processing (AIP) system provides the base of
EMDR therapy (Shapiro, 2001). It uses the trauma as a starting point
(Van der Kolk, 2015) as it processes a new experience and information and
stores it in memory networks that contain related thoughts, images, emotions, and sensations (ibid). A traumatic memory is one that has not been
resolved. It is stored as it is experienced, frozen at that developmental age
and stage when the child first experienced it (Morris-Smith, 2011). This
can be at a crucial period in a child's development, such as when a baby is
left unattended for long periods when hungry or thirsty, feeling abandoned
and numb (Lovett, 1999). Any unresolved traumatic memory from the past
could negatively impact the child's subsequent behaviour and relationships
throughout their life (Shapiro, 2001; Tinker & Wilson, 1999).

Trauma

Trauma is an overwhelming experience that leaves an individual feeling frightened, threatened, and unsafe (Ghnassia Damon, 2008). Shapiro argues that
there are two kinds of trauma – a 'small "t" trauma' (2001:4) or a 'big "T"
trauma' (ibid.). The small 't' trauma is relatively quickly resolved and placed
in its context (Tinker & Wilson, 1999), whereas a big 'T' trauma remains unresolved with an ongoing sense of fear and feeling unsafe (ibid). The big 'T'
traumatic memory is stored frozen in its original form (Shapiro, 2001:4), fragmented and isolated in the different memory networks (Bergmann, 2012).

The use of Bilateral Stimulation (BLS) in EMDR mediates the accessing of
the fragmented and isolated dysfunctional stored memory and links it with
other related memory networks, where it is integrated into a reasonable
memory with no further disturbance (Shapiro, 2001). BLS uses a rhythmic
left-right pattern (Shapiro, 2001; Tinker & Wilson, 1999) that can be achieved
by the stimulation of different senses, i.e., sight, hearing, or touch (Logie,
2012; Shapiro, 2001). Eye movements can track an object, lights, a wand, or
chosen toy in front of the eyes (Logie, 2012; Morris-Smith, 2011), or by alternate tapping (Lovett, 1999) or foot stomping and drumming (Gomez, 2013;

Morris-Smith, 2007; Shapiro, 2001). Van der Kolk (2011) suggests that the BLS activates the brain to integrate different fragments of information related to the trauma with other information stored in the brain. This process occurs naturally for the individual during the 'rapid-eye-movement' (REM) period of sleep whereby the eyes move fast when dreaming and the individual wakes up no longer upset (Lovett, 1999).

Whilst trauma can be experienced by any individual, its impact on a child is dependent on whether they have a consistently attuned parent or adult that is available to reassure and comfort them (Golding & Hughes, 2012; Howe, 2005). Without such support a child can experience a deep upset that can cause emotional and psychological dysfunction. If left unchanged it will impact their development on into adulthood, which could have long-term effects on their brain function and mental health (Rothschild, 2000; Shapiro, 2001; Van der Kolk, 2015).

Dissociation

Children who have experienced trauma may also experience dissociation (Tinker & Wilson, 1999). Evidenced in symptoms such as flashbacks, sleep-walking, nightmares, fears, fluctuating behaviours, lapses of attention, and trances, this can negatively impact their daily functioning (Silberg, 1998). Dissociative behaviours should not be ignored as dissociation is the opposite of the integration of a memory (Morris-Smith, 2011; Struik, 2014). For the child to integrate a traumatic memory, they will need to reprocess it, so that it makes sense to them and, although it will still be a negative memory, it will not trigger dissociation (Spierings, 2016; Struik, 2014). Without such processing the child is at risk of using dissociation to avoid harrowing memories, which could adversely compromise their development (Morris-Smith, 2011; Struik, 2014). For instance, a child involved in a serious car accident where their life and their family's lives were threatened could be adversely affected in many ways, e.g., they might become reluctant to leave the house, unable to tolerate any surprises, or blame the driver, and so develop unhealthy thought patterns in relationships.

Case study: Simon

Simon was five years old when his personal world dramatically changed, following a car accident involving his mother and sister Penny. His mother described how she, his Dad, and sister Penny all doted on him. He was inquisitive and often made them laugh with his jokes. The family did many things together, although at the time of the accident, his father was spending a lot of time at work. So, Mum would take the two children out on day trips. The car had recently been fixed due to a previous car accident when Dad had been driving the car a few weeks earlier.

On one of the day trips at the beginning of the summer holidays, Mum took Simon and Penny out of town to the country to see family friends. She described it as a lovely warm day, during which they had fun with the friends. On the journey back home, Mum stopped for them to pick some fruit. As agreed, Simon and Penny swapped seats and Simon sat in the front. Mum was driving on one of the A roads 'as they usually are less crowded'. When the car was five miles from home, it was hit head-on the driver's side of the car with such severity that the bonnet flew up, obstructing vision.

All three were taken to hospital in separate ambulances. Access to all adjoining local roads were closed, and people were advised on the local radio to avoid the area due to the emergency services blocking off roads. Simon's Mum and Penny were taken to separate hospitals due to the serious life-threatening injuries they both sustained in the accident. Simon was taken to be 'checked over' at the same hospital as his Mum, due to a mark on his neck caused by his seat belt. Simon could not see his Mum in the hospital as she was in surgery. By this time, Simon's Dad was with him and had taken him back to stay with his paternal grandparents.

After the accident, Simon's Mum and sister were hospitalised for several weeks. Dad stayed with Simon's sister who had been seriously injured and had been moved to a different hospital in a nearby city. Simon had regular 'Facetime' contact with his Mum and sister and would visit his Mum with his grandparents. After four weeks, Mum returned home in a wheelchair as she had lost most of the use of both legs. The house was re-modelled to accommodate Mum's mobility issues. Simon's sister returned home two weeks after Mum's return. She had sustained serious, life-threatening injuries with the need for ongoing surgery.

EMDR intervention

Shortly after the accident, the family received brief 'family therapy' together. At that time, Simon started to display troubling behaviours within the family home. A six-week EMDR intervention was recommended for him by the family therapist.

Since the accident, Simon's world had become scary and unpredictable, feeling out of both his and his parents' control. He was struggling with his mother being in a wheelchair, as he found her not to be as available as before the accident. Simon was frightened and confused that his close-knit family, of which he was the beloved baby, had fragmented both physically and emotionally. Each member of the family appeared to experience 'cascades' of trauma (Lovett, 1999:29) initially triggered by the car accident and then subsequent losses and traumas, both medical and personal. His father appeared busy dealing with the aftermath of the accident, ensuring everyone's needs in the family were met, whilst he struggled to cope with the vicarious trauma. His mother and sister were both struggling with PTSD, but had each decided to focus on their physical health. Mum faced the possibility of permanently being unable to walk, and Simon's sister Penny was expected to have ongoing surgery.

I first met the family twelve weeks after the accident. They expressed concerns at Simon's behaviour since the accident. Dad's concern was that '*Simon was having recurrent nightmares, from which he woke up screaming*'. Mum's concerns were in relation to the compulsive behaviours Simon had developed:

> a nervous twitch when any of the family goes to touch him. He licks his fingers and rubs the injury all the time. Also, he puts his fingers at the back of his throat but I try to ignore it.

It appeared that Simon had developed PTSD. This was evidenced in his dissociative behaviours, such as nightmares, obsessive compulsive behaviours, and intrusive thoughts (Lovett, 1999; Tinker & Wilson, 1999).

Simon's history of both positive and negative experiences was gathered from his parents and then with his father and Simon (Morris-Smith & Silvestre, 2007). The child's attachments were also explored at this stage, both in relation to the parents and any other adults (Gomez, 2013; Morris-Smith, 2011). This information can be used with the child to build up their internal resources (Gomez, 2013).

It was agreed that the therapy would take place in the family home to minimise disruption. Dad would be present with Simon during EMDR therapy. Mum agreed to write a narrative of what happened in the accident to use with Simon when processing the car accident (Lovett, 1999; Morris-Smith, 2011). Simon and Dad sat on a blue mat opposite me in the front living room of the family home. Simon was able to identify an emotion and state where he felt it in his body, as well as two things that he thought he did 'well at': these were occasions when he scored a goal at school and when he made a bracelet for 'my Mummy'. I used EMDR with Simon to enhance both positive experiences, with the BLS provided by his Dad who sat behind Simon and tapped his shoulders. We then processed a 'safe place' (Shapiro, 2001) that Simon could recall when he felt overwhelmed. The safe place encourages the child to locate a special external place where he is alone and happy; he is then encouraged to connect with his emotions and feelings in his body, as well as his other senses of sight, smell, and hearing (Tinker & Wilson, 1999). The engaging of the senses, using bilateral stimulation, intensifies the positive feelings, which is then connected to a name or word that the child chooses. The child is then reminded to use his 'safe place' when he feels overwhelmed or frightened outside of the therapy. This demonstrated that Simon could use Dual Attention Stimulation and BLS (Shapiro, 2001; Tinker & Wilson, 1999), both of which are necessary for re-processing traumatic memories. Dual Attention Stimulation is when the individual can focus on an old memory, whilst at the same time being mindful of what is happening to their senses as they follow BLS. Simon confirmed that he had used the safe place when he became upset and irritated by another child at his school.

In order for a child to reprocess a traumatic memory, it is important for the therapist to ensure that the child's memory is aroused sufficiently to process, whilst also remaining in his 'window of tolerance' (Ogden et al., 2006; Porges, 1995), otherwise the child may dissociate and become re-traumatised.

During this period, I used the EMDR protocol with Simon to process a nightmare he had experienced that week. Tinker and Wilson (1999) state that it can be positive for the child if the nightmare is the first negative event to process as it can stop the nightmares, which could encourage the child with the ongoing therapy (1999). Simon drew the drawing below (Figure 18.1), and then he explained the picture and we started to process the nightmare using the EMDR protocol.

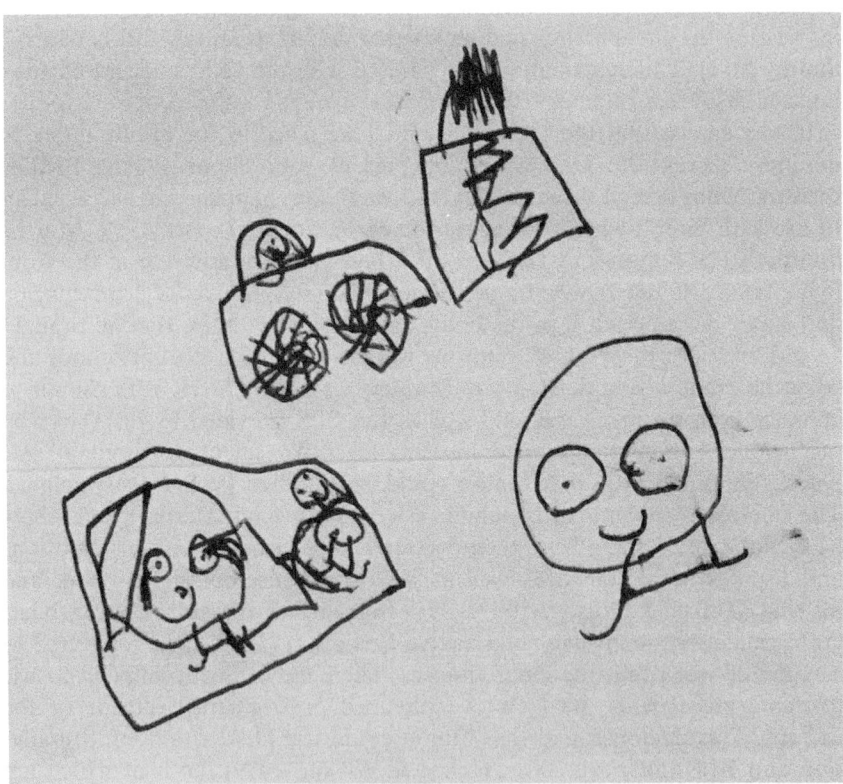

Figure 18.1 Simon's drawing of a recent nightmare

I asked Simon about the picture using the EMDR. What is the worst part of the nightmare? Simon said, 'my house falling down'. I asked Simon how that made him feel. Simon said that he felt 'sad' and chose the saddest face on the smiley scale I showed him. I asked him to tell me what happened. He said that 'Penny, Mummy and Daddy were upstairs. I was on my own in my bedroom, it made me feel sad'. I asked him what he would prefer to think. He said, 'happy family'. I asked him where he felt that in his body and he touched his head and said, 'the head'. Simon said that 'the people were in the car, the wheelchair/car was a monster truck; people in the car die; they had to turn the car, it couldn't stop in time; it's a different car to the one in the nightmare'. Simon said, 'the monster truck crashed into the house and all the parts go into the living room, even the engine, the cars that are broken go the scrap yard, the monster truck gets towed away, the door on the fridge gets broken, then the car gets pushed through there' (he pointed to the right of the living room toward the kitchen) 'the fridge falls over because the door broke on the fridge that made it topple over, because of the big bang'. Lovett (1999) suggests that a nightmare can be indicative of PSTD in a child following a serious traumatic event, such as a car accident. The disturbing fragmented images Simon processed were of him being alone, isolated and afraid, both from the car accident and his beloved mother who was now forced to use a wheelchair. Simon then said he had no more memories. I asked him again 'when you think about the worst part of the nightmare, what do you feel?' Simon said 'sad'. The bilateral stimulation continued with his father sitting behind him, tapping his back. Then I asked Simon again how he felt, and he said 'happy'. I used a scale of smiley to very sad faces, for him to indicate how happy he felt. He picked the 'happiest' face. Before ending the session, I encouraged Simon to go to his safe place, where he could become calm and grounded in the 'here and now'. I also advised Simon's father that the processing may continue and that, if Simon cries in the day or night, Dad should remind him of his safe place and to alternately tap his back slowly, as I explained this would help to calm Simon.

On our last session of EMDR, Simon's mother read out the story she had written about the car accident. Dad used alternative tapping on Simon's back whilst he listened to the story. Simon then fully engaged in the EMDR to process the car accident. After the session, I discussed with both parents my concern that, although Simon had processed the memory of the car accident, he was still suffering with PTSD. Mum raised concern about Simon as his behaviour had become 'oppositional and disruptive' at school, resulting in him 'being given two red cards'. He had also become more challenging at home, 'jiffling and banging' into his Mum; he was also 'dropping to the floor and shouting', 'compulsively licking things' and not wanting to play alone, waking at night and wanting to sleep with his parents. His parents said that such behaviours had not been evident before the accident.

It seemed that Simon was struggling emotionally and psychologically, with many fragmented and confusing fears and emotions following the accident. Whilst Simon had a secure attachment to his parents, it appeared that he had developed an apparent lack of trust in their ability to soothe and help him feel safe. Yet, he was 'acting out' at his parents and clearly communicating some powerful thoughts and feelings. Both parents agreed to my suggestion that I see Simon for individual play therapy at his school.

Introducing play therapy as an intervention

A basic premise of play therapy is that play is the child's 'natural language' (McCarthy, 2008:11), which is 'spontaneous, enjoyable, voluntary and non-goal directed' (Landreth, 2011:4). Within play therapy, play is the child's 'business' and the therapist's 'business' is to provide a safe environment where the child is free to play and not be judged or led in their play. The boundaries are agreed at the beginning of the therapeutic intervention, in relation to the room and its materials and toys, and the time when the session will end, with an agreed five-minute warning beforehand (BAPT Core Competence 22, see Appendix 1). Play therapy is child-centred, in that it is focussed on the child's emotional and psychological needs. There is no expectation that the child should perform or engage in play with the therapist. The child is free to use the session however they choose in relation to the toys and materials provided. As the child relaxes and feels safe in the session, they will spontaneously project (Malchiodi, 2008) any troubling memories held in their unconscious onto the toys and materials. Some of the memories may start in the somatic form with all kinds of emotions and sensations in the body (Rothschild, 2000) but throughout the therapeutic process these will develop into narratives and stories that will help the child to make sense of what is troubling them (Cattanach, 1994). There are no rules about how and when this happens.

A further sixteen sessions were commissioned for play therapy and EMDR (if required) to allow Simon to have the psychological space to explore whatever he wanted to in the session with the toys and materials. I saw him over a five-month period. It was agreed with Simon and his parents that I would see him at school, as he felt safe there and the parents had a good relationship with the school.

Wilson et al. (2001:15) explain that the therapist's focus is on the 'child's feelings, motives and preoccupations' in the child's play. The therapist may use some verbal reflections to the child simultaneously in the session, but the reflections should be non-intrusive to the child's play and should not impede the child's choice and use of different toys and material, nor should they influence the child's exploration or expression. Instead, the therapist has to be attuned to the child's play as they follow the child's lead (Axline, 1964). This is in contrast to EMDR where the child will choose the negative memory that troubles them the most and the therapist, with the child, will try to identify key pieces of information associated with the identified memory.

Simon and I both sat on the same blue mat that I brought with me for the sessions. I provided the same materials for each session: paper and pens, clay, slime, and a sand tray with two bags of toys: one contained cars, helicopters, aeroplanes, tractors, and motorbikes, the other contained people with prams, mythical creatures, and random small and larger containers. I selected the toys and materials carefully in order to provide a variety of toys that Simon might find interesting and 'provide him with opportunities for self-expression' as the toys become an 'extension of the child's self, just as words are an extension of the adult's self' (Landreth, 2011:13). Simon was in control of the toys and stories and could bring as much traumatic material to explore as he could tolerate (Lovett, 1999). Whilst the school provided a room for us to use, the rooms we were allocated would vary in size and also in relation to noise from outside the room. The issue of the room did not distract Simon from his quest to play. He played on my large blue mat and I sat on the edge of the mat, as he tended to use most of the mat to express himself in the play.

Over the first four sessions the themes that emerged from Simon's play were of: 'racing cars crashing', 'catastrophes with aliens invading earth', and 'zombies threatening all the people on earth'. It seemed to me that Simon was distancing himself emotionally from the personal threat of danger, whilst exploring it through guises in his play. It is important to ensure that the repetitive themes shift, otherwise the child is at risk of dissociation and so being re-traumatised (Perkins McNally, 2001). As Simon played with the toys, I used BLS in the form of 'tappers', which were two pulsars that Simon put in his socks. The tappers were connected to a control box, which I held and controlled in relation to the intensity and pace of the pulses. BLS enabled Simon to be calm and focused on his play but also aware of what he was doing in the play.

After eight sessions, a significant shift occurred in Simon's play. He chose to use the sand tray. The themes became more representative of his fears and emotions in relation to the car accident he had experienced with his mother and sister. Perkins McNally (2001) suggests that the sensory element of the sandplay enables the child to be calm enough to focus on otherwise troubling thoughts and ideas. The play took on a more focussed, intense, rapid-moving energy with its own momentum, with accidents involving different sorts of vehicles racing: 'People catapulted out of the car'; 'Mummy and Baby separated'; 'Mummy and Dad are dead'; 'Cars struggling to stop'; 'Baby being abandoned'; 'Super Baby in the pram'. The play became cathartic at this point (McCarthy, 2008) with a renewed surge of energy, a clear focus, and intense emotions expressed when Simon explored 'Mum coming back to life'. The safety of the play therapy allowed Simon to explore the scary themes as they emerged and then to make sense of the impact of them on himself (McCarthy, 2007). The play therapy was about the integration of Simon's fragmented sense of self due to the separation from his mother following the accident, where he had felt abandoned. The EMDR paved the way for the play therapy as Simon was able to use the EMDR protocol to re-process the traumatic nightmares he experienced following the car accident, which then led to the re-processing of his memories from the car accident into a coherent memory, where he could accept that the frightening accident had happened but that he was safe now (Van der Kolk, 2015).

It seemed that the initial trauma of the car accident with his mother and sister became compounded by the disruption in his care, causing him to experience a developmental trauma within his attachment relationships with his parents, as both were 'physically and psychologically' unable to help him understand what was happening (Yehuda, 2016:37). Following the play therapy, I used EMDR with Simon on one more occasion, when he processed his fear that his father would crash their new car. When I later checked with Simon's parents and his school, both agreed that he was 'fine now and back to his old self', in that he was inquisitive, chatty, and fun to be with.

The play therapy intervention, together with the BLS, followed Simon's lead and afforded him the space to explore his subliminal dilemmas, losses, and feelings since the car accident. Cattanach explains that the child chooses the toys that will represent their 'emotions and thoughts symbolically. It is this combination of cognitive sorting of experience and the personal expression which helps the child to integrate and make sense of what has happened in their world' (1994:18). For Simon such play was 'cathartic' (McCarthy, 2008:153) with the catalyst for positive change occurring after he spontaneously explored the themes of 'Mummy coming back to life'. After this, Simon was able to tolerate processing the pervasive fear of a further car accident with his father crashing the new family car.

As part of the ending of the therapy with Simon, I drew a large shield and split it into four parts. I asked Simon a question for each quarter. He then drew or wrote in response to the questions. His answers indicated that he had enjoyed the sessions and drew a picture of both him and me smiling. I asked him what he thought before the accident: he wrote 'happy', and added 'still happy' when I asked him how he felt now at the end of our sessions (see Figure 18.2).

Two weeks before the final session, I spoke to Simon's mother. She said that Simon was in a 'good place at home. He is telling us he loves us more and wants proper cuddles now, before he wasn't showing much emotion after the accident'. At the end of the therapy, feedback from both parents was that the difficulties they had experienced with Simon's behaviour had diminished and were within the range of what could be expected for a five-year-old child. Following my intervention with Simon, the family as a whole entered into family therapy with a family therapist.

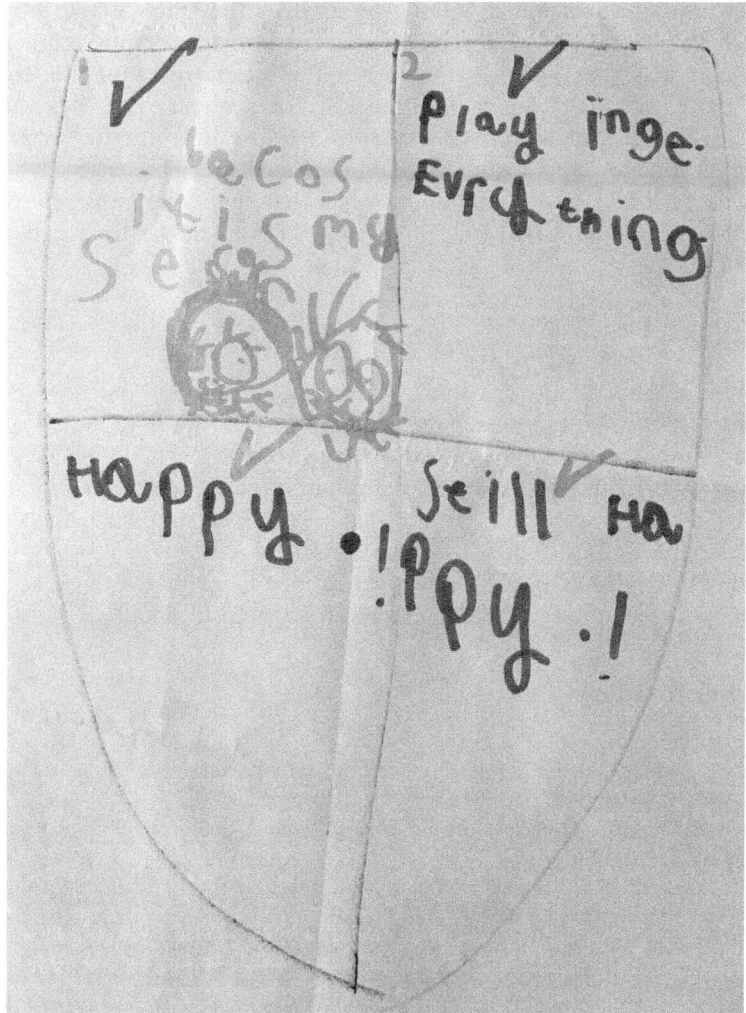

Figure 18.2 Simon's shield from our last therapy session together

Conclusion

In this chapter, I have presented my work with Simon, a five-year-old boy involved in a serious car accident who suffered PTSD. This was evidenced in the form of nightmares, intrusive flashbacks, and also fears about the separation and loss from his mother's care.

Following my intervention with Simon, the family as a whole entered into family therapy again. The use of both EMDR and play therapy at different times in the therapy proved effective at meeting his emotional and psychological needs. EMDR was used at the start of the intervention to help Simon process the car accident he had with his mother and sister and was used again at the end of the intervention for him to process his fear that his father would crash the new car. The play therapy with BLS allowed Simon a space to explore his intense, confusing thoughts, images, and fears following the accident. This enabled him to make sense of his fears and understand that 'his Mum was alive', 'the Baby was back with his Mum', and that 'Dad could be trusted to drive carefully'.

Summary

- Practitioners need to complete accredited training on how to use EMDR with both adults and children.
- It is important to become competent to recognise when a child is traumatised and using dissociative behaviours to cope in the therapy.
- A play therapist should ensure they seek supervision when the themes emerging from the child's play are stuck.
- Play therapy and EMDR can be integrated effectively within one intervention to support a child who has experienced trauma.

Further Reading

emdrassociation.org.uk.
This will provide further information about training and research in relation to using EMDR with adults, children and young people.
Paulsen, S. (2009) *Looking through the Eyes of Trauma and Dissociation*. Charleston: Booksurge Publishing.
The book explains the impact of complex trauma on the individual, through the use of cartoon drawings and diagrams that are underpinned by theory. It describes how the individual's sense of self becomes fragmented through experiencing pervasive trauma and makes useful suggestions on how to help them.
Mills, J. C. & Crowley, R. J. (2001) *Therapeutic Metaphors for Children*. London: Brunner Mazel.
This is an inspiring book for all therapists who use play and art in their work with individuals. It explores the metaphor as a means of expression and then extends it to use as part of the integrative process that allows the individual to make sense of their negative experiences.

References

Axline, V. (1964) *Dibs: In Search of Self*. London: Penguin Books.
Bergmann, U. (2012) *Neurobiological Foundations for EMDR Practice*. New York: Springer Publishing Company.

Bucan-Varatanovic, A. B. & Sabanovic, S. (2017) *EMDR therapy in treating post traumatic stress disorder in an adolescent girl*. Presented at: EMDR Conference, Bosnia & Herzegovina in Sarejavo.

Carriere, R. C. (2014) Scaling up what works using EMDR to help confront the world's burden of traumatic stress. *Journal of EMDR Practice & Research*. 8 (4), pp. 187–195.

Cattanach, A. (1994) *Play Therapy: Where the Sky Meets the Underworld*. London: Jessica Kingsley Publishers.

Colelli, G. (2003) A firefighter with PTSD after the World Trade Center disaster. In: Manfield, P. (ed.) *EMDR Casebook*, p. 187. New York: W. W. Norton & Company.

Crowley, M. (2016) *Opening address*. President of EMDR Association UK & Ireland. Presented at: annual EMDR conference, Liverpool.

EMDR UK & Ireland 'EMDR'. (2018) *Practitioner Accreditation*. Available at: http://emdrassociation.org.uk/training-2/practitioner-accreditation [Accessed 14 February 2018].

Ghnassia Damon, N. G. (2008) Getting to the core: Moving through the language barrier. In: McCarthy, D. (ed.) *Speaking about the Unspeakable: Non-Verbal Methods and Experiences in Therapy with Children*, p. 130. London: Jessica Kingsley Publishers.

Golding, K. S. & Hughes, D. (2012) *Creating Loving Attachments*. London: Jessica Kingsley Publishers.

Gomez, A. M. (2013) *EMDR Therapy and Adjunct Approaches with Children*. New York: Springer Publishing Company.

Howe, D. (2005) *Child Abuse and Neglect, Attachment, Development and Intervention*. London: Palgrave Macmillan.

Landreth, G. (2011) *Innovations in Play Therapy*. Hove: Brunner-Routledge.

Logie, R. (2012) From nightmare to memories. *Therapy Today*. July pp. 28–31

Lovett, J. (1999) *Small Wonders: Healing Childhood Trauma with EMDR*. New York: Free Press.

Malchiodi, C. A. (2008) *Creative Interventions with Traumatized Children*. New York: Guilford Press.

McCarthy, D. (2007) *If You Turned into a Monster*. London: Jessica Kingsley Publishers.

McCarthy, D. (ed.) (2008) *Speaking about the Unspeakable: Non-Verbal Methods and Experiences in Therapy with Children*. London: Jessica Kingsley Publishers.

Morris-Smith, J. (2011) *EMDR for Children and Adolescents Training, Level 1, EMDR Advanced Skills of Child Training*, delivered July 2011.

Morris-Smith, J. & Silvestre, M. (2007) Developmental protocol. In: Morris-Smith, J. (ed.) *EMDR for Children and Adolescents Training, Level 2, EMDR Advanced Skills of Child Training*, delivered November 2011. EMDR Europe.

National Institute for Health and Clinical Excellence 'NICE'. (2018) *The Treatment of PTSD*. Available at: www.nice.org.uk/guidance/cg26/chapter/1-Guidance#the-treatment-of-ptsd [Accessed 14 February 2018].

Ogden, P., Minton, K. & Pain, C. (2006) *Sensorimotor Approach to Psychotherapy*. New York: W.W. Norton & Company.

Perkins McNally, S. P. (2001) *Sandplay: A Sourcebook for Play Therapists*. Lincoln: Writers Club Press, an imprint of iUniverse.com, Inc.

Porges, S. W. (1995) Orienting in a defensive world: Mammalian modification of our evolutionary heritage: A polyvagal theory. *Psychophysiology.* 32, pp. 301–318.

Rothschild, B. (2000) *The Body Remembers. The Psychophysiology of Trauma and Trauma Treatment.* New York: W.W. Norton & Company.

Shapiro, F. (2001) *Eye Movement Desensitization and Reprocessing.* New York: Guilford Press.

Silberg J. L. (1998) *The Dissociative Child: Diagnosis, Treatment and Management* (2nd ed.). Brooklandville: Sidran Press.

Spierings, J. (2016) *An encyclopaedia of interweaves in EMDR therapy.* Workshop at: EMDR Association UK & Ireland Annual Conference, Liverpool.

Struik, A. (2014) *Treating Chronically Traumatized Children: Don't Let Sleeping Dogs Lie!* London: Routledge.

Tinker, R. H. & Wilson, S. A. (1999) *Through the Eyes of a Child: EMDR with Children.* New York: W.W. Norton & Company.

Van der Kolk, B. A. (2011) *Bessel A. van der Kolk Discusses EMDR.* Available at: www.youtube.com/watch?v=Y2cPuv6jKqg [Accessed 14 February 2018].

Van der Kolk, B. A. (2015) *The Body Keeps the Score.* London: Penguin Books.

Wilson, K., Kendrick, P. & Ryan, V. (2001) *Play Therapy: A Non-Directive Approach for Children and Adolescents.* Edinburgh: Harcourt Publishers Limited.

Yehuda, N. (2016) *Communicating Trauma. Clinical Presentations and Interventions with Traumatized Children.* New York: Routledge.

Chapter 19

Relational approaches to play therapy

Supporting adoptive and foster carers and their families

Berni Stringer

Chapter overview

This chapter draws on my experience of working with children needing permanence. I will explore the importance of involving parents and carers (the child's adult) in the journey to regulation, connection, integration and mastery. I draw on my background in play-based models which are integrated into my daily practice. In my experience, an effective intervention opens the child's therapy more fully to parents and carers, empowering them as witnesses to the child's emotional world, promoting and deepening their empathy and increasing attunement with the child. My practice model has been continually developed through reflective and reflexive practice with carers, who are involved at each stage.

Introduction

Children enter care for many reasons but 60% of children in care will have experienced abuse and neglect *in relationship* (DFE, 2016, Table A1). Children harmed in relationship are more fully healed in a relationship with empathic, attuned adults, who support the integration of their experience and life story, enabling them to meet their fullest potential.

Engaging carers in the assessment process

Referrals of looked-after or care-experienced children are often made when a placement is in a state of crisis and has become vulnerable. Although it can feel imperative to act, I will only accept a referral if I have sight of a social work chronology, the Child Permanence Report, other court reports and assessments, review notes and a completed referral form. I have learned that, unless I fully understand the child's history and the imperatives driving the referral, it can become problematic later, with the risk of uncovering unforeseen concerns or lack of clarity in objectives.

Once received, the background information helps me to plot a developmental/experience/impact timeline with carers, using three separate lines of:

- a time and event chronology: as recorded on social work files;
- a developmental timeline: based on Erikson's model of psychosocial development (Erikson, 1950), which helps to 'Learn the child' (Cairns & Stanway, 2004);
- an impact statement: i.e. a consideration of the impact of an event given the child's age and stage of development. This is helpful in considering the 'cumulative harm' (Bromfield et al., 2007) that may have occurred as a result of neglect, repeated abuse and exposure to violence.

Understanding the effect of such experiences on child development and the trajectory of psychopathology is key knowledge (BAPT Core Competences 1 & 2, see Appendix 1) that grounds us in the healing process and promotes compassionate practice. At the point of referral, parents and carers may have experienced considerable periods of distress, leading them to feel less joy or pleasure in the child before them. This exercise can help to promote shared reflective and empathic thinking at this time.

Meet Jay

It is common for foster carers not to have full information about the child's journey. This was the case for Jay's carer. Completing the timeline together establishes a working alliance between therapist and carer/parent and implicitly reinforces their role in the child's healing journey. Read the partially completed timeline in Figure 19.1.

Listening to carers as they share their present experience and completing the timeline with them offers a fuller understanding of the child. Thinking together about the impact line and the 'present need' line helps to set goals and a shared understanding of the task. It helps to increase empathy and compassion in exhausted and anxious adults as they reflect with an attuned other (the play therapist) on the potential impact of harm and how this might intrude into the child–carer relationship. It serves to bring the child's birth family to mind and enables the airing of any residual feelings of ambivalence towards them.

During this exercise, Jay's carers concluded that he had experienced the **confluence** of relational abuse and disrupted attachment, which helped them *understand* and *accept* Jay's rejection of them. This enabled them to frame his behaviour as avoidance of relationship with them and to understand how this leads to frustration and vulnerability in the placement. Acceptance of carer feelings in this shared activity helps carers to feel heard and empowered and promotes rapport and trust, as we respect their

Chronological age	Birth–18 months	18 -36 months	36 months – 60 months
Stage of Development (Erikson, cited Herr, 2008:74)	Trust versus mistrust	Autonomy versus shame and doubt	Initiative versus guilt
Event	Jay born after episode of DV. Known parental alcohol misuse and violence until at 8 months fa' imprisoned for ABH. 2nd baby born. HV concerned- Mo post-natal depression until J 16 months. 16 months - J started nursery. Left late. Often nappy rash. Cried and clingy.	Different friends frequenting home. Jay seen by GP for chest infections. 23 months - hospital admission for burn to arm. 28 months - Treatment for decay in milk teeth. Not talking avoids interactions with staff.	37 months - Mo moved in with own parents. Some good care. Busy household with older adolescents (Mo's siblings) at home. 40 months - J reported by Nursery to be aggressive and non-compliant and stealing food. 46 months - Mo moved in with partner. 48 months - Bruise to arm and cheek referred to LA – accidental CIN plan in place. 54 months - House fire when children left alone. J rescued by services. Smoke inhalation and hospital for 32 weeks. Received into foster care. Six months in placement at point of referral.
Possible Impact			
Present Need			

Figure 19.1 Development/trauma timeline

unique expertise and knowledge of the child. Experience of working with carers and knowledge and understanding of the challenging journey for adopters, promote key competences when working with parents/carers (BAPT Core Competence 7, see Appendix 1).

This process also leads to more focussed and self-aware practice on my part as I hear the carers' unique experience of the child. By exploring the transference, or re-enactment in the child–carer relationship of internalised patterns of past experiences (the child's internal working model), we both begin to understand and rework these internalised relational patterns with the child.

Play therapy is a powerful intervention in a child's life, setting the conditions for symbolic exploration of their experiences in a *unique* but not *exclusive* relationship with their play therapist. Parenting children, particularly when there are challenges, can become what Siegel terms 'Command and Demand' parenting (Siegel & Payne Bryson, 2015:118). To exhort the adult to use play or be playful at this point may feel at best paradoxical – and at worst, impossible. It is important to be self-aware, and to pick up indicators of our own mis-attunement to carers. Exploring the play therapy process, and the meaning of the therapeutic relationship with the carer, can stimulate a review of the carer–child relationship, as the exploration of the difference between 'playing' and 'playfulness' implicitly helps parents to think about the dynamics of their relationship with the child.

Enquiring about the carer's own experience of play is important, perhaps a time they remember playing – who was with them? Was it a solitary process for them? What do they understand about play and child development? This helps carers to begin to commit to the idea of 'just playing' – a helpful idea when family life is challenged. Here one has to hold true to the power of the play process as a therapeutic experience and help the child's adult to understand the play as a metaphor for experience (BAPT Core Competence 6, see Appendix 1). The therapist at this point will be attempting to hear and accept concerns but also begin to engage with the knowledge and understanding of the child and deepen the carer's empathy, whilst being alert to possible contraindications for engaging with the situation; for example, denial of responsibility, intense blaming of the child or risk of immediate breakdown of the placement. In these circumstances, it will be important to focus work within the network of professionals. When there is crisis, the first responsibility is containment. Assessment is a dynamic process and listening well to parental concerns and frustrations can help to calm a situation, help to instil hope and begin to encourage motivation (BAPT Core Competence 18, see Appendix 1).

As we begin to establish our working relationship with parents and carers it is helpful to hold some perspectives in mind: see Figure 19.2 (Maguire Pavao, 2011).

The parenting task as explored by Hughes (2009) shows us that to facilitate optimal development adults must provide physical, psychological and emotional safety for children. This is enhanced by the carer's capacity to self-regulate, and to reflect and act in the moment. The task for carers is to move to repair and engagement in the relationship, offering a safe and positive experience of soothing nurture, structure and attunement. The therapist can help them to make sense of how the child's past may have invaded the present relationship, promoting carer empathy and a protective factor in placement.

| Confirm identity as a caring parent |
| Acknowledge their pain with compassion |
| Shift from control to choice - what do you want to bring to the situation? |
| Who do you want to be in this situation? |
| You alone are not the cause of this situation. You alone cannot solve the situation. |
| You can do your best but not all. |

Figure 19.2 Perspectives for carers

Following completion of the timeline, it is useful to fully explore day-to-day life at home; a helpful tool is the Secure Base Model (Schofield & Beek, 2014). This model explores the circular process of reflective parenting, beginning with experiencing the child's behaviour and considering the need that drives it. I explore the carer/parent thinking, feeling and understanding of the child's behaviour, and encourage them to reflect on their own caregiving behaviour in response to challenges from the child. This leads to thinking with the adult about how the child experiences them.

See for example, the cycle in Figure 19.3.

This is an example of an everyday issue in most families and children usually know their parent is cross 'in the moment'. This small cycle can

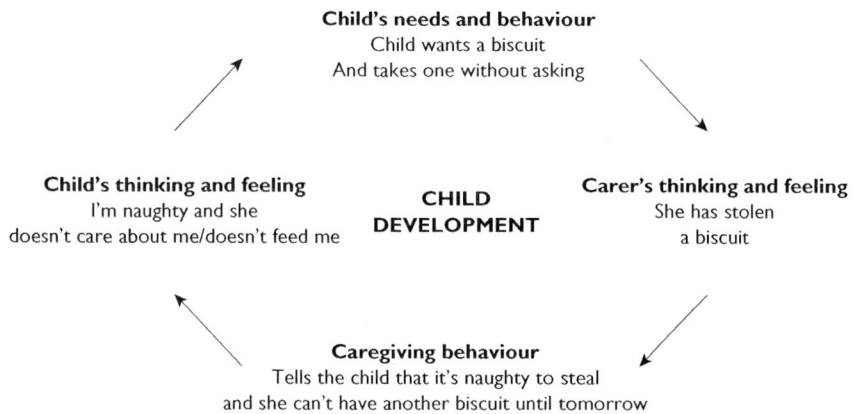

Figure 19.3 Example of child–carer interaction

take on larger meaning for some looked-after children of which the carer, in the moment, may not be aware – leading to the child and carer becoming mis-attuned. With best intentions, parents see their response as pro-social (should not steal) and appropriately educational teaching (lying is inappropriate). In these small daily interactions, it can be difficult to hold in mind the child's world of harm. The gradual erosion of the relationship by these small cycles of challenge, leads to exhaustion and a risk of affirming the child's maladapted – albeit previously useful – responses in relationship.

The play therapist and carer may also have different narratives of the child's behaviour (see Figure 19.4 below). It is important to bring together these two perspectives, present in our different relationships with the child. In my experience, this combined, deeper understanding of the therapist and the carer adds value to the individual work with the child, who experiences the adults working together too. For example, see Figure 19.4:

Behaviour	Parent	Play therapist
Adult hears swearing	Carer feels responsibility to correct teach or punish – i.e. to socialise the child	Experiences a change in mood and affect of the child and remains curious about what the child is feeling
Feelings response	Feels frustrated or not competent – particularly if 10th time today! Gives consequences	Remains curious, notices and comments on perceived feeling of child
Cognitive response	Inappropriate behaviour – needs to learn appropriate behaviour	What do I know about this child's experience, which helps me understand the behaviour?

Figure 19.4 Example of parental and play therapist perspectives

Our support to the child–adult relationship helps the adult to experience a different domain of the relationship – the feelings domain – as the carer moves from frustration to reflection and from sympathy burnout to empathy. The aim in my work is to shift the focus of the placement from containing and modifying behaviour to helping to promote an emotional environment in which the child can have new experiences of being with others. Often this is already happening. When the carer is a secure base for the child, then I think carefully about assuming the child will process experience with me. Often it is more effective to utilise the feelings of security already in place and acknowledge the carer as keeper of the child's story.

This understanding, developed over time, has helped me conclude that working exclusively – or even predominantly – with the child in the play-room does not effectively strengthen the relationship between the child and the adults, and may even implicitly suggest the responsibility for change lies with the child, rather than within the emotional environment.

I do work with children on a one-to-one basis and have experienced how they value the opportunity to be self-determining, heard and understood, and this is an aspect of being a play therapist that I value greatly as a privilege. When the core conditions are in place in the therapeutic relation-ship and felt by the child, the 'essence' of healing relationship is present. However, I hold to the belief that the carer becomes the 'carrier oil' of that experience in the care they too offer. Therefore, even during a long-term individual intervention with a child, I hold in mind that 'advice' and 'prob-lem solving' about day-to-day management becomes less helpful than sup-porting the adult to make an emotional shift in the relationship – for example, from a cognitive problem-solving approach to a more curious and reflective stance about the meaning or messaging of a child's behaviour.

Engaging carers in the intervention

Research into the effectiveness of play-based models such as filial therapy (Guerney, 1964; van Fleet, 2005), Theraplay[1] (Booth, 2009), and Parent–Child Interaction Therapy (Brinkmeyer & Eyberg, 2003; Drewes, 2006) has shown success in increasing parent–child attachment and relationship. Rennie and Landreth (2000) identify an increase in parental empathy, improved family atmosphere and increased self-esteem in the identified child, with subsequent changes in behaviour and play activity (cited in Schaefer & Drewes, 2011).

Adults may feel empowered by learning strategies and often ask what to say or what to do in special play or in specific situations. However, the effects of vicarious trauma can make the application of specific strategies in the moment difficult and the effect short lived. I have found that inviting parents into the playroom to witness play therapy live and to observe the core conditions in process, offers hope to parents that their child can play and 'be' differently. I particularly do this when I have experienced the child in relationship and my experience perhaps differs from the description given by carers. I ask parents in the playroom simply to 'notice' what might be different – or in fact similar – to their own interactions with the child and notice how the child responds. I am not prescriptive about the task. Parents are often very surprised and intrigued by their experience.

Meet Josie

Josie was three years old when she was placed with her prospective adoptive parents. She had experienced neglect and domestic violence from pre-birth and removed to foster care at six months, where she had stayed until placed for adoption. Josie was consistently dysregulated in the day and often throughout the night, screaming and kicking. She had assaulted her parents, who were exhausted, felt out of their depth and at a loss to know what to do. They felt the match was inappropriate and disruption was imminent.

In our first session, Josie seemed confident in the playroom – as children with attachment issues often appear to be. She responded to the non-directive space and invited me into her doll play – 'You be the mummy.' I checked out what sort of mummy she would like me to be and she said, 'a kind mummy', and watched intently as I cared for the baby, occasionally directing me to feed or scold the baby. Towards the end of the session, Josie asked to take off her shoes and socks and bury her feet in the sand-tray. We noticed her feet were 'gone' and 'back', 'there but not there'.

In session two, Josie played this again. She watched intently when I cared for the baby and asked why I was singing, feeding, and playing, to which I responded 'oh … hmmmm … Because that's what kind mummies do …' Josie followed with a series of questions about mummies, checking out what was OK and not OK for babies. She repeated the sand-play. These play sequences continued into the third session.

In these earliest sessions, I was witnessing Josie working hard to under-stand relationship, care, nurture and loss – 'there and not there'. I felt that I had witnessed Josie's ability to reflect and question and that this was important to share with her parents. I was anxious and found myself in a dilemma between Josie's right to privacy and her parents' need to 'see' her. I discussed this in my clinical supervision. With Josie's agreement, her mother and father observed the next session, via a one-way mirror. I asked them to 'notice' her. In effect, they were 'experiencing' or witnessing her.

Josie's parents observed the next four sessions as she engaged in nurture play, sand box and conversation. It was during one of the observations that Josie asked if she would stay with 'this Mummy and Daddy' forever. I asked if this is what she wanted and she affirmed she did. A powerful experience for her parents to witness and hear.

After extended play observations, my responsibility is no longer a teaching one, but becomes facilitative, to explore what parents have noticed and what meaning they have made of the child's play. What we came to understand was that, in the stress of introductions and moving in, her parents had come to know the distressed Josie. They had not witnessed her other abilities. Observing Josie experiencing the core conditions helped her parents witness her in a different way and they 'fell in love' with her, felt hope and motivation to sustain the placement. At this point we moved to a filial process, with Josie's parents more fully understanding and ready to accept the concepts of filial therapy (van Fleet, 2005).

Early in my practice, it felt like magic happened in the playroom! However, I have come to understand that the conversations prior to inviting the child into the playroom, the playroom environment and the presence of the core conditions (Rogers, 1959) come together to provide an environment where all feelings can be explored and accepted. It begins with the very earliest reflections on the lived experience of the child in the trauma timeline and continues with the regular 'touch base' emails and conversations I have with parents and carers who support the individual process.

My own learning

Play-based models have proven results in supporting children and their adults. Skills can be taught as we invite adults to engage in 'knowledge acquisition' (Bloom et al., 1956), i.e. to receive and recite information and then enact this with feedback in observed play sessions.

However, it is in the observation sessions and feedback conversations that adults can move from a passive to an active learning stance, even if they are not yet 'doing'. In the case of Josie, witnessing Josie created a 'disorientating dilemma' (Mälkki, 2012; Mezirow, 2009) for them. Offering enquiry and reflection helped move her parents – they had seen other possibilities – to be emotionally open to possibility and change, where they had previously felt hopeless, helpless and angry.

When change like this occurs, there is a shift in me as the therapist as I become 'uncertain' in my own knowledge and increasingly open to reflection with the adult. My role has now shifted from sharing knowledge or giving support – both power positions – to engaging with the adult in an intersubjective space. Shared evolved understanding offers an ongoing framework within which parents and carers can be empowered at an affective level to care for their children in attuned and congruent ways, based in deep empathy.

In effect, we experience a transformational shift from a position of 'knowledge application' such as an understanding of child development or attachment theory and analysis, e.g. 'What attachment style is this child?', to the possibility of creating and co-constructing ideas and thoughts and applying understanding and remembering (Pohl, 2000). In our enquiring with parents, when constructing a trauma timeline or witnessing a child's play, we can support by listening, reflecting, reframing and accepting, so that parents can shift to creative and playful interactions with their children. The difference between playing and being playful begins to emerge.

Josie's parents saw skills in her that they had not witnessed previously, and this gave them hope. Hope helped them to regulate the profound anxiety, caused by feeling they had made a terrible mistake and helped them to move to deep empathy for her feelings of confusion and loss. In relationship with me, co-constructing an understanding of her experience moved them to explore what she needed and how they provided it. This brought awareness of differences in their parenting styles, which had added to confusion to Josie's experience of home life. Her parents' witness of the play therapy process facilitated a change in the emotional environment of home.

The learning from this work early in my filial career helped me understand the importance of offering extended observations to parents, supported by post-session thinking and reflection with them. When parents then offer sessions themselves, they have already begun the process of change in the family/parenting environment.

Committing to paper

When carers begin play sessions at home, I continue to have an email exchange with them. This effectively begins a regular weekly dialogue about the emerging understanding, increasing empathy and playfulness in the family. This may happen for a number of sessions.

Here is an example taken from a regular email exchange after Jay's carer Sharon had undertaken a filial process. This was Jay's eighth special play with his carer.

SHARON: Jay was excited to be doing special play, he walked into the room surveyed all the toys and went straight to the toolbox and began to hit it with the hammer. The play with the toolbox lasted a few minutes then he went to the playdough. He remembered the last time we played with the playdough.

THERAPIST: This is good news …! Jay is building memories with you as he links one session to another.

SHARON: I used the dagger to help get the playdough out which he copied but unfortunately he was a bit rough and started to flick pieces out which flicked into my eye then his. I stopped him and offered to help him, but he threw it down … went into mini rage and threw toys and said he wanted to stop playing.

THERAPIST: Offers of help seem to be difficult for him? What are your thoughts about that? Could you just acknowledge 'Mummy is here to help if you want me to'.

SHARON: I said I understood he was cross because I had stopped him from using the dagger and that he found it difficult when I offered to help but that Mummies can help and that makes things easier for little boys. He did calm down and began to play with the baby doll.

THERAPIST: OKAY!!!! Your empathy has done the trick! WOOHOO!!

SHARON: He moved closer to where I was sitting on the mat and moved the baby on to his knee, commenting 'make you sit on my knee'. I said that he was gentle with the baby, which he liked; he then said, 'baby sad needs milk'.

THERAPIST: My goodness – wow – this is wonderful! How do you feel about this Sharon? What is he showing you? Is it safer to do this in play because he has some degree of control and feels safer?

SHARON: I asked how baby was feeling after the milk and Jay said 'better.' He put plasters on the baby and began to feed the baby again and said to baby 'baby needs noony' (his word for dummy).

THERAPIST: What were you saying Sharon? You have to take care not to prompt him and continue to track the play and comment on feelings.

SHARON: (response to therapist comment): At this point Berni I was not saying anything, he said everything very quickly and the whole thing was over in minutes.

SHARON: Jay put down the baby, picked up his tool set and asked me to hold his feet whilst he played.

THERAPIST: Wow! Children are amazing aren't they!! How did that feel for you? Is he allowing himself to be vulnerable?

SHARON: He then moved closer to me and asked me to hold things for him but not to play. Jay then moved to sit on my knee and asked me to hold him, moving my arms to hold him closer, he then said 'mummy let go' but when I relaxed my hold he moved my arms back round him he did this about 3 times.

THERAPIST: Oh Yay!! FANTASTIC! He really is exploring with you isn't he – what are your thoughts about this?

SHARON: (response to therapist comment): I think that it is good he can now express his feelings and now seeks out affection. He does this in and out of filial, he will do this with Steve and Jack as well. When Jack and Jay watch TV together you hear him say 'hold me Jack' and they cuddle on the settee together. I think he is trying out things with the pushing away, is he questioning will I want him back if he pushes away from me?

SHARON: At the end of the session he did not want this to end so I said that I would make a teddy bear picnic if he played for a few minutes in garden to let me do this which he agreed to. Jay enjoyed the teddy bear picnic teasing me with the little biscuits and pretending to feed his teddy bear.

THERAPIST: How are you feeling about this session Sharon? Sounds like you had a really good time! Are you enjoying him? He certainly seems to be enjoying you Sharon ... clearly you are providing a safe enough environment for him to explore and play well.

SHARON: *(response to therapist comment)*: I am enjoying having Jay at home more, we had a difficult time with Jay last week. He was not sleeping well at night time and was not having a sleep every day in the afternoon. As the week progressed his tolerance levels were getting worse. We feel he enters a destructive cycle of behaviour which he can't get out of and normally can only be broken by an intensive play with me.

In this exchange, the carer and therapist are engaged in 'upstairs brain thinking' (Siegel & Payne Bryson, 2015:35), which supports the carer's cognitive understanding and emotional processing about their child. It is committed to paper in an email trail and so always available to parents to reflect on.

When children are in one-to-one play therapy

Individual play therapy usually only begins after I have completed a timeline and the Secure Base conversation. I begin each or alternate sessions with 'talk time' of ten to fifteen minutes with the child and carer together. Here we can review the week and share what has gone well, or what has been a challenge, and think together a little bit.

The child may be playing and seem not to be attentive; however, I believe they are in a more relaxed state and likely to be able to 'hear' their parent more effectively. Talk time provides a useful grounding for the play therapist to stay in touch with the day-to-day experience of the family and the follow-up time for the child in the playroom enables further time for reflection through playing. Individual play therapy with the child in the room remains core to my practice, but the overall outcome is enhanced by regular communication and enquiry with carers and parents.

Summary

- In this discussion, I have proposed a full and inclusive role in the play therapy process for parents and carers of children needing permanence.
- I suggest that this begins during the assessment phase, by co-constructing a trauma timeline and thinking reflectively about the child's experience, using a known model of psychosocial development.
- Carers' involvement continues with their extended play observation and careful discussion of what the parent has witnessed.
- With empathy and reflection as the key principles in the relationship, we can shift to deeper and effective change in the relationships between the therapist and carer and carer and child. This reduces the need for skills teaching and direct parenting advice.

- Change occurs in me as I shift to a deeper understanding of the lived experience of the family and this ensures I remain humble in the process, reducing the power base of traditional professional roles.
- The play therapist becomes less prominent in the child's life, as the carer's involvement in therapy leads to a felt change for the child, contributing to deep repair in their closest relationship.

Note

1 Theraplay is a registered service mark of The Theraplay Institute, Evanston, IL, USA.

Further reading

McKee, D. (2015) *Not Now Bernard*. London: Anderson Press.
This is a children's favourite and adults can appreciate it as a comment on day to day life when caring for children. It is playful way of making important points about attending, noticing and attunement in relationships with children, and a cautionary tale too!
Pullman, P. (2010) *His Dark Materials Trilogy*. London: Harper Collins
This was a recommended text when I began training. This trilogy is a child centred adventure that amplifies the creativity, courage and resilience of children who recover from fear and harm.
Raiten-D'Antonio, T. (2007) *The Velveteen Principles*. London: Health Communications.
As a child I loved *The Velveteen Rabbit* (Williams, 1922). It was my first experience of magic and becoming 'real'. Raiten-D'Antonio's book, based on the original story, offers a reflection on the principles of kindness, generosity and loving and the journey to finding 'self'.
Rogers, A.G. (1995) *A Story of Harm and Healing in Psychotherapy*. New York: Viking.
I have read and re-read this book. It is the story of one woman's journey to her therapy career and an account of her own experience of therapy which can harm. There are wonderful descriptions of play in the playroom as her child client takes his own journey to healing, witnessed by his therapist.

References

Bloom, B.S., Engelhart, M.D., Furst, E.J., Hill, W.H. & Krathwohl, D.R. (eds.) (1956) *Taxonomy of Educational Objectives, Handbook I: The Cognitive Domain*. New York: David McKay Co Inc. Available at: www.nwlink.com/~donclark/hrd/bloom.html#three_domains [Accessed 30 September 2017].
Booth, P. (2009) *Theraplay*. (3rd ed.) San Francisco, CA: Jossey-Bass.
Brinkmeyer, M. & Eyberg, S.M. (2003) Parent–child interaction therapy for oppositional children. In: Weisz, J.R. & Kazdin, A.E. (eds.) *Evidence-Based Psychotherapies for Children and Adolescents*. New York: Guilford. pp. 204–223.

Bromfield, L.M., Gillingham, P. & Higgins, D.J. (2007) Cumulative harm and chronic child maltreatment. *Developing Practice.* 19 pp. 34–42.

Cairns, K. & Stanway, C. (2004) *Learn the Child: Helping Looked after Children to Learn.* London: British Association for Adoption and Fostering

Department for Education. (2016) *Table A1 in Children Looked after in England Year Ending 31st March 2016.* London: DfE.

Drewes, A., Carey, L.J. & Schaefer, C.E. (eds.) (2006) *School-Based Play Therapy.* New York: John Wiley & Sons Inc.

Erikson, E.H. (1950) *Childhood and Society.* New York: Norton & Norton.

Guerney, B. Jr. (1964) Filial therapy: Description and rationale. *Journal of Consulting Psychology.* 28(4) pp. 304–310.

Hughes, D. (2009) *Principles of Attachment-Focused Parenting.* London: W. W. Norton & Company. Available at: www.danielhughes.org/p.a.c.e. [Accessed 30 September 2017].

Maguire Pavao J. (2011) How many people does it take to adopt a child? Video lecture. Available at: https://youtube/KqnShliWV4M [Accessed 30 September 2017].

Mälkki, K. (2012) Rethinking disorienting dilemmas within real-life crises: The role of reflection in negotiating emotionally chaotic experiences. *Adult Education Quarterly.* 62(3) pp. 207–229. American Association for Adult and Continuing Education

Mezirow, J. (2009) Transformative learning theory. In: Mezirow, J. & Taylor, E.W. (eds.) *Transformative Learning in Practise: Insights from Community,* p. 18. San Francisco, CA: John Wiley & Sons Inc.

Pohl, M. (2000) *Teaching Complex Thinking: Critical, Creative, Caring.* Cheltenham: Hawker Brownlow.

Rennie, R., & Landreth, G. (2000) Effects of filial therapy on parent and child behaviors. *International Journal of Play Therapy.* 9(2) pp. 19–37.

Rogers, C. (1959) A theory of therapy, personality and interpersonal relationships as developed in the client-centered framework. In: Koch, S. (ed.) *Psychology: A Study of a Science. Vol. 3: Formulations of the Person and the Social Context,* p. 184. New York: McGraw Hill.

Schaefer, C. & Drewes, A. (2011). The therapeutic powers of play and play therapy. In: Schaefer, C. & Drewes, A. (eds.) *School-Based Play Therapy* (2nd ed.) Hoboken, NJ: John Wiley & Sons Inc. pp. 41–61.

Schofield, G. & Beek, M. (2014) *The Secure Base.* London: British Association for Adoption and Fostering

Siegel, D.J. & Payne Bryson, T. (2015) *The Whole Brain Child Workbook.* Euc Clare, WI: PESCI Publishing USA.

van Fleet, R. (2005) *Strengthening Child-Parent Relationships through Play.* Sarasota, FL: Professional Resource Press Canada

Chapter 20

Working with parents and carers
Child Parent Relationship Therapy

Trudi Cowper

Chapter overview

In this chapter, I will present my involvement in delivering a Child Parent Relationship Therapy (CPRT) group filial therapy programme over the past five years. I will begin with a brief overview of the model and describe how I have adapted it for my particular practice context. I will describe how CPRT supports parents to focus on their existing strengths and discuss the use of video recording and peer feedback processes within the group to encourage skills development. I will use examples from practice to illustrate how the CPRT approach helps parents to identify and respond effectively to their children's emotional needs. Case examples have been anonymised and are presented with parental permission.

Introduction

Child Parent Relationship Therapy (CPRT) is a ten-session filial therapy model created by US play therapists Garry Landreth and Sue Bratton (2006). This group course was a development of Guerney's Filial Therapy approach (1964), which was designed to teach parents (or carers) child-centred play therapy skills to use in special playtimes with their child. In this latter approach, a play therapist may demonstrate sessions for the parent with the child and provide live supervision of parent/child play sessions as part of the process. In Landreth and Bratton's group model, only the parents attend and the filial therapist facilitates a safe and welcoming parent group where experiences are shared and specific skills are taught each week (for which a folder of handouts and worksheets are provided). Weeks 1–3 focus on introducing both the toys and the main therapeutic play skills such as empathic listening and allowing the child to lead the play. From week 4 the parents begin their weekly play session at home with one of their children and they are required to video them, as extracts are viewed by the group each week. The therapist provides supervision of their skills, encouraging the other group members to notice and support each other's development. Weeks 4–10 of the course focus on the group's sharing of experiences, video supervision of play sessions and further skills development. These skills include: empathic and esteem-building responses, therapeutic limit-setting, encouragement and internal motivation (rather than the external evaluation of praise), and a general enthusiasm for playfulness and imaginary play. The filial approach takes the view that the parent can be the most effective therapeutic agent of change for their child, and that the parent/child relationship will naturally be enhanced in the process. The efficacy of CPRT is well supported by numerous US research studies, which emphasise it as a valuable application of a play therapist's skills and knowledge to family work that has the potential for inter-generational and social change (Landreth & Bratton, 2006). The filial approach and CPRT particularly evidence the play therapist's skill in working with parents and carers (BAPT Core Competence 7, see Appendix 1).

The rationale for a group method, as well as being practical and cost effective is that, more significantly, the parents will offer support and encouragement to each other, with many parenting struggles being normalised and addressed in the process. Importantly, the therapist promotes these connections between parents. (Note: Where I have used the term 'parent' in this chapter I will be including other carers of a child such as grandparents, step-parents, aunts and uncles, all of whom have attended this CPRT service. However, the approach could also be used for foster carers, for example.)

Context of project

After delivering two pilot CPRT courses for TGP Cymru, a children and families charity in Wales, finance was gained to deliver further courses in Cardiff from 2014 for four years. The first year was co-delivered with a play therapist colleague and subsequent years by myself as course leader, also undertaking all administrative tasks, phone calls, and visits and promoting the course to other professionals. Each group had a maximum of six parents. Our funding was from the Welsh Government-funded Families First programme (Welsh Government, 2017) in Cardiff, which aims to reduce child poverty and inequalities in education, health, and economic outcomes for children, by focusing on early intervention and preventative measures. Cardiff, while an affluent area of Wales, is also an area of significant deprivation. It is ethnically very diverse in comparison with the rest of the country and the city is also an initial accommodation and dispersal centre for asylum seekers (Cardiff & Vale of Glamorgan Integrated Health & Social Care Partnership, 2017). A high proportion of parents who have attended CPRT are white Welsh, but there have also been parents from other ethnic backgrounds, including those seeking asylum. In my experience it is usually mothers who attend, but fathers have also come to CPRT, both single fathers and those in parent couples.

Contra-indications to the use of CPRT include: parents with more complex mental health needs that would impede their ability to hold play sessions regularly and to focus on their child, or the child having issues or experiences that would be unmanageable for the parent. (Landreth & Bratton, 2006). For intermediate difficulties, I also offer 1:1 or dyad delivery rather than a group and this also works well. What is lost from a group approach is compensated by a service tailored to the individual family's needs. Otherwise, CPRT takes the relatively inclusive stance of viewing play as a basis for child/parent communication and parental acceptance of their child, effective regardless of socio-economic or cultural background (Landreth & Bratton, 2006). At the time of writing, in my CPRT practice I have worked with 17 groups and numerous individuals or dyads: a total of over 90 families.

Referrals process

Referrals to our service are often made by a professional, usually from health services or other statutory or voluntary agencies. Increasingly, there have been self-referrals from parents, which generally come as phone or email enquiries. Mostly, parents are concerned about an emotional or behavioural issue they feel their child has and indicate that their relationship is not as positive as it could be. After a follow-up phone call where we can briefly discuss parents' expectations and outline the course, I invite parents to a CPRT 'taster' session of around two hours. This will include an introduction to the course, a play session video clip, discussion of some of the skills, and a presentation of the toys. This establishes the tone of the course and the commitment involved, generating initial connections and emotional safety within a group. I then have a 1:1 meeting with interested parents at home to discuss their family in greater detail. Parents who have attended a taster have been those most likely to commit to and complete a ten-week course.

Play and emotional development

We now understand from neurological research how babies need to learn with the help of their parent or a significant other to regulate their emotional states, to begin to develop a positive sense of 'self' and acquire useful knowledge about human interaction. Gerhardt (2008) also identifies the significance of parents' abilities to verbally feedback children's emotional states, in the development of the child's 'verbal self' at ages 2 and 3. She adds that the ability to put feelings into words even helps the left and right brain to become integrated, leading to emotional security in adulthood. Having an attuned parent who is able to symbolise their feelings accurately in words helps the child to differentiate between states, to express their feelings, and to navigate them around others.

For many parents, once children become verbal it can be common to rely on verbal communication, slipping gear into an adult mode of reasoning and relating and to assume a more developed understanding. We can rapidly move away from the 'mirroring', and what Gerhardt calls 'psycho-feedback' (Gerhardt, 2008:25), which often happens naturally between the parent and baby, rather than developing that form as the child grows older. It may also be, of course, that the parent was unable to provide this type of emotional regulation for their baby initially, or that it was hindered in some way. CPRT encourages parents to revisit these early forms of parent–child communication. When a parent uses therapeutic play skills, their child is not *expected* to communicate verbally but can do so exclusively with toys and art materials if they wish. The parent learns how to respond to any communication the child makes, verbal or non-verbal, as in this example from a parent/child play session:

> Harry, aged 4, requested that his Dad crawl around on all fours in their play session. Harry then did the same and crawled underneath the Dad where they both remained, quite still for a few moments, somewhat like a baby bear taking protection and comfort from his father's physical presence and emotional availability to his child. This was a spontaneous occurrence amongst other more typical play of cars and figures. It illustrates the child/parent play sessions as enabling the child to get their needs met in a child-centred way. Harry did not need to decide consciously that this kind of physical closeness was what he wanted, much less to verbally request it. He knew that his father was willing to play under his direction and that he could be spontaneous without any justification.

Here, the parent takes responsibility for understanding and meeting the emotional needs of their child and the child learns a healthy way of seeking contentment and connection.

When parents on a CPRT course have accurately and empathically reflected their children's feelings to them, both in and out of the play sessions, the child has often responded in ways such as a delighted: 'Yes! Mummy! You feel me!' or a sudden recognition of: 'Yes! I *am* angry!' as if a light has been switched on inside of them by their parent. One child said to his parent outside of a play session, 'Mummy, tell me what I am feeling!' They have the knowledge that their parent is likely to recognise further emotional experiences they will have, to truly notice *'me'*, to sort their jumbled bodily sensations into a coherent, worthy, and accepted 'self'.

Many parents who come to CPRT say, quite reasonably, that they would like their child to understand and express themselves better. CPRT helps *parents* to understand their child's needs and feelings, or to recognise and articulate the understanding that they already have about their child and, in the process, develop the child's ability to express emotions and to seek healthy emotional regulation.

The toys and how they help

Within the CPRT model, it is suggested that parents are given the task of assembling their own set of play equipment for their child at the beginning of the group process. As most parents accessing our service have low household incomes and other pressures to deal with, we decided not to ask the parents to gather the toys themselves. Instead, the charity provided each parent with a special box of toys, funded from the overall project budget. The parents can keep the toys on completing the course to encourage them to continue with the play sessions. Parents may add relevant items to their box such as baby doll's clothes or put together an additional toy box for later sessions with one of their other children.

The toys selected are like a mini kit of those that can be found in a play therapy room. As outlined in the CPRT course materials, they encompass a small number of the following categories:

Nurture and real-life toys such as a baby doll, baby bottle, a picnic set, a fierce and a more benign animal puppet, domestic and wild animal figures, toy mobile phones, a doctor's kit.
Aggressive toys such as a soft foam dart gun, two foam swords, handcuffs.
Creative/expressive materials such as art and craft materials, scissors, glue, musical instruments. (Landreth & Bratton, 2006:171–173)

Parents are shown the toys at the taster session and this provides an early opportunity to identify any toys that may cause them anxiety. Commonly these will be: the gun, sword, handcuffs, or scissors for fear of provoking aggression or harmful behaviour in a child. The baby bottle can also concern parents who are worried about unmanageable 'regressive' behaviour. Both the bottle and the doll may worry parents who feel that their son will reject these toys (and therefore the session and parent) on the basis that they are 'girls' toys'. The course creates a space for parent and child to explore assumed gender roles and frequently there is surprise at the kinds of play that may result, which challenges these notions and can be freeing for both parent and child. Here is an opportunity for the filial therapist to explore the value in having these items in the play session and to remind the parents that this special time will be different with their use of therapeutic skills and undivided focus on their child. Here, I can give parents examples of children developing self-control, altering their physical position to avoid hurting a parent in their play, and of using the baby doll to consider perhaps their own babyhood and their place in the family. We also recognise the appeal for children in returning to hide-and-seek play and their delight in being discovered, truly *seen* as they might be as an infant. With the parent's calm understanding, the child is permitted to examine some previously inexpressible feelings, which become normalised and steadied by the person they need the most. This method is effective because it originates within play, where the child and their world is important and accepted by the parent. It is not just about one-way parental control. The parent experiences the benefit of this two-way communication for themselves: a frequent comment from them at the end of a course is of the calmness they feel as a result, as well as reporting this observation in their child. A sense of fulfilment and of belonging to each other seems to be regenerated.

The toys are the most engaging, interactive way to inspire discussion amongst parents about imaginative play, and it is important to emphasise that they can be used in various ways, within safe limits that the parent will establish (in keeping with the permissive play therapy principle). The significance in CPRT, however, is that the toys and the therapeutic elements allow the child to explore complex issues and to consider them alongside their parent or other care-giver, as this example shows:

> One parent on a CPRT course was Bethan, a mother of two daughters: Sophie aged 6 and Georgia aged 4. Georgia was diagnosed with global developmental delay, which affected her mobility. Sophie seemed frequently angry and upset about the amount of care Georgia required from her parents. After Georgia fell and hit her head one day, needing a trip to hospital and stitches, Sophie was particularly resentful and cross about the attention and presents Georgia got from family and friends at school and did not seem concerned for her sister, which her mother found difficult to deal with. In their play session shortly afterwards Sophie played with the doctor's kit, eventually pretending that she had a head injury and having Mum play at being the doctor attending to her 'wound', which she did empathically. This led to Sophie picking up a scalpel-like toy and asking, 'What's this? Did they use this on Georgia?' This implied a curiosity that she had not expressed previously and Mum gave Sophie some information about the treatment Georgia had received. With Bethan's full, non-judgemental attention on Sophie and her needs, they both experienced a calm exploration of Sophie's feelings about the incident that was not possible for her at the time when her emotions were high. Sophie then had Mum be the patient while she cared for her as her doctor. Mum experienced Sophie's nurturing qualities, which could not easily emerge

amongst her sister's needs. After the course Bethan said that Georgia had been found a place at a special needs school and that she was surprised when Sophie expressed regret at her sister leaving the school they attended together.

Video recording

A major feature of the CPRT approach, as opposed to other filial models, is that the therapist does not usually conduct any play sessions with the children to demonstrate play therapy skills, but the parents are required to video their home play sessions and bring them to the group for sensitive feedback from both the therapist and the rest of the group. Parents report that they learn from each other's videos and it is an invaluable tool for the therapist to highlight different skills used with the group (Landreth & Bratton, 2006:27–28). Our charity loans the parents a small video camera for this purpose and thus avoids the need for parents to use their own mobile phones.

Both the group process and the use of video rather than live demonstration sessions with the children by the therapist enhance the view of the parent as the expert on their own child and enables the parent to take the lead in their play sessions rather than have the therapist initiate demonstration sessions or observations. For some parents who have had a lot of professional intervention in their family lives, or who live with anxiety or depressive episodes, the tendency to feel disempowered by learning a new skill can be more acute. Even relatively confident parents report after the course that preparing to show their first video was uncomfortable but that this was relieved after the first viewing and feedback.

For this reason, I took the decision to view sections of all participants' videos each week. A suggested format for CPRT is to ask for two volunteers each week to bring in their videos. However, I decided that, as there were often cases of high anxiety or stress, where a parent may be especially vulnerable to perceived criticism, this could be addressed for all the parents at the same time by viewing sections of all their videos at every course session. Parents can all be reassured with positive comments about both their acquisition of the play skills and their personal manner with their child. It also offers the filial therapist a good indication each week of where each parent is at in terms of their comprehension and application of the skills, which can also develop on seeing each other's play sessions. Although more time-consuming, it can reduce the amount of time needed for emphasising specific skills when they are demonstrated in the videos and are integrated with the skills learning. The parents will have different strengths and it is useful for them to be able to notice these in each other, making comments on each other's videos such as, 'You remembered all that stuff about tracking what they're doing', or 'You were really calm when you put in the limit about the gun'.

Although I feel this method can be particularly therapeutic for families who have had previous directive interventions from professionals, there have been some exceptions to this. I have at times used the alternative filial therapy approach of demonstrating sessions with a child and of also observing play-times between a parent and a child, rather than using video. This has been a useful method of assessment where the parent or child may be particularly vulnerable, where parental abilities are uncertain, or where video/audio recording is too inhibiting for parent or child. In all other cases, however, parents will experience taking the lead in their child's well-being as early as possible, an element of freedom that they, in turn, will be permitting their child in play.

Supporting a parent's sense of competence

It is important that all the unique child/parent relationship-enhancing attributes that the parents already possess are encouraged, that I accept the parent as an individual and value their autonomy as a parent. The therapist works to ensure that parents are esteemed within the group as having insights and skills to offer everyone else. So many times, for a first showing of their play session, a parent will enter the CPRT room declaring that their play session was 'terrible' or 'I did it all wrong'. After acknowledging to parents the obvious challenge and commitment involved in agreeing to show a video of themselves with their child to relative strangers, we all view it and can clearly identify all the skills they are working hard to put in place. Without fail, all of the many parents I have worked with in CPRT have allowed their child to lead the session from the outset and been able to apply many other skills too, often more than I would expect.

In a group, I will also share some of my own experiences and struggles as a parent, including play sessions I have had with my son and how they enhanced our relationship. This element of self-disclosure, which is encouraged in CPRT (Landreth & Bratton, 2006), is a departure from the use of self that a play therapist may generally be used to, but can be liberating for parents in the group. At times, I have shared my uncertainty with parents as to how I might have responded in a situation that one of them has handled instinctively and in a way that only a parent can. This can be both humbling for the therapist and empowering for the parent. Ryan and Courtney (2009) explore the beneficial use of congruence in both play and filial therapy practice, benefits that I have also experienced in my practice and that can be integrated with a chosen filial therapy model. My following reflections on a CPRT session illustrate the helpful use of congruence by a parent in her play session with her son:

> During a play session a child threw the blanket with toys on up in the air in anger: should the parent put all the toys back in a gentle, empathic way while calmly reflecting? Should they empathically set

a limit? The reality is that there is a variety of different responses that could be helpful. The therapist's work is to support the parent to feel confident in deciding on an approach for themselves, using their therapeutic skills. In this example, the parent kept her attention on her son rather than the toys and calmly reflected the child's anger and sadness about himself. She then verbally shared her feelings of love towards him. The boy calmed down very quickly and began to play again. The parent had contained and responded to her child's difficult, perhaps lonely, feelings rather than simply empathising or setting a limit. She felt it important to let him know at that point how she felt about him and it was an instinctively helpful response that could not easily be 'taught'. Here, as therapists, we can support a parent to make their own informed choices about ways of congruently responding to their child and thereby deepening the attachment relationship.

The skills are so new or profound to some parents that their initial application can produce a startling impact on themselves and on the child. Often a joy and calmness overcomes the child that takes the parent by complete surprise, an occurrence described by one parent as 'magic'. Perhaps in some cases we could even surmise that, if the 'psycho-feedback' stage of the parent/infant relationship had been hindered, filial therapy can go some way in restoring it.

Role-play and other approaches to skills learning

Another suggested method for teaching skills is for pairs of parents to role-play a parent and child to practise the skills. Many parents who come to our service, especially those unused to further training or even being in a group, can feel too inhibited to 'pretend' in front of others. In my experience a parent can show by their video each week that they are adequately implementing what they are learning. Although paired role-play can increase a person's confidence and I do use it when it seems helpful, I have found it more effective to use a group approach to skills learning. As an alternative, parents can be given time to become more comfortable in contributing to group discussions and to respond as a group to scenarios as 'parent' that I may act out as 'child'. I regularly use video examples of myself and other play therapists with a child. Parents will often use a phrase or a tone of voice in their play sessions that they have seen on a demonstration video, quite appropriately, and then develop their own style as time goes on. The play sessions have been described by some parents as 'a way in' for them to their child's play, and these examples provide a safe place to start. Here we find another cue for the filial therapist to use and adapt CPRT materials to suit the parents in the group, gaining a feel for what could work best ('Effective work with different client groups': BAPT Core Competence 25, see Appendix 1).

The learning experience

I ran a few courses for a while in an old secondary school and one parent told me that she had been a student there. I asked what it was like, returning here to do the course. She said it was a bit odd at first and that she had walked down the corridor, recalling that 'Mr Jones' office had been there and Mrs Evans' over there'. It made me think about how being in that building might affect her experience and about all our varied learning journeys. As play/filial therapists, we inevitably reflect on the experiences and vulnerabilities that shape us, but this is not the case for everyone. When we embark on learning with others, we do not know what their corridor looks like (or what Mr Jones and Mrs Evans were like for that matter either).

At times, something unexpected occurs in the group, perhaps the sharing of a recent bereavement, sudden bouts of prolonged laughter as the stresses of the week unravel, or the arrival of a parent with a young child when their childcare arrangements for that day have fallen through. At these times I ask myself: 'What is the most useful thing I can do for the group right now?' It is likely that I will not follow the provided structure of the course to the letter, but will consider the therapeutic needs of the group members at that moment as best I can. For this reason, although I believe that every course that I deliver is absolutely Child Parent Relationship Therapy and retains its core values and skills learning, each one is also as different as the parents who join it.

Ending the group process

In the final session we explore further what has changed for the parent and the child, and many parents reflect on unexpected changes in themselves. A frequent comment on feedback forms at this stage is that the parent feels themselves to be calmer and able to respond to their child and defuse difficult situations. They feel that their child is happier and they feel closer. We celebrate by sharing lunch or cakes and parents receive certificates. Some parents are unused to receiving certificates and this provides tangible evidence of the effort and motivation they have shown in strengthening their relationship with their child. As well as revisiting initial parental concerns in the last two sessions and asking for feedback about the course and perceived changes, I use the short form Child-Parent Relationship Scale (Pianta, 1992), which I will have asked the parent to complete at the start of the course. These will generate discussions on the parent and child's journey and I offer parents a follow-up 1:1 session. All parents who complete the course have reported improvements in their relationship with their child and the behaviours that were concerning them.

In CPRT, parents are prioritising their child's emotional development and their relationship with their child. This emerges in the play sessions, in other episodes of family life as they generalise the use of their therapeutic skills, and in the CPRT group where they take the time and courage to consider their life as a parent, trying to see the world through their child's eyes. They do this amongst a multitude of demands on themselves. Even finding the time and energy for a half hour play session with your child can be a challenge in a society where there are always other tasks to be done, information to process, numerous messages about parenthood to consider. However, in CPRT, play therapists have a means to encourage and raise the confidence of parents that they are the most powerful resource their children have.

One mother said to me, early on in a CPRT course, 'I see now, it's me who can change, not my son that needs to'. Parents find resources within themselves; rather than feeling reliant on external help, they discover their own impact on their children. The discovery extends to the children too. Some contact I have had with parents, months and even years after a CPRT course, revealed that children will often request 'special playtime' with their parent if time has lapsed between sessions and they feel a need for it: they seek out their parent and the play space they have experienced together.

A mother ending a CPRT course said that previously she had not enjoyed being a mum but that now she did; a father commented that he felt newly hopeful for his family's future; other parents suggest that all parents should do a course like this, that it should be as commonplace as antenatal classes. With filial therapy we can see the mutual benefits of this approach for parent and child, including a realisation of the potential in their relationship, a discovery that can produce profound results.

Summary

- CPRT provides a structured time-limited group process for teaching filial play skills for parents.
- Groups can address the needs of a diverse range of parents and can be adapted as necessary to deliver to specialist populations or to individuals and dyads for more vulnerable parents or to meet specific needs.
- Parents undertake 30-minute play sessions at home each week that are videoed and reviewed by the whole group to support skills development.
- CPRT empowers and motivates parents as they take the lead in their therapeutic sessions with their child.

Further reading

Guerney, L. & Ryan, V. (2013) *Group Filial Therapy: The Complete Guide to Teaching Parents to Play Therapeutically with their Children.* London: Jessica Kingsley Publishers.
A 20-week whole-family model with advice and practical resources for the filial therapist.

Landreth, G.L. (1998) *Parents as Therapeutic Partners: Listening to Your Child's Play.* Lanham, MA: Jason Aronson Inc.
Case examples of parent/child play sessions and parent/therapist discussions.
Rogers, C. (1986) *A Therapist's View of Psychotherapy.* London: Constable & Company Ltd.
Person-centred therapy with adults: the chapter 'Characteristics of a helping relationship' is particularly helpful.
Sunderland, M. (2007) *What Every Parent Needs to Know.* London: Dorling Kindersley.
An accessible resource for parents/carers and therapists on a child's early years and the development of secure attachments.
Van Fleet, R. (1994) *Filial Therapy: Strengthening Parent-Child Relationships through Play.* Sarasota, FL: Professional Resource Press.
A handbook of a single-family filial therapy model.

Useful video resources

Child Parent Relationship Therapy (CPRT in Action) (2013) by Sue C. Bratton and Garry L. Landreth [DVD]. Center for Play Therapy, University of North Texas.
Choices, Cookies and Kids: A Creative Approach to Discipline (2014) by Garry L. Landreth [DVD]. Center for Play Therapy, University of North Texas.
Play Therapy in Action – An Introduction to the Core Skills of a Play Therapist (2009) produced by BAPT [DVD]. Available at: www.bapt.info/play-therapy/training-dvd/

References

Cardiff & Vale of Glamorgan Integrated Health & Social Care Partnership. (2017) *Cardiff and the Vale of Glamorgan Population Needs Assessment for the Social Services and Well-Being (Wales) Act 2014.* Available at: www.cvihsc.co.uk/wp-content/uploads/2017/02/Population-Needs-Assessment-1.pdf [Accessed 11 January 2018].
Gerhardt, S. (2008) *Why Love Matters: How Affection Shapes a Baby's Brain.* East Sussex: Routledge.
Guerney, B. (1964) Filial therapy: Description and rationale. *Journal of Consulting Psychology.* 28 (4) pp. 303–310.
Landreth, G.L. & Bratton, S.C. (2006) *Child Parent Relationship Therapy (CPRT): A 10-Session Filial Therapy Model.* New York: Routledge.
Pianta, R.C. (1992) *Child-Parent Relationship Scale- Short Form.* Charlottesville: University of Virginia.
Ryan, V. & Courtney, A. (2009) Therapists' use of congruence in nondirective play therapy and filial therapy. *International Journal of Play Therapy.* 18 (2) pp. 114–128.
Welsh Government. (2017) *Families First Programme Guidance,* April 2017. Available at: http://gov.wales/docs/dsjlg/publications/cyp/170419-families-first-programme-guidance-en.pdf [Accessed 11 January 2018].

BAPT play therapy core competences

The effective deployment of skills and knowledge in play therapy are of the up-most importance to clients, families, the public and the profession. Play therapists must ensure that their practice is based on clear and coherent competence. The core competences of play therapists are defined in three main areas: knowledge and understanding, personal development, practice skills and a list of personal qualities that are a pre-requisite of good practice. A play therapist's core competences are:

Knowledge and understanding

1. Knowledge of theories of child development
Understand some of the key theories of healthy child development processes within the context of familial and social diversity; and be able to discuss these in relation to observed behaviour.

2. Knowledge of developmental psycho-pathology
Understand the clinical needs of specific groups of children affected by disrupted development; drawing on theories of attachment, mental health, social and emotional wellbeing, disability and trauma. Understand the emergence of psycho-pathology within human development.

3. Knowledge of ecological systems and social constructionist theories of society
Understand how the wider systems of family, community, culture and social/government policy impact on children, young people and families and be able to integrate systems thinking and analysis into therapeutic practice with individuals.

4. Knowledge of theory and practice of play therapy
Understand the theory and practice of play therapy, including the humanistic child-centred approach. Understand models of the change process in a play therapy intervention.

5. Knowledge of different models of play therapy, including integrative approaches
Understand and integrate different models of play therapy including directive, non-directive and developmental approaches.

6. Knowledge of theories of play development and of the functions of play
Understand theories of normal and abnormal play development, the role of play and the use of play as a therapeutic metaphor.

7. Knowledge and practice of working with parents/carers
To have the ability to articulate/translate play therapy practice/process and, if appropriate, to engage with the child's parents/carers in the therapeutic process.

8. Knowledge of the legislation and policy context for play therapy
Understand current legislation and policy relating to the practice of play therapy in the context of health, education and social care in the UK, both public and private sectors, including child protection and safeguarding.

9. Knowledge of theories of anti-discriminatory practice in play therapy
Understand principles of anti-discriminatory practice in relation to children, young people and their families within the context of a diverse society.

10. Knowledge of contemporary research and practice
Demonstrate knowledge and understanding of contemporary practice and research in play therapy. Understand evidence-based practice principles.

Personal development

11. Possession of the essential personal qualities for a play therapist
Demonstrate identified personal qualities of a play therapy practitioner to promote public protection and ethical practice (see Personal qualities of a play therapist).

12. Application of ethics and values in practice
Understand ethical practice relating to play therapy to ensure protection of children, young people and families and the public – as detailed in Ethical Basis for Good Practice in Play Therapy. Conform to the required standards for clinical governance laid out by BAPT.

13. Maintenance and effective use of clinical supervision
Use clinical supervision to promote and ensure ethical play therapy practice and the protection of the public. Use clinical and/or managerial supervision to review and consider own strengths and limitations; operate and practice efficiently within own levels of competence and within limitations of role. Comply with BAPT's recommended guidelines for clinical supervision.

14. Utilisation of personal therapy and support for development
Integrate personal therapy and developmental support in an appropriate and effective manner. Demonstrate ability to be self-reflective and to integrate learning into therapeutic practice to ensure effective and ethical standards of practice and promote public safety.

15. Maintenance of continuing professional development
Maintain Continuing Professional Development in accordance with BAPT requirements, for promotion of high standards of play therapy practice.

16. Maintenance of basic skills in independent business practices
Demonstrate and maintain skills needed to manage their own independent business, including effective financial management, compliance with regulations for self-employment, management of personal data, procedures and policies to ensure public protection, health and safety etc.

Practice skills

17. Engagement and facilitation of a therapeutic relationship
Demonstrate effective engagement and facilitation of the therapeutic relationship with clients and significant others.

18. Assessment of need
Understand and be able to undertake assessment of the emotional, psychological and social needs of clients; and to formulate appropriate therapeutic objectives.

19. Planning and contracting for play therapy practice
Formulate clear, meaningful and appropriate therapeutic contracts, including therapeutic aims, objectives, boundaries and rules.

20. Intervention and provision of direct therapeutic service
Intervene and provide play therapy to achieve identified therapeutic objectives; monitor and evaluate the effectiveness of play therapy interventions and adapt skills and techniques to a diverse range of children, young people and families.

21. Provision of well-planned therapeutic endings
Provide planned and coherent opportunities to enable work with clients to end in a therapeutic manner.

22. Maintenance of rules and boundaries within play therapy practice
Maintain clear professional, personal and therapeutic boundaries.

23. Maintenance of confidentiality and privacy
Maintain the confidentiality and privacy required by clients and significant others; meeting both legal and ethical standards, including data protection

requirements. Recognise the limitations of confidentiality in relation to safeguarding children and vulnerable adults.

24. Clinical record-keeping and writing skills
Accurately record play therapy interventions, working within the requirements of data protection legislation. Communicate effectively in writing through clinical records, written assessments and reports of therapeutic progress.

25. Effective work with different client groups
Work in an effective anti-discriminatory way with a diverse range of children, young people and families, considering the individual's identity and cultural needs.

26. Communication skills
Communicate effectively, through non-verbal and verbal expression, with clients and significant others. Use a range of therapeutic, person-centred skills, including active listening, empathic responding, questioning, paraphrasing, tracking, reflection and summarising.

27. Inter-personal communication through use of creative media
Demonstrate and facilitate a range of verbal, non-verbal and symbolic communication using a variety of play and creative media with children, young people and families.

28. Maintenance of effective inter-professional relationships
Collaborate and communicate with other professionals; demonstrate effective inter-professional working for the benefit of children, young people and families. Work within agency policies and procedures and work effectively as part of a team around the child, young person and family.

29. Develop and manage a play room/play therapy environment
Take responsibility for the development and safe management of the play therapy environment/play room, in line with health and safety standards. This includes selection and maintenance of play materials, risk assessment of the environment and taking appropriate steps to ensure continuing safety; ensuring privacy during sessions, preserving confidentiality in use and storage of therapeutic materials produced in sessions.

30. Effective work in different settings
Contribute effectively to the work of organisations, demonstrate understanding of agency functions and priorities. Consider the dilemmas of integrating play therapy practice within organisational contexts. Work independently, set priorities, plan and manage own workload and organisational tasks efficiently.

31. Application of evidence based research to play therapy practice
Identify and critically evaluate relevant current research evidence and integrate into play therapy practice. Demonstrate that play therapy practice is

informed by contemporary evidence-based research. Demonstrate an understanding of research methods and the application of research methods within clinical contexts. Application of evidence-based approaches in the evaluation of play therapy outcomes and effectiveness to assure quality of service delivery and enhance the evidence base for play therapy.

Personal Qualities

Empathy

To empathise with the emotional and psychological expressions, experiences and needs of clients and significant others.

Sincerity

Commitment to being sincere and genuine to self and others.

Honesty

To act truthfully and with integrity towards self and others.

Respect

To acknowledge and show acceptance towards other people's understanding, experiences and abilities.

Ethical

To be committed to ethical practice and able to comply with the ethical code and values defined by the British Association of Play Therapists.

Knowledgeable

To be able to apply knowledge, evidence and experience critically.

Self-awareness

To assess, review and consider own competences, strengths and weaknesses as a play therapist.

Self-responsibility

To operate and practise efficiently within own level of competences.

Congruence

To be authentic and genuine in conduct with clients and significant others.

Compassion

To be emotionally warm, caring and concerned towards others.

Critical reflection

To critically reflect upon the emotional, social and psychological world of clients, significant others and the Self, and to integrate reflection into practice.

Commitment to professional development

To continue professional development as a play therapist in a responsible and effective manner.

Commitment to personal development

To be reflexive, to integrate personal insights into future practice, to continue personal development in a responsible and effective manner.

BAPT's ethical basis for good practice in play therapy

The establishment of dynamic Ethical Principles for play therapists' work-related conduct requires both a personal commitment and acceptance of responsibility to act ethically and to encourage ethical behaviour by students, supervisors, supervisees, employees, colleagues and associates.

These Ethical Principles are intended to guide and inspire play therapists towards achieving the highest ideals of the profession. Ethical Principles, as opposed to Standards or Codes, do not represent obligations in their own right. However, all play therapists are obliged to consider their practice with direct reference to each of these Ethical Principles.

Principle A: responsibility

These Principles are aspirational but are considered good, ethical practice for a play therapist. Play therapists need to be motivated, concerned and directed towards good ethical practice. They are required to take responsibility to maintain these standards and play therapists should always accept responsibility for their professional behaviour and actions. Play therapists are concerned about the ethical compliance of their own practice and their colleagues' professional conduct. When ethical conflicts occur, play therapists attempt to resolve these conflicts in a responsible manner. Play therapists are also aware of their professional responsibilities towards their clients, society and to the communities in which they work.

Principle B: beneficence

Play therapists strive to benefit those with whom they work, acting in their best interests and always working within their limits of competence, training, experience and supervision. This principle involves an obligation to use regular and on-going supervision to enhance the quality of service provision and to commit to enhancing practice by continuing professional development. An obligation of the play therapist is to act in the best interests of clients and this is the paramount consideration for play therapists, since clients are generally non-autonomous and dependent on significant others. Ensuring that the client's best interests are met requires monitoring of practice and outcomes and, accordingly, BAPT has set down standards for supervision which all members of BAPT should follow.

Principle C: non-maleficence

Play therapists are committed to not harming those with whom they work. Because play therapists professional judgements and actions may affect the lives of others, they are aware, concerned and committed to guard against personal, financial, social, organisational, emotional, sexual or political factors that may lead to a misuse of their influence or exploitation of those with whom they work. This may involve not providing services when unfit to do so due to personal impairment, including illness, personal circumstances or intoxication. Play therapists have a responsibility to challenge the incompetence or malpractice of others and to contribute in investigations or adjudications concerning the professional practice and/or actions of others.

Principle D: fidelity

Play therapists establish relationships of trust with those with whom they work. Play therapists honour and act in accordance with the trust placed in them. This principle obliges play therapists to maintain confidentiality and restrict disclosures of confidential information to a standard appropriate to their workplace and legal requirements.

Principle E: justice

Play therapists recognise that fairness and justice is an entitlement for all persons. This obliges play therapists to ensure that all persons have fair and equal access to, and benefit from, the contributions of play therapy and to equal quality in the services being conducted and offered by play therapists. Play therapists exercise judgement and care to ensure that their potential biases, levels of competence and limitations of their training and experience do not directly or indirectly lead to unjust practices.

Principle F: respect for people's rights and dignity

Play therapists respect the dignity and worth of all people and the rights to privacy, confidentiality and autonomy. Play therapists who respect the autonomy of those with whom they work ensure accuracy of advertising and delineation of service information. Play therapists seek freely the informed consent of those legally responsible for clients and, where possible, assent from clients, engage in clear and explicit contracts, including confidentiality requirements and inform those involved of any foreseeable conflicts of interest. Play therapists are aware that special safeguards may be necessary to protect the rights and welfare of clients who are non-autonomous and dependent on significant others.

Principle G: respect for people's needs and relationships

Play therapists respect the needs of individuals, including emotional, psychological, social, financial, educational, health and familial needs. Play therapists who respect people's needs and relationships are aware that clients may be dependent upon significant others and that autonomous decision making may not be possible. Play therapists respect the client's relationships and ensure that, where possible, those in significant relationships to the client are included in the decision making processes.

Principle H: self-respect

Play therapists apply all of these principles to themselves. This involves a respect for the play therapist's own knowledge, needs and development. This includes accessing opportunities for personal and professional development. There is a responsibility to use supervision for development and to seek training for continuing professional development (see BAPT's Continuing Professional Development documents). Ensuring play therapists are appropriately safeguarded by insurance is also a requirement for this principle.

Sample contract

(See Chapter 3, The role of clinical supervision in play therapy practice, by Carol Platteuw)

Supervision contract between supervisor and supervisee

The frequency of the supervision will be ....

The cost of the supervision is £......... per hour.

The supervision will take place at ....

The supervisor is contactable in between sessions for case discussion if something needs to be considered urgently on ....

The supervisor is willing to read sessional notes in advance of supervision but would need them forwarding in advance by email 3 days before supervision.

Supervision is offered in accordance with the BAPT code of ethics.

The supervisor will keep brief notes of issues discussed within supervision sessions. The notes remain the property of the supervisor though in exceptional circumstances (child protection or legal issues) access to these notes may be required. All such notes and records will be securely stored in compliance with GDPR regulations, until ....

The supervisee will take responsibility to ensure they have a valid enhanced DBS check, have sufficient insurance to cover their play therapy work, maintain their membership of their professional body and adhere to the Code of Ethics.

A minimum of one month's notice is required to terminate the contract.

Signed .... Date.....................................

Signed............................... Date.....................................

Index

Note: CC refers to the corresponding Core Competence in Appendix 1, page numbers in italics refer to figures

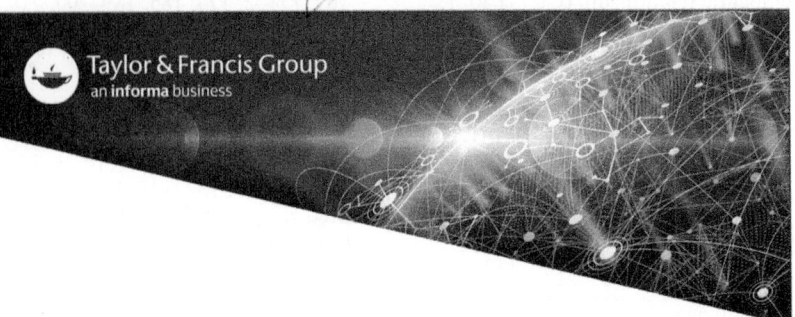
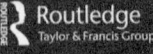
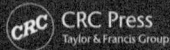